# CONTESTED SPACES:
## ABORTION CLINICS, WOMEN'S SHELTERS AND HOSPITALS

*Pour Martin, toujours*

# Contested Spaces:
# Abortion Clinics, Women's Shelters and Hospitals

Politicizing the Female Body

Lori A. Brown

**ASHGATE**

© Lori A. Brown 2013

All rights reserved. No part of this publication may be reproduced, stored in a retrieval system or transmitted in any form or by any means, electronic, mechanical, photocopying, recording or otherwise without the prior permission of the publisher.

Lori A. Brown has asserted her right under the Copyright, Designs and Patents Act, 1988, to be identified as the author of this work.

Published by
Ashgate Publishing Limited
Wey Court East
Union Road
Farnham
Surrey, GU9 7PT
England

Ashgate Publishing Company
110 Cherry Street
Suite 3-1
Burlington
VT 05401-3818
USA

www.ashgate.com

**British Library Cataloguing in Publication Data**
Brown, Lori A.
 Contested spaces : abortion clinics, women's shelters and hospitals : politicizing the female body.
 1. Architecture and women--Canada. 2. Architecture and women--Mexico. 3. Architecture and women--United States. 4. Hospital architecture. 5. Abortion services--Canada. 6. Abortion services--Mexico. 7. Abortion services--United States. 8. Architecture--Psychological aspects. 9. Feminism and architecture.
 I. Title
 720.8'2-dc23

 ISBN: 978-1-4094-3741-3 (hbk)
        978-1-4094-3742-0 (ebk)
        978-1-4724-0430-5 (epub)

**Library of Congress Cataloging-in-Publication Data**
Brown, Lori A.
 Contested spaces : abortion clinics, women's shelters and hospitals : politicizing the female body / by Lori A. Brown.
      pages cm
 Includes bibliographical references and index.
 ISBN 978-1-4094-3741-3 (hardback) -- ISBN 978-1-4094-3742-0 (e book)
 1. Architecture and women--North America. 2. Architecture--Psychological aspects--North America. 3. Abortion services--North America. 4. Health services accessibility--North America. I. Title.
 NA2543.W65B76 2012
 720.82--dc23

2012028079

Printed and bound in Great Britain by the
MPG Books Group, UK.

# Contents

*List of Figures* *vii*
*About the Author* *xi*
*Preface* *xiii*

1 **Introduction** 1

2 **Social and Spatial Practices** 21

3 **Legal Frameworks Understood Spatially** 43

4 **Case Studies and Spatial Awareness** 71

5 **Landscapes of Access: United States, Canada and Mexico** 95

6 **Conclusion** 193

*Bibliography* *211*
*Index* *231*

# List of Figures

| | | |
|---|---|---|
| Fig 1.1 | March for Women's Lives April 25, 2004 Washington D.C | 2 |
| Fig. 1.2 | Pre-Easter anti-abortion protestor sidewalk queue in Louisville, KY April 2012 | 3 |
| Fig. 1.3 | Pre-Easter anti-abortion protestor sidewalk queue in Louisville, KY April 2012 | 4 |
| Fig. 1.4 | Pre-Easter volunteer clinic escort queue in Louisville, KY April 2012 | 4 |
| Fig. 3.1 | US abortion timeline 1870–1970 | 44 |
| Fig. 3.2 | *Roe v. Wade* | 45 |
| Fig. 3.3 | Hyde Amendment | 46 |
| Fig. 3.4 | *Hill v. Colorado*. Plan and perspective diagrams illustrating legislated spaces | 50 |
| Fig. 3.5 | *Madsen v. Women's Health Center*. Plan diagram illustrating legislated space and noise restrictions | 51 |
| Fig. 3.6 | *Schenck v. Pro-Choice Network of Western New York*. Plan and perspective diagrams illustrating legislated spaces | 52 |
| Fig. 3.7 | Key spatial terms | 54 |
| Fig. 3.8 | FACE law | 55 |
| Fig. 3.9 | Canada abortion timeline 1800s–1988 | 58 |
| Fig. 3.10 | *R v. Morgantaler* | 59 |
| Fig. 3.11a | Abortion in Canada | 60 |
| Fig. 3.11b | Abortion in Canada | 61 |
| Fig. 3.12 | Mexico abortion time line 1850–2007 | 63 |
| Fig. 3.13a | Abortion in Mexico | 64 |
| Fig. 3.13b | Abortion in Mexico | 65 |
| Fig. 4.1 | Event Matrix. A chart of most of the activities of the CWLU in 1972 | 75 |
| Fig. 4.2 | Jane newspaper publicity | 76 |
| Fig. 4.3 | Abortion is a personal decision | 77 |

| | | |
|---|---|---|
| Figs 4.4, 4.5 & 4.6 | Women on Waves. Exterior and interior views of the abortion boat | 81 |
| Fig. 5.1 | USA county with and without providers | 96 |
| Fig. 5.2a | USA providers per state | 98 |
| Fig. 5.2 b | USA providers per state | 99 |
| Fig. 5.3a | USA restrictions by state | 102 |
| Fig. 5.3b | USA restrictions by state | 103 |
| Fig. 5.4 | Southern region synopsis | 105 |
| Fig. 5.5a | Mississippi clinic distances | 112 |
| Fig. 5.5b | Mississippi potential clinics | 113 |
| Fig. 5.6a | Mississippi poverty statistics | 114 |
| Fig. 5.6b | Mississippi location of religious centers | 115 |
| Fig. 5.7a | Mississippi hospitals | 116 |
| Fig. 5.7b | Mississippi pharmacies | 117 |
| Fig. 5.8a | Mississippi pharmacy data | 118 |
| Fig. 5.8b | Mississippi pharmacist replies | 119 |
| Fig. 5.9a | Kentucky clinic distances | 122 |
| Fig. 5.9b | Kentucky potential clinics | 123 |
| Fig. 5.10a | Kentucky poverty statistics | 124 |
| Fig. 5.10b | Kentucky location of religious centers | 125 |
| Fig. 5.11a | Kentucky hospitals | 126 |
| Fig. 5.11b | Kentucky pharmacies | 127 |
| Fig. 5.12a | Kentucky pharmacy data | 128 |
| Fig. 5.12b | Kentucky pharmacist replies | 129 |
| Fig. 5.13 | Midwestern region synopsis | 131 |
| Fig. 5.14a | South Dakota clinic distances | 136 |
| Fig. 5.14b | South Dakota potential clinics | 137 |
| Fig. 5.15a | South Dakota poverty statistics | 138 |
| Fig. 5.15b | South Dakota location of religious centers | 139 |
| Fig. 5.16a | South Dakota hospitals | 141 |
| Fig. 5.16b | South Dakota hospitals; South Dakota pharmacies | 142 |
| Fig. 5.17a | South Dakota pharmacy data | 143 |
| Fig. 5.17b | South Dakota pharmacist replies | 144 |
| Fig. 5.18a | Nebraska pharmacy data | 145 |
| Fig. 5.18b | Nebraska pharmacist replies | 146 |
| Fig. 5.19a | North Dakota pharmacy data | 147 |
| Fig. 5.19b | North Dakota pharmacist replies | 148 |
| Fig. 5.20a | Western region synopsis | 150 |
| Fig. 5.20b | Western region synopsis | 151 |
| Fig. 5.21a | Utah clinic distances | 155 |
| Fig. 5.21b | Utah potential clinics | 156 |
| Fig. 5.22a | Utah poverty statistics | 157 |
| Fig. 5.22b | Utah location of religious centers | 158 |
| Fig. 5.23a | Utah hospitals | 160 |
| Fig. 5.23b | Utah pharmacies | 161 |

| | | |
|---|---|---|
| Fig. 5.24a | Utah pharmacy data | 162 |
| Fig. 5.24b | Utah pharmacist replies | 163 |
| Fig. 5.25 | Newborn security anklet | 183 |
| Fig. 5.26 | Detail, newborn security anklet | 184 |
| Fig. 6.1 | Composite maps for Mississippi | 196 |
| Fig. 6.2 | Composite maps for Kentucky | 198 |
| Fig. 6.3 | Composite maps for South Dakota | 200 |
| Fig. 6.4 | Composite maps for Utah | 202 |
| Figs. 6.5–6.8 | New locations for clinics: Shopping malls, military bases, jails, public and high schools | 206 |
| Fig. 6.9 | New locations for clinics: churches | 208 |

## About the Author

At the intersections of architecture, art, geography, and women's studies, Lori Brown's work emerges from the belief that architecture can participate in and impact people's everyday lives. As an architect and artist, her design, speculative work, and teaching all engage with the larger idea of broadening the discourse and involvement of architecture in our world. Focusing particularly on the relationships between architecture and social justice issues, she has currently placed emphasis on gender and its impact upon spatial relationships. Three projects she is currently working on include a retro-fitted bus providing medical care for rural areas in upstate New York, a collaborative project with a Turkish colleague focusing on women's shelters in Turkey from the perspective of government policies influencing their locations to the spatial issues that women and children have as shelter inhabitants and co-organizing a mentoring program for women and minority architects in New York City and central New York state. In addition, she curated, organized and participated in *feminist practices*, an international group of women designers and architects whose work engages feminist methodologies which was recently published as an edited book, *Feminist Practices: Interdisciplinary Approaches to Women in Architecture*, by Ashgate in December 2011. She has been awarded artist residencies at Macdowell, Jentel and Caldera and her work has been exhibited widely and has been published in *306090*, *gender forum*, *Journal of International Women's Studies* and *ACME*, the journal of critical geography. In 2008 she was awarded the American Institute of Architects Diversity Best Practice Honorable Mention and a commendation for the Milka Bliznakov Prize for the *feminist practices* exhibition. She is an associate professor at Syracuse University where her teaching builds upon her interdisciplinary interests and goals of challenging the gendered academic landscape with alternative pedagogical methods. She is a registered architect in the state of New York and a member of the American Institute of Architects.

# Preface

> *The architect's only option is to find a course for revolutionary praxis outside the traditional boundaries of [her] field.*[1]
> 
> Joan Ockman, Architecture, Criticism, Ideology

Frustrated with the lack of political engagement in my discipline, I decided I had to work on a topic unavoidably political in order to force architecture to do and say *something*. From the moment this project began, I stepped outside my comfort zone eventually realizing I had to let the research direct the path this project would take. It was a risky endeavor taking many years to complete but I can honestly say I am glad I have taken the time and made the investment in something so challenging. One result from this interdisciplinary project is that I will forever approach my work differently ever more committed to the political engagement of architecture. The project has also provided me opportunities to meet others both within and outside my discipline doing quite exciting and challenging creative spatial research.

The nascent stages of this project began somewhere during the middle of my tenure track process after a long conversation with a friend and former colleague Andrew Klamon. I must thank him for that important brainstorming session. The beginning research would not have been possible without Katie Walsh, a former student and now friend. Thank you for never doubting the project and working fearlessly on it even when others had questions. I must also thank the Macdowell Colony where during this phase of initial research I was provided time, amazing space (and food) to think, read and begin to formulate ideas about the project combined with thought-provoking colleagues asking important and difficult questions.

The research, which began more as a series of public talks comprised of mapping and visual explorations, emerged intermittently. These events provided opportunities requiring me to propel the project forward where I was also able to receive much needed feedback. I would like to thank the following for their invitations: Matrilineage Symposium Women and Arts at Syracuse University, Linda Alcoff former director of Women Studies at Syracuse University, Rebecca Gardner and her Women and Art Seminar at DePaul University, Emma Wilcox and Evonne Davis at Gallery Aferro, Jeannine DeLombard and the F. Ross Johnson-Connaught Distinguished Speaker Series at the Centre for the Study of the US University of Toronto and the Third International and Interdisciplinary Conference on Emotional Geographies, University of South Australia Adelaide, Australia.

I would also like to thank Meta Brunzema and Jonnell Allen Robinson for their conversations once the project was underway. Jeannine DeLombard, *again*, for all her thoughtful suggestions, editing and time in Toronto. Barbara Opar, Syracuse University School of Architecture librarian, for her ability to find things I swore I just was unable to find! I would like to thank Duke University's Sallie Bingham Center for Women's History and Culture Library Archives and the Mary Lily Travel Grant; the Director, Laura Micham, and Kelly Wooten, Librarian, for all of their support while doing archival research in their collection. I must thank Leslie Kanes Weisman for her ongoing support and for putting me in touch with Merle Hoffman, founder of Choices Women's Medical Center and a pioneer in the women's healthcare and abortion movement.

I must also recognize and thank Roberta Feldman. She was the first person to emphatically and convincingly suggest all these years of research and work should become a book. I would also like to thank her for the additional suggestion of interviewing providers across the country in order to bring a more personal and on-the-ground perspective to the project. She was of course right.

I also must thank my local Planned Parenthood and the years of volunteering at the New York State Fair. It was always so interesting to discuss sexual health and hand out condoms to passers-by, especially those teenagers who always thought they were secretly grabbing condoms by the handful! Of course we knew but let them anyway ... These experiences provided education and insight into current women's health issues and the public's reaction to these issues. I must also thank Charlotte Taft, Director of the Abortion Care Network. Her ongoing work in abortion rights is truly inspiring and I was able to meet many providers because of her. I would also like to thank those at *Everysaturdaymorning Blog*, http://everysaturdaymorning.net/. The work they do escorting women and their family and friends in Louisville, Kentucky is truly amazing. Their fearlessness and publicly candid, thought-provoking reflection on abortion by those literally on the front line protecting women accessing their legal right is inspiring. I also thank Estelle Carol, Coordinator for the CWLU Herstory Project and her help in locating images from the days of Jane. In addition, thanks goes to Dr. Rebecca Gomperts, founder of Women on Waves. Her project made me see the potential of spatial tactics and the power one has to change the world. I am truly indebted and inspired by her work.

I would also like to express my gratitude to my former dean at Syracuse University, Mark Robbins, for his continued support through several faculty grants in helping make research for this project possible. I would also like to thank both Mark Linder and Francisco Sanin, former and current graduate chairs, for supporting the project through years of graduate research assistants. I would like to acknowledge all of these students who have provided countless hours of help on this project. They are: Lindsey MacDonald, Ariana Douso, Laura Swartz, Chris Netski, Vera Tong, Daina Swagerty, David Caballero, and finally and especially Janet Lee, who has been instrumental in creating the included drawings, diagrams and maps.

In deep gratitude do I recognize and thank Val Rose, the commissioning editor for the book. I am forever grateful for her belief and patience in this project. This book would not have been possible without her commitment and ability to see potential in the research and the value it would have across several disciplines.

I absolutely must thank all of those fearless and committed people in abortion and women's shelter work who agreed to be interviewed. Your willingness to share with me your experiences, struggles and successes continue to amaze me. I am moved by your lives work and commitment to women's reproductive healthcare and the survivors of domestic violence. I only hope I do justice to your conviction, power and voice.

I would also like to thank my family and friends in Syracuse and elsewhere with special heartfelt appreciation to my father Joseph Brown and my brother Michael Brown, Ann Husaini, Susan D'Amato, Kelin Perry, Kim Steele, Alison Mountz, Samantha Herrick, Susan Branson, Cynthia Hammond, Özlem Erdoğdu Erkarslan, Craig Watters and Jane Rendell. Your continued support, friendship and rigorous intellectual engagement help me strive to be a better feminist and person.

And lastly, to Martin. You have endured quite a bit during this second book. Words cannot express the love and gratitude I feel for all your support during this very long process; all the long dog walks, delicious meals, cups of tea, shopping and domestic upkeep you provided while I was in my office, glued to my laptop for days and weeks at a time. I would also like to thank you and acknowledge all the graphic consultations and book cover designs you have created. Thank you, thank you, thank you! This project would never have been completed without you and all your love, encouragement and belief in what I do and stand for. *Merci beaucoup mon cheri.*

**NOTE**

1    Rendell 2006: 191.

# 1

## Introduction

2011 was a watershed year in the United States for the reduction of women's reproductive rights at the state level. With more than 1,100 provisions introduced by legislators, the end of the year saw 135 of these provisions enacted. This is a marked increase from the 89 in 2010 and the 77 in 2009. Of these enacted last year, 68 percent restrict abortion access. These restrictions took many forms including time sensitive abortion bans, longer waiting periods, ultrasound requirements, varying insurance restrictions including complete prohibition of insurance coverage for abortions in a few states, stricter clinic building regulations, limits to medication abortion, reduction in family planning and abstinence-only education requirements.[1] Combine these new restrictions with the first three months of 2012 where the required contraception coverage in President Obama's healthcare mandate and certain states' transvaginal ultrasound abortion requirements have made significant headlines with outbursts from both political sides.[2] These examples are further evidence that there is a continued backlash against women's health needs and the ability for women to have full autonomy over their own healthcare decisions. Women are clearly not fully participatory citizens with complete control over their own bodies as these issues make evident.

As a feminist architect, I seek intersections between architecture and the political in order to provoke change both out in the world and within my own discipline. This book emerged from the desire for architecture to be political, something it is not good at being, and to deal with issues that are inherently politicized within our contemporary culture. Working on a few design competitions foregrounding particular gendered spatial relationships including a floor of single-room occupancy units for homeless women in downtown New York and a housing competition for a single mother and her child allowed me to conceptualize idealized spatial needs and test these through design. As well I seek and find local partnerships in need of design expertise and work with these various groups on a pro bono basis helping them realize their spatial needs. A few of these yet-to-be-built design projects include a renovation of a hospital chapel, the Library of

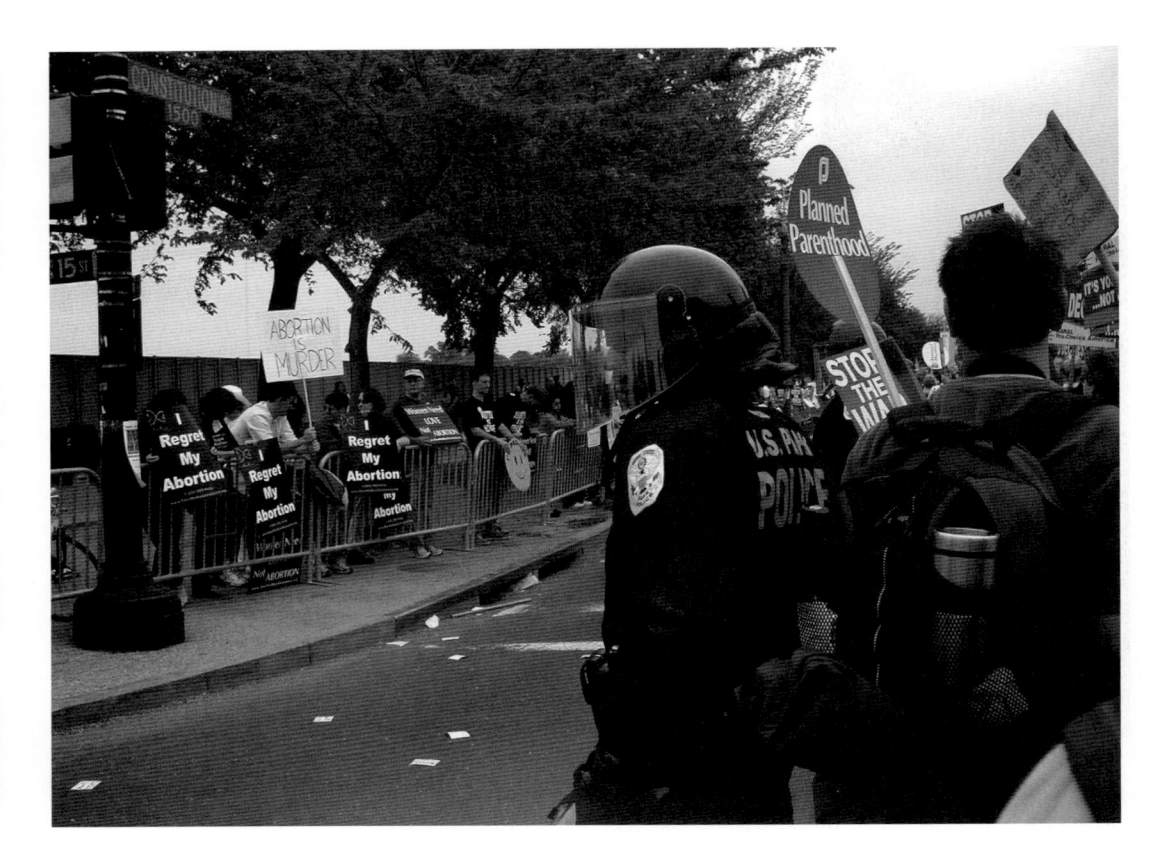

Fig 1.1 March for Women's Lives April 25, 2004 Washington D.C. Source: Lori A. Brown, 2004

Feminism for the Matilda Joslyn Gage Foundation, the renovation of the ground floor of an elderly housing tower for the Syracuse Housing Authority and the recently completed renovation of a kitchen, dining room and storage spaces for a local women's shelter. In each of these cases, my role was one of collaborator and partner envisioning how their spaces could be much better suited to their needs, sometimes with minor alterations and other times with more radical reconfigurations. These building projects fulfill a desire to work locally but there continues to be a drive to work toward larger-scaled social and political projects hoping to produce greater societal changes.

When considering what spaces are inherently contested and politicized, abortion clinics seemed like an obvious choice. Integral to abortion is how clinics intersect with public space and the First Amendment of the US Constitution guaranteeing an individual the right to freedom of speech and peaceful assembly.[3] As polarizing an issue as abortion is in various parts of North America, abortion provides an interesting platform to think through complex relationships of space, a woman's body, varying degrees of federal and state control, the fluid and ever-shifting terrain of reproductive healthcare access, potentials of design thinking in transforming spatial relationships and ways to radically rethink these issues to provoke change.

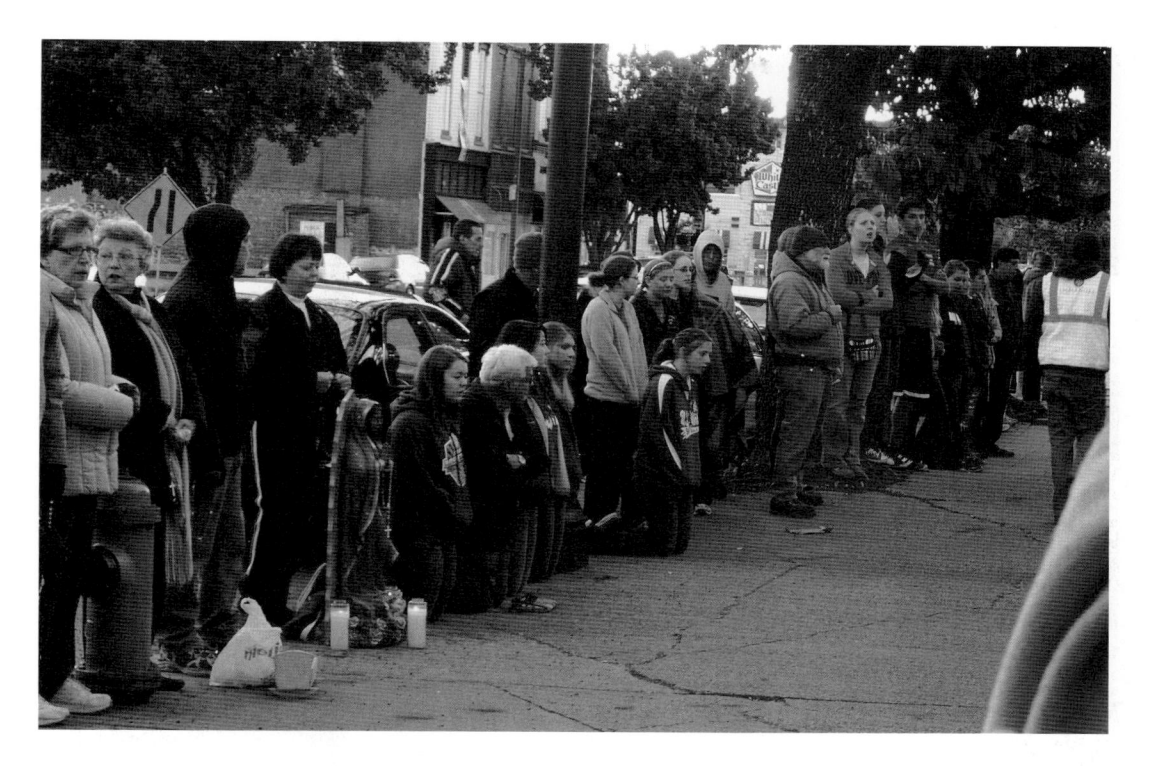

Another series of related questions more specific to the discipline of architecture include: What is the value of design thinking for the greater public in terms of abortion and public space? What role could architects have in exploring overlooked spaces like abortion clinics and women's shelters? How can design positively impact access? Although not explicitly aligned with the types of non-places theorized by the anthropologist Marc Augé, these types of spaces have an affinity coinciding with what he states: "[n]on-places could be seen, approaching them from another vantage point, as the heirs to everything that has created discomfort or annoyance in the history of human spaces."[4] Although the spaces of abortion and women's shelters are themselves not the creator of discomfort, the idea of these spaces definitely fall within this idea and the physicality of their existences clearly create discomfort for a large segment of the population.

Another motivation for the research is to reinsert architecture back into contemporary culture and the built environment of everyday space. As I have recently written, I am interested in foregrounding the expanding types of practices at varying scales occurring within architecture today. Practices calling into question or critically dismantling power dynamics, those giving voice and representation to people who are often silenced or not represented, others helping to bring communities into action through collaborative design processes and those practices revealing the deeply embedded sociopolitical relationships structuring our spaces are all part of the larger idea of how I am defining practice.[5] This research falls within these broader definitions.

Fig. 1.2 Pre-Easter anti-abortion protestor sidewalk queue in Louisville, KY April 2012
Source: Nelson Helm, 2012

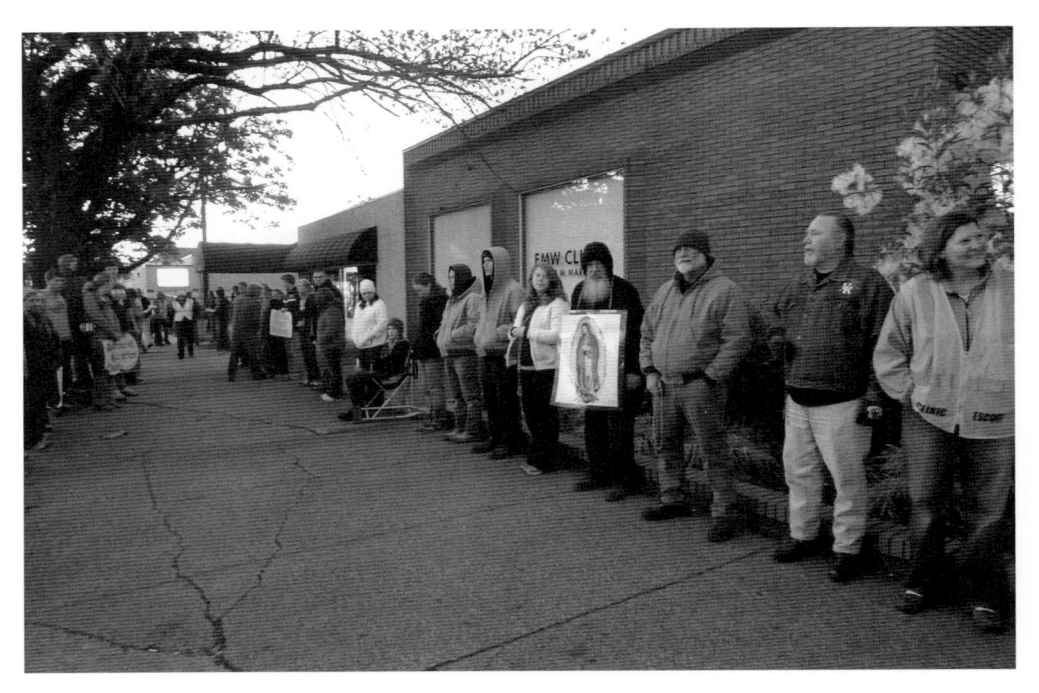

Fig. 1.3    Pre-Easter anti-abortion protestor sidewalk queue in Louisville, KY April 2012
Source: Nelson Helm, 2012

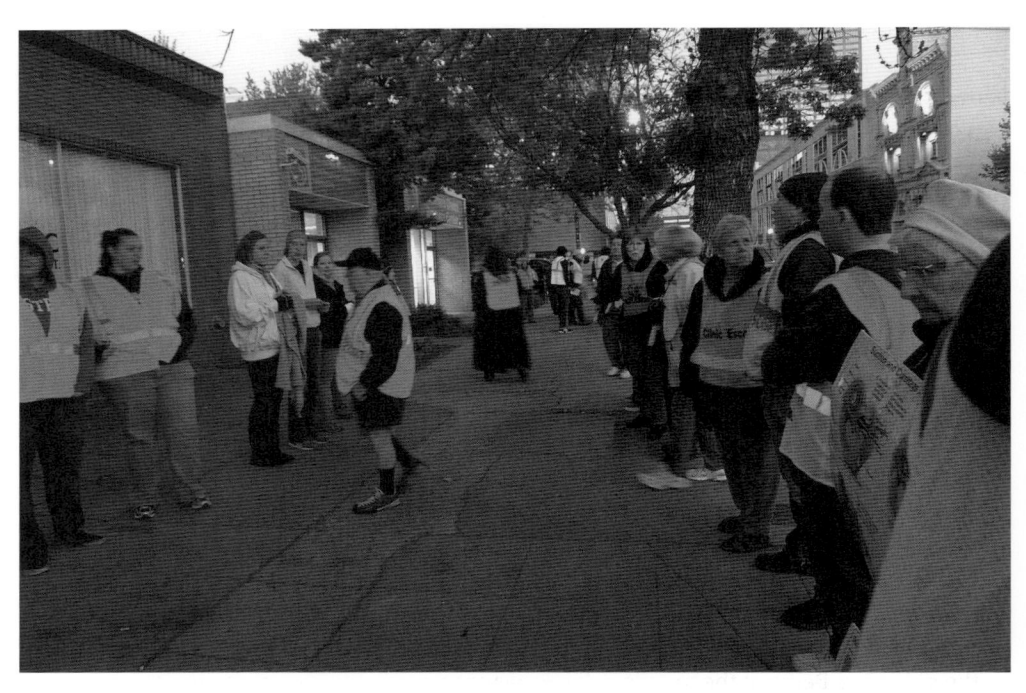

Fig. 1.4    Pre-Easter volunteer clinic escort queue in Louisville, KY April 2012
Source: Nelson Helm, 2012

What does it mean for the practice of architecture that architects are only directly engaged with from 2 to 5 percent of all building construction?[6] Where does this leave the discipline that is supposed to design and be responsible for the world's built environment? Although Fisher's introductory essay for *Expanding Architecture Design as Activism* is really focused on public-interest architecture, I believe the point he makes is pertinent to the larger argument regarding the lack of architecture's political and public presence, even absence, for those who are not wealthy—for the 99 percent. Or in other words, everyone but a limited few.

Architectural and cultural critic Reyner Banham's "A Black Box" criticizes architecture for its entrenchment within itself and the solipsism the discipline instills and perpetuates from the very beginning of architectural education, especially within design studio pedagogy and culture. The discipline, as he argues, operates on such a narrow value-system with "unspoken—or unspeakable—assumptions on which it rests." Architecture, no longer acknowledged as the "dominant mode of rational design," is seen as the "exercise of an arcane and privileged aesthetic code." He goes even further lambasting architecture as too proud and too accepting of a "parochial rule book [that] can only seem a crippling limitation on building's power to serve humanity." However, he ends the essay with a glimmer of hope that if architecture would allow itself to be "opened up to the understandings of the profane and the vulgar, at the risk of destroying itself as an art in the process …"[7] architecture may find an engaged existence in the world.

Architecture that engages in contemporary issues contributes to concerns out in the world. In *Architecture and Participation*, the editors skeptically question the general coinage of participation as an uncritical engagement with the user. Instead they are interested in exploring the "politics of participation," the "contested" terrain that participation opens up within participatory processes and the unexpected results from such a process. In the editors' framing of the book, "participation is not always regarded as the guarantee of sustainability within a project but as an approach that assumes risks and uncertainty."[8] These uncertainties and places of potential conflict "forc[e] it to engage with issues that in the long term will make architecture more responsive and responsible." This results in both an "alternative means of production … [that] leads to alternative aesthetics and spatialities." This type of participation suggests an "expanded field for architectural practice; it is a means of reinvigorating architecture, bringing benefit to users and architects alike."[9] As one of the book's editors, Jeremy Till, argues in his essay "The Negotiation of Hope," one result of architecture's denial of the political is its need to present itself as knowledgeable and specialist and the more it focuses on aesthetics over the user, the more and more detached architecture becomes from everyday needs and the "social life-world."[10] Focusing on space that is so highly politicized and contested, this research does precisely the opposite. I as the architect seek to find openings and gaps of possibility for re-inserting architecture into places ignored by the discipline. Being at the margins offers a way to exert productive pressure to improve our environment.

## THE PROJECT'S EMERGENCE

I think it is important to briefly mention how the scope of the project evolved because it speaks to a honing of research and potential impact of the book. When I first began preliminary research on the space of abortion, I imagined working with my regional Planned Parenthood and their local affiliates. I proposed interviewing patients, doctors and staff to better understand how people experience and live through their spatial constraints. At the time I was most interested in two particular aspects of these spaces. One was the patient's movement and flow through public space and how a person navigates the potentially complicated landscape outside clinic doors in the legally defined public realm. The second was how the clinic's spatial interior organization influenced a patient's experience from the moment she entered through the front doors into the waiting room until her name was called and her experience while "in the back." I was aware that my proposal had gone through at least a few of Planned Parenthood's bureaucratic layers and after waiting for a year and half, I finally received a no.

Not happy about their decision at the time, I did not want to give up on the project because although it was not entirely clear what I would now be researching, I felt that there was something important and necessary in looking at a type of space that most architects ignore. The "no" required I rethink and refocus the research and I realized the issues I needed to investigate really begin at the state level. Although abortion was legalized in 1973 through the Supreme Court *Roe v. Wade* decision, state legislatures have ultimately become the arbiters of access. A clear example can be seen by Mississippi and South Dakota, two of the most restrictive states in the country for abortion access. Each state legislature has publicly declared their goal to make their state what they refer to as "abortion-free" with absolutely no providers.[11] One can see through years of proposed and passed legislation both states are incredibly close to doing so.

As a result of these interests and the confluence of events, the project began to more broadly examine each state's influence and manipulation of reproductive healthcare laws and what impact they were having on a woman's right to physically access abortion. This required that I begin to think about the project on a much greater scale, no longer at the localized site of an individual clinic but at the scale of the state and how the state's legal exploitations of certain issues could produce drastically negative affects spatially on the ground. This also led me to look more closely at the most restrictive states, to better understand the impact these restrictions produce in terms of access, expense and time for a woman seeking care. I also interviewed independent providers to further demonstrate how these abstract laws impact real life situations and provide personal examples to parallel the data I was collecting.

In addition, two major shifts occurred within the research. First, the scope of the project expanded to include all of North America in order to provide a more diverse and in-depth reading of these contested spaces. Canada and Mexico are dramatically different in their histories, policies and regulations of abortion and provide provocative comparisons expanding the research. Second, women's shelters and hospitals were added to the research. Although not explored to the same degree, these two additional spatial groups broaden ideas of what it means for spaces to be both contested and regulated and reveal different ways of conceptualizing potentials of altering and/or disrupting the problems within each. There is something to be learned from the comparison of these spaces as they each deal with contestation and securitization in different yet related ways.

Abortion is still a hot-button issue, publicly debated and policies throughout North America continue to change. Clinic security is more and more a concern but varies significantly according to geographical location. Women's shelters require a great degree of security and privacy protocols affect all aspects of a woman's life while in residence. The philosophy of how and where to locate women's shelters and whether they remain secret and hidden within a city are currently being debated. I will discuss a number of groups that are testing different spatial models and what the merits of a more open and less-hidden shelter means not only for the residents but also the communities where they are located. In addition, every community has a hospital. Similar to both abortion clinics and women's shelters, geography of location matters for hospitals too. Security measures vary greatly from those where one can just walk right in and go directly to a patient's room without ever being asked for any identification to other hospitals where upon entering one is required to first register with the front desk's security officer, provide government-registered identification and receive a temporary identification sticker to affix to your clothing before ever being allowed access to a patient's room. There is a far greater degree of security in maternity and psychiatric areas of hospitals where concerns of child abduction or potentials for a patient to cause harm to herself or others requires higher degrees of securitization.

## THE ROLE OF PUBLIC SPACE IN THE RESEARCH

One of the initial issues that drew me to this research was the intersection of a highly politicized and charged space being contested out in the public realm. Utilized and active public space is vital for a democracy to work. The most recent examples of this can be seen during the Arab Spring in 2011 and the ongoing Occupy movement. All the many protests, calls for democracy and accountability of public and corporate figures continue to take place out in the public, occupying our public spaces. Although across the US, local city governments have reacted by shutting down numerous public spaces in a myriad of contorted and problematic ways, the point to be made is that what makes these most recent movements so powerful and influential is that they occur *in the public and are visible*.

Public space is critical in different ways for abortion clinics and women's shelters. Anti-abortion protestors regularly exercise their first amendment freedom by protesting out in front of abortion clinics across the United States. They are protected under law to be able to do so. It is part of the freedom individual citizens of this country have to be able to publicly speak out against issues one is against. As will be discussed in Chapter 3, both state and federal courts have ruled both in support and in opposition to certain abortion rights cases weighing free speech against abortion access. This has produced a variety of legislation controlling and manipulating physical boundaries around clinic properties and people's bodies. Domestic violence requires the public and publicity to raise awareness and garner public attention. Because domestic violence is so privatized, it is only through the making of it public that change can come about.

The distinctions created through many of these rulings rely on the problematic gendered division of public and private space historically associating men with the public realm and women with the domestic realm. But as the geographer Nancy Duncan has so elegantly articulated, these binaries, entrenched within political philosophy, law, popular discourse and general spatial practices, are used to legitimate oppression, regulate and exclude sexuality and sexual difference, and preserve more traditional structures of patriarchal and heterosexist power.[12] Privacy, the basis of the Supreme Court's *Roe v. Wade* decision legalizing abortion in the US, is deeply entrenched within "Western political theories of freedom, personal autonomy, patriarchal familial sovereignty and private property."[13] Unlike in abortion, privacy is a legal hindrance creating difficulty and often delays for state intervention in domestic violence cases. The need for more privacy can be traced back to the ascension of the European nation-state.

Through the increased autonomy of the family, state authority became further separated from and limited over the family unit. Over time, the right of family privacy became institutionalized. Duncan posits that although there are spatial elements to many of these social and political issues, "the solutions to these problems are not purely spatial or environmental ones."[14] This is also the case with this research.

As Duncan has noted, not all spaces are so easily divided into public or private realms.[15] I would first like to briefly lay the theoretical groundwork that further establishes the public realm's development prior to discussing how two leading feminist theorists have challenged these ideas. In the writing of critical theorist Jürgen Habermas who has examined the evolution of the public realm, his history first demonstrates how the emergence of this space during Greek antiquity was both exclusionary and gendered; one predicated on citizenship, a male land- and slave-owning privilege. It is interesting to note during antiquity "[t]he public sphere was constituted in discussion … forms of consultation and of sitting in the court of law … as well as in common action …."[16]

During the Middle Ages within feudal society, the attributes of lordship were referred to as "public" since the idea of lordship required a public representation, one exhibiting status that others must see. "[R]epresentation pretended to make something invisible visible through the public presence of the person of the lord …." This was further reinforced by one's attire, demeanor, forms of discourse and noble conduct.[17]

With the development of early capitalist trade, a new social order begins to emerge. The public sphere as we more commonly know it begins to take a more recognizable form during the rise of the bourgeois. Public meant state-related; one where the manorial lord's authority became the ability to police people under his purview. With the traffic in goods emerged the traffic in news. Although in the beginning restricted only for merchants, news eventually became a commodity to be exchanged as well. This initial public sphere, apolitical in form as argued by Habermas, is the literary precursor to contemporary public space. These were the spaces of coffee houses, salons and table societies where people, both noble society and the bourgeois, came together to discuss the latest news and cultural events. Although initially not political, these spaces of discussion quickly became more focused upon public criticism and political discourse.[18]

Comparing the differences in the development of these spaces in Britain, France and Germany, Habermas notes in both Britain and France a "parity of the educated" occurred with a larger inclusion of the middle class taking place in Britain. In France, unlike in the other two countries where only men were allowed access, the salons "like the rococo … were essentially shaped by women."[19] In Germany, social inclusiveness was a priority. In all cases, this "social equality was possible at first only as an equality outside the state. The coming together of private people into a public was therefore anticipated in secret, as a public sphere still existing largely behind closed doors."[20] According to Habermas, once "privatized individuals … ceased to communicate merely about their subjectivity but rather in their capacity as property-owners desired to influence public power in their common interest, the humanity of the literary public sphere served to increase the effectiveness of the public sphere in the political realm."[21]

Of the many feminist critics of Habermas's work, there are two I would like to briefly highlight. The first, critical theorist Nancy Fraser, argues that Habermas's ideas about the public sphere as one based on discursive interaction, where citizens debate common issues separate from and critical of the state, are absolutely relevant to critical theory. However, she writes that his idea is "not wholly satisfactory" and requires further questioning in order to more fully address the limits of "actually existing democracy." In her essay "Rethinking the Public Sphere," Fraser responds to Habermas's intention of presenting a new form of public sphere to retrieve its critical function.[22] She establishes a different history shedding insight onto several key omissions by Habermas. The first of these being that although Habermas argued this public space was open and accessible to all, where "inequalities of status were to be bracketed … discussants … to deliberate as peers" in fact it was not like this in practice. Gender served as exclusion to participation. For example in France the new republic public sphere was established in "deliberate opposition to that of a more woman-friendly salon culture …."[23] In addition, in Britain and Germany the societies, clubs and associations were all based upon this new bourgeois class formation. They were incredibly exclusionary and served as "training grounds" for the rising "universal class" that would eventually come to power. Embedded within this structure is the separation of public and private realms where bourgeois women were becoming associated with the newly defined private domestic realm. Fraser cites research by Mary Ryan foregrounding many ways that nineteenth century North American women found to be engaged in political life. These counter-civil societies were located within women-only associations and reform societies and initially began within the private sphere of their homes; these women created ways to be engaged publicly. What Ryan demonstrates is that there were many counterpublics: "nationalist publics, popular peasant publics, elite women's publics, and working class publics ... and [they] were always constituted by conflict."[24] Habermas does not recognize any of these constituencies.

Fraser argues against the following four assumptions Habermas makes and suggests an alternative approach to public space. First, it is possible for the public sphere to be bracketed in order that deliberation can happen as equals and political democracy necessitates societal equality. Second, a single "comprehensive public sphere is always preferable to a nexus of multiple publics." Third, public discourse should only focus on the common good and discourse should deny the inclusion of "private interests" or "private issues." Fourth, a "functioning public sphere requires a sharp separation between civil society and the state."[25]

Her alternative comprises "a plurality of competing publics to better promote the ideal of participatory parity" in contrast to Habermas's single public space. She acknowledges when there are societal inequalities, the less powerful groups will not have the same power of voice and representation as the dominant groups and this will be further exacerbated if there is only one public sphere that all must engage. She refers to these new spaces as *"subaltern counterpublics"* signifying "they are parallel discursive arenas where members of subordinated social groups invent and circulate counterdiscourses, which in turn permit them to formulate oppositional interpretations of their identities, interests, and needs." These new publics increase discursive space and contestation requiring that their once unheard voice must be publicly acknowledged and debated.[26]

The political theorist Iris Marion Young puts forth a different idea about public space. In discussing the public sphere, it is interesting to note that she first defines publicity as a space or a precise indoor or outdoor location "for communicative engagement and contest" open to all. Combined with the idea of location is also one's ability to invite the public to this space for such activities requiring one's access to public media in its various forms. Second, publicity refers to a plurality of citizens "with varying interests, priorities, values, and experiences." Due to the multiplicity of citizens or actors as she refers to them, the public is exposed to a diversity of viewpoints and attitudes and as a result, the public "has little control over how the public will take up, interpret, and act in relation to what they see and hear." The third aspect of publicity refers to the type of expressions made public. These need to be made in such a way that they can be understood by anyone.[27]

In contrast to both Habermas and Fraser, Young actually argues for a public sphere that incorporates some elements from both of their two theories. She agrees with Habermas' idea that:

> *a single continuous public process or "space" is necessary if the idea of public sphere is to be helpful in describing how a diverse, complex, mass society can address social problems through public action. The scope of activity, interaction, contradiction, and conflict requires an open flow of communication across neighborhood, region, and associational networks.*[28]

In addition, Young also agrees with Fraser's idea of subaltern counterpublics as a way to create space "where members of subordinated groups develop ideas, arguments, campaigns, and protest actions directed at influencing a wider public debate, often with the goal of bringing about legal or institutional change."[29]

Young believes democratic theory and practice requires both the single public sphere argued by Habermas and the subaltern counterpublics defined by Fraser. Both are needed because without the ability of smaller groups to organize and publicize their concerns, the unified public will exclude and disenfranchise some actors. Where Young then diverges and reframes the argument is through the way she defines democracy. She questions a democracy where "élite decision-makers are elected and subject to the rule of law" because this definition does not address the influence of regular citizens. For her, the connection between citizens and the powerful is critical for exerting influence on democracy. Although the commonly referred adage of democracy "rule by the people" acknowledges this connection, it does so, she argues, on a superficial level. Democracy, for her argument, is "a process that connects "the people" and the powerful, and through which people are able significantly to influence their actions. Democracy is more or less strong and deep according to how strong are these connections and how predictable that influence."[30]

This primary connection is the public sphere. A healthy public sphere is a space of "opposition and accountability … and policy influence."[31] Political actors through their various methods can help instigate change. Their power resides in the ability to uncover, expose, publicize and even shame powerful actors. In so doing, ordinary citizens' use of the public sphere is one way to "limit power and hold powerful actors accountable." Because power hides in often hard to find places, it is even more critical for diverse citizen groups to do their utmost to expose power abuses. As she states "[c]reative acts of civil disobedience often force power to become naked."[32] Through politicizing their discoveries, inequalities can be disrupted. But the powerful actors will not make it easy and will do their upmost to control the public message. She acknowledges that it takes great will by the excluded to get their message heard and for these reasons, the public sphere will "be a site of struggle—often contentious struggle."[33]

Because protest has for decades been a part of the abortion debate, the way we understand and use public space is critical to rethinking access to reproductive healthcare. Citizen actors on both sides of the issue have been exerting political pressure. So much so that now anti-abortion groups have been successfully influencing state legislatures across the country creating ever more restrictive and unbalanced laws. Although legal on paper, abortion is becoming more and more difficult to access for poor women of color. Young's ideas of civic action and even disobedience are critical to a thriving democracy, but what happens when one set of actors are so successful in curtailing women's legal rights to autonomy and control over their own body? What happens when the state intervenes too much? What needs to be done then?

## CONTESTED AND POLITICIZED LANDSCAPES

As an architect, I am aware that there is typically little overt discussion about the cultural responsibility we have in designing the built environment. Of course there are those of us who advocate strongly on the side of considering whom we are designing for. However, more generally, there is a tacit acknowledgement that we are designing for users, these users have specific needs and we, as architects, are to decipher and translate their needs into formal realities. One of the inherent problems in this scenario is that this process tends to rely upon a strict degree of abstraction. By removing real people and even real problems from this causal relationship, it makes it far easier to pursue designing form without regard for who or how it will be used. As mentioned earlier, Banham raises issue with architecture's disconnect to the world's problems and admonishes architecture as a discipline only of aesthetic production.

It is imperative to reconnect a primary aspect of architecture to the role of cultural and material production or stated in a different way, to meaning. In this discussion design and architecture will be used interchangeably. Anthropology defines design as spatialized cultural ideas reflecting "cultural ordering" and operating as a "communication system." As anthropologist Setha Low has written, "[d]esign is … a culture-making process in which ideas, values, norms and beliefs are spatially and symbolically expressed in the environment to create new cultural forms and meaning."[34] In these terms, design can either be man-made or a response to ecological factors. Design is reactive to and legible through certain specific social and political contexts. One's reading of culture influences how one spatializes a response or in other words, produces architectural form. Design as a form of "culture as meaning system," symbolizes. Cultural and social ideas become embedded at a variety of scales including the domestic, the institution and the city. All spatial relationships "reflect sociopolitical, economic, and cultural changes …."[35] They are markers of time, place and power.

Intersecting with ideas of cultural representation are expressions of place and landscape. Although place is a geographical location connected to people and economic activities, social theory's definition of place refers to a group of spatially connected people that are able to negotiate "cultural identity, state power, and capital accumulation."[36] Place reflects culture, is shaped by it, and in turn shapes it. During the fourteenth century, European landscape painting operated as symbols of power relations. These paintings were not facts. Today the term landscape is understood as the representation of social and material practices; "the architecture of social class, gender, and race relations imposed by powerful institutions."[37] Often the term stands for "a contentious, compromised product of society." When cited today, landscape evokes representations of social controls and unbalanced economies. As sociologist Sharon Zukin writes, cultural geographers "regard all landscapes as symbolic, as expressions of cultural values, social behavior, and individual actions worked upon particular localities over a span of time."[38] For her the direct correlations between material and cultural aesthetic practices and how they are shaped and influenced by economic and political powers translate into research about landscape—"the major cultural product of our time."[39]

The contested landscapes this book explores seek to make explicit political, cultural and social influences. These connections will be discussed further in Chapter 5 when examining women's shelters, hospitals and specific regions where clinics are located. It is important to note that these differing landscapes are legible in particular ways and at distinct scales: from their physical locations within a city, legislated lines providing literal zones of "safety," state restrictions legalizing and perpetuating cultural and social influences to undisclosed and hidden shelter locations. Forms of political landscapes reveal multi-layered complexities embedded within the three categories of spaces the book examines.

## INTERSECTIONS

In *The Production of Space*, Henri Lefebvre differentiates ways space operates within systems of power. *Representations of space* are abstract and conceptualized operating as a verbal and intellectual system of signs and are "the most dominant space in any society (or mode of production)."[40] Scientists, urbanists, planners and social engineers are all a part of the representations of space. *Representational space* is lived through associated non-verbal images and symbols, users and inhabitants. This space is "the dominated and … passively experienced space which the imagination seeks to change and appropriate."[41] Bodies of government or systems of justice are signified spatially through their various legislative buildings and courts of law. Additionally there is social space that includes production of labor, social hierarchies and biological reproduction.[42]

Architecture's potential, for the argument of this research, resides more not within representational spaces but in what de Certeau calls its tactical abilities. De Certeau distinguishes between tactics as actions that are independent from the law and strategies that follow and conform to abstract models.[43] Explaining further, he states that a strategy "seeks first of all to distinguish its "own" place … of its own power … it is an effort to delimit one's own place in a world bewitched by the invisible powers of the Other. It is also the typical attitude of modern science, politics, and military strategy."[44] Conversely, a tactic "is a calculated action determined by the absence of a proper locus … the space of a tactic is the space of the other … It must vigilantly make use of the cracks that particular conjunctions open in the surveillance of the proprietary powers. It poaches in them … It can be where it is least expected … a tactic is an art of the weak."[45] The ability, as Young argues, to gather divergent publics together for debate and conversation in order to influence political institutions, can be witnessed through more temporal and tactical efforts. Like the counterpublics that organize together, these temporal moments like protests, clinic escorts, women's safe houses, advocation for legislative change, and so on, have the ability to target specific issues and public spaces to raise awareness around particular concerns or events through placing pressure, politicizing through publicity and even possibly shaming of public figures. It is here where the possibility lies—potentials for public space around reproductive healthcare clinics, women's shelters and even hospitals for counterpublics to exert force and influence change. Whether this entails outright counter demonstrations, escorting or exerting political pressure on state power, these de Certeauian tactics have historically proven to undermine representations of space.

Architecture, in this project, refers to two larger sets of inquiries, both impacting the emotional and physical geographies in and around clinics, women's shelters and hospitals. The first, and most straight forward, is the obvious relationship between the literal building, its siting and access, what one passes through to enter the building and security required to ensure safety. The second set requires a broader framing of architecture and its engagement with the larger political, social and geographic sets of concerns that inherently affect how space is not only designed but also, and more importantly for the sake of this research, registers in the everyday world with everyday people: architecture as the register of these antagonistic forces. This second set of issues includes the economics around spatial production, the exclusionary tactics of such production and the direct impact legislation has on the occupation of the built environment.

Intersections between architecture, feminist geography, art as well as other spatial practices are important for establishing the framework of the book. Having written earlier about these important influences, feminist methods provide multivalent approaches, recognize problems are always complex and layered and are inherently political acts of engagement. Feminist methods seek to both disrupt power structures and reveal power inequalities.[46] Questioning "universal" knowledge and what may first appear as neutral claims, feminist methods contribute through contextualizing and repoliticizing knowledge and knowledge production.[47] Feminist scholarship is interested in issues of subjectivity, identity and the body and how sexual difference reflects power relations. People are "culturally shaped and historically and spatially positioned."[48] As art historian Griselda Pollock has so articulately stated:

> the organizing unities of feminism, women, theory and so forth, which helped us to locate a point of dissidence and critical difference from official knowledge and established social forms, have themselves to be politically fractured. Feminist stands here for a political commitment to women and to changes that women desire for themselves and for the world. Feminism stands for a commitment to the full appreciation of what women inscribe, articulate, voice and image in cultural forms: interventions in the field of meaning and identity form the place called "woman or the feminine." Feminism also refers to a theoretical revolution in ways in which terms such as art, culture, woman, subjectivity, politics and so forth are understood … Feminist readings are made from the spaces of politicized and theorized feminist subjectivities and social positions. These are necessarily plural … contemporary feminism is acutely aware of conflicts, diversity and resulting tensions between the political alliances signified by feminism and the real divergences and distances between the socially constituted women who make up the movement.[49]

Doing feminist research, as feminist geographer Pamela Moss has written, influences all facets of the research process. One is more aware of the multiple contexts of where research occurs, the situatedness of the researcher, how one collects and analyzes information and the social constructions of gendered spatialities.[50] The philosopher Sandra Harding has written that these broader definitions of feminist research and methodology remind us that it is not only the research questions asked but also those that are not asked that become influential in understanding the larger research potential. As well, she articulates one important component of feminist research is that it is generated from the experiences of women. These experiences are critical for the larger concerns of "social life in general." For "[w]omen should have an equal say in the design and administration of the institutions where knowledge is produced and distributed for reasons of social justice …."[51] Asking "[h]ow can politicized inquiry be increasing the objectivity of inquiry?"[52] she responds that these "social values and political agendas" are believed to expand the scope and breadth of research and provoke "greater care in the conduct of inquiry …."[53] Feminist empiricism argues that the "context of discovery" is equal to the "context of justification." One potential of this way of thinking is "for eliminating social biases that contribute to partial and distorted explanations and understandings."[54] As stated earlier, we are all products of our environments; "what we do shapes and constrains what we can know."[55] I feel it is important to locate this body of work within this larger context. I hope this expands the scope and breadth of spatial practice while foregrounding women's experiences.

## METHODOLOGY

> *How can we use our educational apparatuses and institutions to make social change—how we can reinvigorate "our capacity as agents to act as well as to know otherwise, to intervene in the world as well as the academy, to have an effect."*[56] *(Gayle Greene)*

As I mentioned at the beginning of this chapter, the research emerged from the desire to force architecture to confront the political. Not only am I interested in expanding the discipline to be more politically engaged and relevant to the general public but also I aspire to raise awareness about our built environment, the influences directly shaping it, how these influences affect people's lived lives, look for places of potential and speculate upon ways to intervene within and into these spaces in order for them to be more inclusive and diverse. No space is neutral. Place and space are created through various agents of power and influence. As sociologist Heidi Gottfried has written "[r]esearch is inherently political, structured in hierarchies of power among researchers, between sponsors of research and researchers, and between researchers and the subjects of their research."[57] She further posits that if feminist practice is to "question social relations based on power" then feminist research has to offer resistance and challenge academic power and all its many effects in order to create alternatives to it; "[r]esearch itself can be a vehicle for consciousness-raising."[58]

Although I have previously partnered with many groups and underrepresented communities as an architect, this is the first time interviews are a major portion of a creative research project. I believe it is important for me to be understood as an advocate and supporter of the work abortion providers do and that I am present to hear and tell their side of the story. The research works to create a space of collaboration and conversation with the participants and hopes they see these interviews as a way for their voice to be heard and represented.[59] The media fully portrays the anti-abortion side of the debate but not near enough is presented and reported in support of abortion and the impact state legislation is actually having on access. As Jennifer Hyndman has been quoted, "many feminist and other geographers do fieldwork precisely to critique, deconstruct and reconstruct a more responsible, if partial, account of what is happening in the world."[60] This is precisely what I hoped to accomplish through interviewing and spending time with many providers across the United States.

Once the research changed focus and began to examine the differences among state abortion legislation, it became apparent that I needed to look more closely at the most restrictive states. Because this research spans many years, some of the state data collected is no longer the most current. However, I think the data still provides representation of the most salient and key issues. In order to have a broader understanding of these issues and to think more creatively about ways access could be increased, pharmacies became one way to expand this idea. If pharmacies stocked and sold the morning-after pill or emergency contraception (EC), then this is one earlier and additional space along the reproductive healthcare line of access. As a result, my research assistants and I called all the pharmacies in South Dakota, North Dakota, Mississippi, Kentucky, Nebraska and Utah to determine if they stocked and sold the morning-after pill. We posed as women in need of the prescription and documented the responses of all pharmacists we were able to speak with. These results are represented in Chapter 5.

It was important to be able to speak with on-the-ground providers in order to gain a more realistic understanding of how a state's various laws impact and influence a women's ability to access an abortion and how a provider's clinic deals with the ongoing onslaught of protestors. I interviewed only independent providers in some of the most restrictive states as well as others in less restrictive states. Prior to arriving at an area, letters of introduction were mailed to local clinics including an overview of the research, information about myself and my university affiliation with my website and business card about four to six weeks in advance. I would then follow up with a series of phone calls in hopes of setting up an appropriate time to meet someone at their clinic. Typically this step would take several rounds of phone messages before being able to speak directly with a clinic director or doctor. Although all doctors and clinic directors agreed to allow me to use their real names and locations, I have decided not to disclose them due to the highly politicized and charged nature of abortion in this country. I feel strongly I need to provide anonymity out of respect for what they do. The research has undergone IRB approval from my university. After consulting colleagues in other disciplines who research in other sensitive and politicized areas, they all agreed this would be the best way to protect my interviewees. Location is assigned by region of the country and no names are mentioned when discussing interviews.

The research presented in this book is really a hybrid of sorts. As an architect I have most often worked through drawings and models. Due to this subject matter and the goals of the research, mapping and diagramming seemed more appropriate and better suited in conveying the data collected. Most often I write alongside the maps and images as a way to further explore their information. Another goal was to create graphic representations merging data from many websites to create more legible and easier to understand information. I hope this is in fact what happens as you read through the book.

Chapter 3 focuses upon the legal frameworks around abortion in all three countries. Several major and influential court rulings are discussed in more detail with a series of diagrams demonstrating the spatial implications for each. A discussion of the differences and similarities of the three concludes this chapter. Chapter 4 presents a series of case studies for abortion, women's shelters and hospitals. These were selected for a variety of ways they creatively and sometimes unexpectedly engage space and access. From domestic spaces, motels, offices, pharmacists to clinics, the different way space was produced and accessed is a primary concern in this chapter. A few of the examples date to before abortion was legal to other more present day examples as well as some of the interesting changes happening in the location of women's shelter. Chapter 5 focuses on the landscapes of access for all three countries as well as a discussion around security and how security can be used as a space of potential. This chapter includes many maps and diagrams of the data collected through the calling of pharmacies and of state restrictions. Chapter 6 concludes the book thinking through the ways the research can have potential effects for these contested terrains.

## NOTES

1. Guttmacher Institute 2012.
2. For more information please see Pear 2012a, Grady 2012, Goodstein 2012, Pear 2012b, Eckholm 2012.
3. "The United States Constitution." 1789.
4. On the Move 2009.
5. Brown 2011. There are also many recent, edited books that are focusing on similar issues. A few include Awan et al. 2011, Kossak et al. 2010, Lepik and Bergdoll 2010, Petrescu 2007, Jones et al. 2005.
6. Fisher 2008: 9.
7. Banham 1999: 294, 297–9.
8. Jones et al. 2005: "Introduction," xiv.
9. Jones et al. 2005: "Introduction": xv, xvi.
10. Jeremy Hill, "The Negotiation of Hope," in Jones et al. 2005: 29, 31.
11. Although somewhat dated, please see Frontline's 2005 documentary *The Last Abortion Clinic* on Mississippi's state legislative efforts to do this.
12. Duncan 1996: 127–8.
13. Duncan 1996: 128.

14  Duncan 1996: 127–8.
15  Duncan 1996: 129.
16  Habermas 1989: 3–4.
17  Habermas 1989: 7–8.
18  Habermas 1989: 14–29.
19  Habermas 1989: 33.
20  Habermas 1989: 34–5.
21  Habermas 1989: 56.
22  Fraser 1990: 57–8.
23  Fraser 1990: 59.
24  Fraser 1990: 60–61.
25  Fraser 1990: 62–3.
26  Fraser 1990: 66–7.
27  Young 2000: 168–9.
28  Young 2000: 171.
29  Young 2000: 172.
30  Young 2000: 173.
31  Young 2000: 172–3.
32  Young 2000: 175.
33  Young 2000: 174–6, 178.
34  Low 1988: 188.
35  Low 1988: 187–90.
36  Zukin 1991: 12.
37  Zukin 1991: 16.
38  Zukin 1991: 16–17, 18.
39  Zukin 1991: 22.
40  Lefebvre 1991: 39.
41  Lefebvre 1991: 39.
42  Lefebvre 1991: 26–46.
43  de Certeau 1984: 29.
44  de Certeau 1984: 35–6.
45  de Certeau 1984: 36–7.
46  Brown 2011: Introduction and Conclusion.
47  Duncan 1996: 245, 247.
48  McDowell 1999: 7–8.

49  Pollock 1996: xv.
50  Moss 2002: 3.
51  Harding 1987a: 7. I think the introduction should be 'a' and the conclusion should be 'b'.
52  Harding 1987b: 182. I think the introduction should be 'a' and the conclusion should be 'b'.
53  Harding 1987b: 183.
54  Harding 1987b: 183.
55  Harding 1987b: 183, 184, 185.
56  Gottfried 1996: 14.
57  Gottfried 1996: 14.
58  Gottfried 1996: 16.
59  Although I had not read Linda McDowell's book *Gender Identity & Place Understanding Feminist Geographies* in its entirety prior to interviewing, many things she discusses resonated with me in regards to how a feminist conducts research and what sorts of methods feminist more generally use to promote collaborative and non-manipulative relationships with their participants. Please see her "Postscript: Reflections on the Dilemmas of Feminist Research" for more.
60  Sparke 1996: 212.

# 2

## Social and Spatial Practices

My first academic introduction to the idea of relationships between space and gender was when I arrived at graduate school for architecture and was exposed to Beatriz Colomina's edited book *Sexuality and Space*. Resulting from an interdisciplinary symposium, the book brings together a collection of critical thinkers whose scholarship intersects the "relationships between sexuality and space hidden within everyday practices ...."[1] Her book's introduction proposes a few positions that were influential to me at the time: "the politics of space are always sexual, even if space is central to the mechanisms of the erasure of sexuality" and "space is ... a form of representation."[2] What I was not aware of nor realized until many years later was that these ideas were not new but were part of a much larger body of work from disciplines such as geography, anthropology, art, sociology and women's studies. As Colomina recognized, work on sexuality by feminist theorists was a "glaring absence ... conspicuously ignored in architectural discourse and practice."[3] That was in 1992 and now, 20 years later, there still remains an absence within contemporary architectural discourse.[4]

Several of the contributors to that edited collection would come to be influential in my intellectual development but none more so than the philosopher Elizabeth Grosz. She was the first person I seriously read working within the categories of gender, sex, space and power relations. Because I could *see* the spatial relationships she was writing about, there was an immediate connection made between my architectural training and ways space reinforced specific power relations and social constructions of identity. As an architect, my education and practice working with real, material and spatial relationships allowed Grosz's work to be quite accessible since she writes in spatial terms. I was able to enter into and visualize the physicality and spatial influences she was theorizing about.

Grosz's contribution for *Sexuality and Space*, "Bodies-Cities," references the reciprocal relationships between bodies and cities and how each informs and influences the other. For her, the body is "concrete, material ... indeterminate, amorphous, a series of uncoordinated potentialities ..." and the city is "a complex and interactive network which links together ... imaginary and real, projected or actual architectural, geographic, civic, and public relations."[5] Grosz writes she is interested "in exploring the ways in which the body is psychically, socially, sexually, and discursively or representationally produced, and the ways, in turn, bodies reinscribe and project themselves onto their sociocultural environment so that this environment both produces and reflects the form and interests of the body."[6] She argues against this binary or one-way relationship between bodies as the cause and cities as the effect or the city mirroring the body and the idea that the "state parallels the body."[7] Design is not a one-way system but in fact the body; its needs, desires, mobilities and interactions inform the evolution of how spaces and places are created. Bodies directly impact the evolution and network of spaces and in turn, are affected by such spaces. Grosz argues against the use of the human body, typically gendered male, as representative of the body-politic because this results in the universal ideal to be rendered male; the body-politic is then by association masculine.[8]

Instead, she proposes a different model combining both the body and city as "mutually defining" producing an "interface, perhaps a cobuilding." This is not to be thought of as a total model or system but one that generates fragments, "sub- or microgroupings" one that is more about "disparate flows ... events or entities ... brought together or drawn apart in more or less temporary alignments."[9] In many ways, she is describing what already happens at varying and indeterminate scales reflecting ever-changing economic and sociopolitical fluctuations.

Grosz also asks "how different cities, different sociocultural environments actively produce the bodies of their inhabitants as particular and distinctive types of bodies, as bodies with particular physiologies, affective lives, and concrete behaviors."[10] She argues that cities organize, orient, divide, connect, socialize and regulate bodies. This happens differently in cities around the world at varying economic levels for all genders.

## THE SOCIAL AND SPATIAL

Like Grosz, other feminist theorists write about and speculate upon relationships between the body, sexuality, social relations and space. This chapter will discuss a variety of people whose work intersects with one or more of the following topics: space and the body, public–private dichotomies, the home and architecture. The chapter will conclude considering the spaces of possibility for this research building upon this body of literature.

In her edited collection *BodySpace Destabilizing Geographies of Gender and Sexuality*, Nancy Duncan contextualizes and situates the book in terms of social relations and states "[f]eminists are ... exploring the far-reaching implications of a new epistemological viewpoint based on the idea of knowledge as embodied, engendered and embedded in the material context of place and space."[11] This "situated knowledge" is one based in awareness of social, cultural and geographical sets of relationships and are spatially "constructed and negotiated" and integral to place. Like Grosz, Duncan believes that space is both controlling and confining of power and yet has the potential to disrupt these power relations.[12] The cultural geographer Affrica Taylor states space is "political currency" and therefore will always be fought after. "Securing space, in whatever form, is a political act: whether through invasion of territories; colonization; dispossession; appropriation; representation; the disciplining of knowledge; or the purchase of real-estate. The occupying of space is an assertion of power, and continual displacement is power's spatial effect."[13] One registers these power grabs and displacements every day in myriad ways and in differing degrees. Be it through protesting out in front of abortion clinics hoping to persuade or even prevent women from entering, women and their children having to seek temporary shelter outside their home for reasons of safety and security, to the state forcing a woman to undergo a transvaginal ultrasound in order to access her legal right to abortion, the space of the public, the domestic and the body are continually contested, invaded and fought over for control.

As geographer Linda McDowell describes, place is constituted through relations of power that define rules and boundaries, who is welcome and who is excluded. These places are "contested, fluid and uncertain."[14] Another geographer, Elizabeth Kenworthy Teather, defines the sense of place as "the link between place and meaning" that can be different for each individual and hard to codify.[15] What happens when we begin to consider relationships between gender and place? How does gender influence our experience and reading of place? As political theorist Linda Alcoff has stated "gender 'is not a point to start from in the sense of being a given thing but is, instead, a posit or construct, formalizable in a non-arbitrary way through a matrix of habits, practices and discourse.'"[16] To take this idea one step further, theorist Judith Butler calls gender a "cultural performance—the effect of a set of contested power relations." She believes gender is never stable but always contested.[17] Gender is powerful, can undermine the status quo and changes based on proximities and associations of different social and political groups.

Emodiment "captures the sense of fluidity, of becoming and of performance ... question[ing] the relationship between anatomy and social politics."[18] As geographer Robyn Longhurst notes it is interesting that certain aspects of the body with all its untidy, fluid-producing possibilities is typically not included. The body abstracted is a cleaner and easier idea to argue rendering it "incorporal, fleshless, fluidless, little more than a linguistic territory ... reduced to systems of signification."[19] She argues ignoring the "messy" body with uncertain boundaries renders certain issues "invisible and/or ... illegitimate by the hegemons in the discipline."[20] She continues by stating:

> *Although it now is permissible, even desirable, within feminist and postmodernist discourse to acknowledge something of ourselves and our political locatedness in the production of our texts ... it is still permissible only to acknowledge and reflect on certain things about ourselves—things we are supposed to unproblematically know and understand such as our gender, ethnicity, and/or age. Many things remain off limits—too private, too "inappropriate," too messy, to put into our epistemic "master" pieces.*[21]

Longhurst believes that a potential of embodiment could lead to investigations between bodies and cities that are "mutually defining"[22] as Grosz has suggested. I mention Longhurst's work in relation to two aspects of this book's research: abortion and domestic violence. Within both of these domains, what happens to the body, whether it is violated and to what degree the body is violated, oscillates between complete and total abstraction through verbal and written description to a total and inaccurate manipulation of meaning through images. People want to ignore and disregard this content. People do not want to see a woman after she has been assaulted because it is disturbing. In the same way, anti-abortion protestors know that when they protest with their fallacious images of fetuses they make people pause and feel uncomfortable. That is precisely their point. However, I would like to believe that if there were more honest and real discussions and depictions of these issues within the media, the public might find they would have a different relationship to abortion and domestic violence and would be more willing to engage in real and productive discussions about the issues.

**The Body and …**

Society scrutinizes and regulates the body constantly. Others register the body through the many different spaces and varying scales the body occupies.[23] As mentioned earlier, these are socially and politically constructed relations continually in flux. Referencing Michel Foucault, McDowell summarizes his ideas about the body and his careful historical analysis demonstrates how science, moralities, legal and other structures as well as personal and interpersonal beliefs "produce the forms of sexed Embodiment that they regulate." Bodies are created and acted on through "discursively constructed institutional settings."[24]

These shifting scales offer an interesting intersection with both abortion and women's shelters. Abortion and domestic violence occur in the most private of space, the space of a woman's body. However, both intersect with the public when debated, legislated and accessed. This inversion of something so personal and private being debated within the realm of the public is a strange and troubling paradox. In the sense that through the making of *publicness* the issues around each are ultimately manipulated and changed into something no longer about women's bodies, women's choice, or women's safety but are used to benefit the different political parties own agendas.

**… Pregnancy**

I feel it is beneficial to include a brief discussion about a selected body of research within feminist geography and philosophy discussing the pregnant body. I am interested in how these theories influence the reading of the body in space. This work is important because it provides an alternative reading and understanding of a woman's body in space and how society comes to engage a woman who is pregnant. I recognize there is no equivalent in spatial experience to a nine-month pregnant body compared to, say, a six-week pregnant body but these authors provide important insights that are worth noting and thinking about further for the evolution of this research. Although clearly not physically visible in the same ways, a woman knows she is pregnant at a certain point whether she visibly appears to be so or not. This knowledge informs how she navigates space and how others engage her in space.

Drawing from her own experience as well as others, Iris Marion Young's essay "Pregnant Embodiment Subjectivity and Alienation" discusses the relationship between a woman to that of her pregnant body. As she notes, subjectivity as a part of pregnancy is absent from discourse so her essay seeks "to let women speak in their own voices." Pregnancy, Young writes, does not belong to the mother; her body is but a container for the developing fetus. She is in a "condition" where she must take the utmost care of herself. Pregnancy is temporal; a period where the woman "experience[s] herself split between past and future."[25] This experience challenges how she understands her body's boundaries where there are no longer distinct separations between what is legible within the body, herself, and outside the body. Due to these uncertain boundaries, her ever-expanding pregnant body undermines and challenges how she experiences her body and the space around her. The pre-pregnant body image is retained yet now movement occurs with a pregnant body. The boundaries one thought one had are no longer the same.[26]

Because the pregnant body is desexualized by culture, there is a temporary separation from the "sexually objectifying gaze that alienates and instrumentalizes her when in her nonpregnant state." She notes that some women have felt approval from strangers while visibly pregnant.[27] I would argue that actually the opposite occurs for women seeking abortion. This happens at least on two different levels. First is the physical encounter with scrutiny. A woman going to an abortion clinic is under direct surveillance by certain publics standing outside those doors trying to speak to her as she makes her way to the front door. Second is the result of legislation where, through the use of state power, a woman's body is legislatively controlled resulting in physical limitations and diminishment to and sometimes prevention of her ability to make her own personal and autonomous decisions.

One last point I would like to highlight Young makes is in relationship between women's reproductivity and medicine. For most of medicine's history, women's reproductive processes were not included within the field of medicine nor needed to be. However, once subsumed within the field of medicine, these processes became considered diseases needing treatment. Young makes the argument that this legacy defining "pregnancy and other reproductive functions as conditions requiring medical therapy … has not been entirely abandoned."[28] This paternalistic idea of requiring treatment, of taking control over a woman's body has greatly influenced the abortion debate once the procedure became illegal by the time of the Civil War. Clearly there is a connection between medical therapies and the practice of abortion and even to the medicalization of domestic violence. The medical establishment wants control over how these issues are diagnosed, labeled, reported and treated. This will be discussed in more detail in the next chapter, especially in regards to the establishment of the American Medical Association (AMA) in 1847 and the subsequent impact the AMA had on women's reproductive health.

Robyn Longhurst's research with pregnant women reveals that for many, their pregnant bodies in public become a concern both for themselves and others. As the body becomes more visibly pregnant some women find that their normal public behaviors are less and less socially acceptable. Whether they are unhappy with their bodies and therefore do not want to be seen in public preferring privacy instead, she notes many pregnant women have mentioned that once they enter public space, they feel as if their fetus is a public concern. Their "bodily space is frequently invaded" through the gaze of others and even the touching of their stomachs by complete strangers.[29] They feel under surveillance and often just a vessel for the fetus whose wellbeing is more of a concern than that of the woman. One of her interviewee's journal entry noted that "[s]ometimes I feel as though being pregnant automatically deprives me of any individual identity and personal space … because I've got a 'bump' it seems that I've become public property …."[30] Pregnant teenagers elicit even further recrimination when out in public. This is of course socially, culturally, economically and politically influenced. As Gail Reekie as noted, "[t]he body of the pregnant teenager exposes the limits of what is culturally thinkable about proper sex and motherhood."[31]

Although women seeking abortions in the first trimester are not visibly pregnant, they experience some of the same pressures and expectations as a woman further along in their pregnancies. These experiences become exacerbated when they must pass a line of anti-abortion protestors in front of a clinic, file for judicial bypass if underage or be insulted because of the many state restrictions they must endure. The state intervenes at varying stages along the process of seeking reproductive healthcare. In many states, the wellbeing of the fetus has usurped not only the wellbeing but also the rights of the mother.

**PUBLIC AND PRIVATE DICHOTOMIES**

Designing spaces requires architects to think through multiple possibilities of spatial relationships before arriving at a solution. The public–private division is one of the most commonly considered and ubiquitously referenced. Within architectural education, this spatial dichotomy is introduced early on to beginning design students so they begin to understand basic spatial differences of public and private realms. Typically discussed in the most generic and basic of ways, these terms are presented as simple abstracted ideas making the division between the public and private appear to be straightforward and neutral. The public is associated with exterior and large gathering areas and the private is associated with interior and more personal spaces.

Clearly a critical problem with this type of introduction to public and private space is that it establishes these spaces as oppositional and easily divided into clear and distinct spatial binaries. This overly simplified description renders these spaces in the most banal of ways. It prevents a young designer from understanding space as complex, mired in complicated relationships that are messy, not so easy to name or so clearly divided into distinct zones of use. Nor does it take into account how gender, race, economics and political entities influence and shape space, things outside architecture yet inherently a part of producing architecture.

As Linda McDowell has written, the public–private distinction is an Enlightenment idea and one integral to the right of the individual. As the modern democratic state emerged, the divine right of kings was replaced by the equality of the individual citizen. More specifically she notes this public–private distinction has its roots in John Locke's *Second Treatise* where he differentiates between civil society and political power. Within political power, he believed this included husbands' rule over their wives, "having a "foundation in nature" as men are "the abler and stronger." This "natural" subordination … is based on ties of sentiment, and blood."[32] As the family became separated from the public sphere, women became prohibited from this world outside the home while men were able to freely associate out in public. The separation between public and private produced a clear gendered division with men accorded access to public space while women were relegated to the private domestic realm. Since these spaces were constructed as inherently "natural" spaces of difference, it was common for these distinctions to become institutionalized. Although this binary is still evident today, many feminists have worked tirelessly to dismantle and define differently these ideas.[33]

One result of this separation between the public and the private is the abstraction of each removed from the personal. Duncan cites Young's work on this division as one relying on an "opposition between public and private dimensions of human life, which corresponds to an opposition between reason, on the one hand, and the body, affectivity, and desire on the other." Duncan extrapolates Young's ideas further stating that this then produces an "ideal of universality and impartiality … based upon a model of an individual abstracted from any real context …" Yet we all recognize this model does not exist and is in fact a "fiction."[34] Fraser deconstructs the public/private distinction arguing that these terms are "cultural classifications and rhetorical labels. In political discourse, they are powerful terms that are frequently deployed to delegitimate some interests, views and topics and to valorize others."[35] Designing with these distinctions only reinforces and perpetuates the interests of some over others and continues to operate at such a level of abstraction that effectively removes any spatial specificity or any nuanced readings of difference that could emerge from these spaces.

So how to intervene and disrupt this binary? How to conceptualize a different space? One such powerful suggestion has been through the theorizing of a "third space." McDowell references Homi Bhabha's ideas of this third space as one based in the "non-synchronous temporality of global and national cultures open[ing] up a cultural space—a third space—where the negotiation of incommensurable differences creates a tension peculiar to borderline existences." He describes third-space residents as:

> the subjects of cultural difference do not derive their discursive authority from anterior causes … where differences are effects of some more totalizing, transcendent identity to be found in the past or future. Hybrid hyphenisations emphasise the incommensurable elements as the basis of

> *cultural identities. What is at issue is the performative nature of differential identities: the regulation and negotiation of those spaces that are continually, contingently, "opening out," remaking the boundaries, exposing the limits of any claim to a singular or autonomous sign of difference— be it class, gender or race ... difference is neither One nor the Other, but something else besides, in-between.*[36]

Nancy Duncan also argues for a drastic rethinking of this deeply rooted public/private division. She believes there needs to be de-territorializing and more "progressive geographies" created that are open-ended and empowering to provide resistance to the normative and homogenizing policies currently in place. She references Seyla Benhabib's idea that "[a]ll struggles against oppression ... begin by redefining what had previously been considered 'private,' non-public and non-political issues as matters of public concerns, as issues of justice, [and] as sites of power."[37]

## THE HOME

As has been mentioned previously, the home has been rendered historically as private female space. The home's identity is one in stark contrast to the representation of urbanity and public life.[38] It has been noted by many that this domestic space, where we all live in one form or another, is idealized and imagined, associated with feelings and memories. These all reference a real space and connect over time and place. The home is a place "where personal and social meaning are grounded." It is a place accompanied by a range of emotions.[39] This idea of home, "the 'reality' and the symbolic meaning of the home combine to produce the construction of a particular version of a home in different ways in different societies."[40] Each of us conceives of home differently although there are overlaps of similarity culturally and socially produced. These social relations require movement across public and private spatial divisions and help undermine this dichotomy.[41]

Another important influence in constructing the identity of home has been its separation from developing capitalist economies during the nineteenth century. During industrialization, the idea of the home as this haven, separate and safe from the city, became inscribed into Western ideology. The home's religiosity and sacredness became ever more apparent throughout the late eighteenth and nineteenth century. As the center of love, nurturance, and family, the home as overseen by the mother was a place of peace and a constant refuge from the competitive city.[42] McDowell cites the Victorian critic John Ruskin who espoused and reinforced these views through his writings. In *Sesame and Lilies* he writes that the:

> *very true nature of home—it is the place of peace—the shelter not only from all injury, but from all terror, doubt and division. In so far as it is not this, it is not home; in so far as the anxieties of the outer life penetrate into it, and the inconsistently minded, unknown, unloved, or hostile society of the outer*

*world is allowed by either husband or wife to cross the threshold, it ceases to become home.*[43]

With this idea of home, what happens to sexuality? As noted by Johnston and Longhurst, Foucault revealed that overtime attitudes of sexuality have greatly changed. There was a frankness and tolerance of the illicit during the seventeenth century with little need of sexual secrecy. However, by the nineteenth century this began to change and sexuality was relegated to the home. Foucault writes "[the conjugal family took custody of it and absorbed it into the serious function of reproduction." They write, "[i]t became unacceptable, among Victorian bourgeoisie at least, to talk about sex. The only legitimate space for sex it seems was parents' bedrooms."[44] The Victorian wife was to serve all her husband's needs from sex on demand and clean laundry, to preserve making and roast meat dinners. "[S]ex was a necessary obligation owed to men and not one which women were permitted to talk or think as owed to themselves."[45] Even though the Victorian era existed from the mid nineteenth to early twentieth century and although the sexed body is now prevalent throughout most media outlets worldwide, this repressiveness towards sex is still pervasively and culturally embedded. We continue to see this today through government-supported abstinence-only education programs and the controversy over contraception coverage.

Home is a complicated space. From the outside, it appears as this loving, happy and peaceful place. But once we begin to look inside, like Pandora's box, we may be shocked by what we discover the home can really be. As no space is neutral, the home is full of contradictions and uncertainties and is often a primary site of violence and oppression against women.[46] Furthermore, the design of homes further reflects and reinforces certain power dynamics, gender relations and expectations of an idealized nuclear family.[47]

## HOME AS A SITE OF DOMESTIC VIOLENCE

Home, considered to be the realm of the female, is also a place controlled by patriarchal systems of power and as such have been known to be a space that can deny women and children their autonomy and safety. As Duncan mentions, "'[a] man's home is his castle' … reveals the important historical link between masculinity, patriarchal autonomy and its spatial expression in the form of private property."[48] These legal and therefore political definitions of privacy produce gendered spatial relationships and often reproduce inequalities. Because home is private space and consequently less regulated by the state, this place becomes a site that can hide power inequalities making it difficult to monitor and ensure a woman's safety inside her own home.[49]

Domestic violence is a serious problem both in the United States and abroad. According to womenslaw.org, "[a]bout 95 percent of victims of domestic violence are women. Over 50 percent of all women will experience physical violence in an intimate relationship, and for 24–30 percent of those women, the battering will be regular and on-going."[50] The 2010 United States Centers for Disease Control National Intimate Partner and Domestic Violence Survey found that women are far more likely than men to encounter sexual violence, intimate partner violence and stalking; 1.3 million women were raped in 2009 and 18.3 percent of women compared to 1.4 percent of men have been raped sometime during their life.[51] The Canadian government has stated, "[g]ender-based violence is perhaps the most wide-spread and socially tolerated of human rights violations. It both reflects and reinforces inequities between men and women and compromises the health, dignity, security and autonomy of its victims."[52]

The home can be a space of conflict and contestation and is often "the most common site of violence."[53] Geographer Rachel Pain has researched and written extensively about geographies and fear of violence and has noted experiencing sexual violence drastically alters a person's spatial perception and mobility. Violence, no matter at what point in a person's life it occurs, changes one's life. When violence occurs within private space, one result may be larger perceptions of security are broken.[54] It has also been observed, "women's emotional and practical reactions to the possibility of violence are wide ranging. Most women exhibit spatial confidence as well as spatial restriction and fear … [and] are influenced by spatial, temporal and social contexts."[55] Women are taught from a very young age how to self-impose spatial constraints for their own protection and these continue to be reinforced over time.[56]

Because domestic violence takes place within the privacy of one's home, it remains an invisible problem. As acknowledged earlier, due to the home being privatized space it is difficult to regulate. At times serving to hide the abusers, this space allows the abusers continuing control of both the space and the bodies of their survivors. Control comes through different guises and one way abusers seek to manipulate their victims is through isolation. When not allowed to leave, the home can become a space that separates the person from support networks, social services and law enforcement.[57] This further illustrates concerns around privacy "which often function ideologically to delimit the boundaries of the public sphere in ways that disadvantage subordinate social groups."[58] The "rhetoric of privacy … has historically been used to restrict the universe of legitimate public contestation." As Fraser writes:

> [t]he rhetoric of domestic privacy seeks to exclude some issues and interests from public debate by personalizing and/or familializing them; it casts these as private-domestic or personal-familial matters in contradistinction to public, political matters … the result is to enclave certain matters in specialized discursive arenas and thereby shield them from general public debate and contestation. This usually works to the advantage of dominant groups and individuals and to the disadvantage of their subordinates. If wife battering, for example, is labeled a "personal" or "domestic" matter and if public discourse about this phenomenon is canalized into specialized institutions associated with, say, family law, social work, and the sociology and psychology of "deviance," then this serves to reproduce gender dominance and subordination.[59]

Although restrictions on participation in the public may no longer exist, there may still be, as Fraser describes above, other restrictions like domestic privacy further restricting a woman's ability to contest domestic violence. Domestic privacy becomes a way "through which gender and class disadvantages may continue to operate subtextually and informally, even after explicit, formal restrictions have been rescinded."[60]

Created to provide survivors a safe space to go until more long-term housing can be found, shelters were often spaces created by activists to help women who had experienced domestic violence and had no other place of refuge. Shelter spaces act as "a site of resistance against the imprisoning strategies of the battering partner." Providing temporary housing, food, and support social services, it is not uncommon for childcare and job training to be a part of, or nearby to these places as well.[61]

Duncan writes why she believes shelters are not always the best solution to domestic isolation and violence. For her, funding is generally always a concern; often there is limited space or no space at all because the shelter is full; some women must travel great distances to find a safe place; there may be possible language or cultural differences of women seeking shelters; and probably the most important issue is a cultural one. People seeking aid from strangers may feel shameful that they are going outside their own private family structure; they may be embarrassed and even stigmatized to do so. The communal living and sharing of resources is also a difficult transition to make and people must parent in public while in shelter residence.[62]

Interested in challenging the boundary between public and private, Duncan's own research of marginalized groups including abused women and sexual minorities works to reveal how these groups counter this spatial division. "The destabilizing of this boundary is a countervailing force working to open up not only private space but to reopen public space to public debate and contestation." She focuses on these two particular groups because for her, they have found some ways "for resisting the spatial framework and dominant spatial practices of Anglo-American society."[63] Duncan argues for a real opening up of the private realm as a way to make visible the invisible. "[P]rivate issues need to be deterritorialized ... more thoroughly public(ized) and legitimated as appropriate to public discourse. As Benhabib puts it, 'the struggle to make something public is a struggle for justice.'"[64] Duncan argues for a "multi-pronged attack" on the many ways space and behavior are manipulated and regulated; what she calls an "outing of everybody." In this way, the public–private dichotomy becomes less rigid and stable and publicly questioned through outlets such as the media, the courts, and social movements. What she hopes for is a "deterritorialization ... creation of open-ended, proliferating and inclusive sites of empowerment and resistance against exclusionary, reterritorializing processes ...."[65] This is reminiscent of Fraser's subaltern counterpublics where smaller, less institutionally powerful actors are able to exert pressure for change.

Although incredibly important in filling a need in communities across the country, many shelters rely on volunteer efforts of labor and financial resources to remain open. Where the state is failing the public, citizens are stepping in and providing resources and support where networks are lacking. McDowell notes a connection in the 1980s when the state become ever more dependent on women's volunteer labor with what was called "rolling back the state" and the reduction of services the state was providing.[66] Women stepped up when the government stepped out.

I have witnessed this with my own volunteering at a local shelter. I provided architectural expertise for a recent capital improvement project. Although I freely entered into this relationship precisely because I wanted to donate my time and knowledge to a local organization, I realized I became conflicted the longer the renovation project went on. This internal conflict arose from gradually understanding there are certain expectations donors have that establish limits of possibilities. To be more precise, I bumped up against the vision I had presented for the project and donors' expectations of what the project "should" be. Thankfully this happened once construction had begun. Although I do not know where all the money came from that allowed the project to happen, I was aware that a significant portion was through donations and grants. At some point it was made clear that these renovated spaces could not be nicer than any donor's own spaces. This comment revealed what I perceived to be as a nasty underbelly to work in areas like domestic violence. It is all right for things to get better but you know what, they can't get *that* much better because then they may be *too* good for those who are using them.

This experience has made me question my role within these larger structures of power. A few issues I have been thinking about include what role does pro bono work have in perpetuating imbalanced power structures and patriarchal models and how does one come to understand value with something that is free. Clearly I became complicit in these power structures without even realizing it. All I had hoped to do was make these spaces better for shelter residents and in the end became incredibly frustrated as the process revealed other things about pro bono work.

I have realized institutions, whether they are for the greater good of neglected constituents or not, maintain and work within certain structures of power. In this case, directors, employees, donors, paid labor and volunteer free labor begin to define a rather clear hierarchical landscape. And value. Well, people do not seem to value something that is free, or they value it a whole lot less. This is problematic because in order for the exchange to be productive for all parties, value and the acknowledgement of value must be present or a part of the "contract" for all involved. Important lesson learned. Next time, I will require a fee for services provided. It may be drastically reduced but there must be something of value exchanged by both parties for the transaction to be equitable and respected.

## ARCHITECTURE

Beginning in the early 1970s coinciding with the women's movement, feminist architects and designers began to challenge the more normative assumptions of the built environment such as space is neutral and design is an objective and purely rational discipline.[67] Many during this period called for more equal representation of women in the profession or a more drastic overturning of the patriarchal discipline altogether.[68] Others feminists in planning and architecture during the 1970s and early 1980s were critical of gender's impact on space. They revealed that so many of the designers were men producing space used by women. During this time these feminists criticized many of the inherent spatial discriminations women encountered.[69]

One aspect of this feminist history that most interests me is the intersection of activism with spatial politics and design. Three examples present different tactics in intervening into and within existing patriarchal systems of design and practice. The first was by a group of 75 women, the Fifth Street Women, in New York City who took over an abandoned building on New Year's Eve in 1971. In solidarity they declared that because their city does not provide for them they collectively took over a building to create the things they need "essential to women—health care, child care, food conspiracy ... [and a] feminist center ..." Through this taking of space, they were acting politically to change society.[70]

The second is the Woman's Building in Los Angeles that opened in 1973 housing the Feminist Studio Workshop, the first independent school for women artists by Judy Chicago, Sheila Levrant de Bretteville and Arlene Raven. The Women's Building included galleries, performances, a bookstore and travel agency, a café and the offices for the National Organization for Women. Named in honor of the structure built for the Chicago World's Columbian Exposition by architect Sophia Hayden, this 1893 Italianate Renaissance loggia-lined structure located in Jackson Park[71] exhibited cultural work by women from around the world.[72] The Los Angeles Woman's Building was an internationally recognized center for women's art and creative endeavors and was open until 1991.

The third is the London Matrix Feminist Design Co-operative begun in the early 1980s comprised 25 women working together for over 14 years. As an offshoot of the New Architecture Movement, this group of female architects questioned the more traditional role of architects campaigning for their unionization.[73] Matrix was invested in how theory could influence practice and their work included book projects and building design. Coalescing around the writing of *Making Space: Women and the Man-Made Environment*, an architectural collective was established. Non-hierarchal in structure, all members were paid equally and their client base would draw from those who would not typically have access to architectural services. Matrix was committed to not working with individuals or companies.[74] The primary focus of their design practice was state-funded and socially based projects including housing. In addition, Matrix was a member of the state-funded Association of Community Technical Aid Centres (ACTAC) providing design and technical advice to voluntary organizations.[75] Invested in partnering and empowering groups, they worked collaboratively with clients facilitating a more transparent and engaging design process.[76]

In the early 1980s, Leslie Kanes Weisman passionately argued that although space is a cultural artifact, it often does not accommodate for a vast majority of its users. The built environment profoundly affects people's lives and "[w]omen must demand public buildings and spaces, transportation, and housing, which support our lifestyles and incomes and respond to the realities of our lives, not the cultural fantasies about them." For her, "[o]ne of the most important tasks of the women's movement is to make visible the full meaning of [women's] experiences and to interpret and restructure the built environment in those terms."[77]

Architectural historian Dolores Hayden's 1981 provocation "What would a non-sexist city be like?" questions "[i]s it possible to build non-sexist neighborhoods and design non-sexist cities?"[78] How would such spaces be different from what we have right now? She makes a strong argument that housing does not support the needs of employed women. Daily logistical problems working women encounter are not private problems but societal ones the market will not effectively change. She mentions several international alternative housing examples from Copenhagen, Hamburg and London and traces a brief American history of experimental socialist and utopian housing communities that challenged the more normative structures of housing. Hayden proposes the HOME model, Homemakers Organization for a More Egalitarian Society. Re-conceptualizing private life and public responsibilities, this new structure calls for a reordering of home and work, making women's lives better. This is a feminist cooperative housing model promoting shared responsibilities by all family members for domestic labor, shared spaces for such needs as childcare and house-keeping, reduction of household energy consumption and creating spaces that promote more sociability and less segregation by race, class and age. Hayden argues that if the divisions between public and private space become a socialist and feminist priority of the 1980s and if the divisions between domestic labor, domestic space and a woman's workplace are transformed, women have a much better chance of becoming "equal members of society."[79]

In the 1990s, the influence from other disciplines including cultural and social theory, art, film, philosophy, psychoanalysis and women's studies broadened the discourse in architecture and offered other ways to think about and critique architectural practice. Bringing these outside theories into architectural discourse enabled an intellectually based critique of design, architectural production, representation and occupation. Feminist theory, subjectivity and representation became particularly influential in thinking through some of these issues and power dynamics.[80]

As Jane Rendell has discussed, people such as Jennifer Bloomer through both her writing and creative practice sought other ways to understand and explore the feminine through architectural production. "Bloomer's work demonstrated that the feminine can be a radical element in architectural practice."[81] Her work reveals how signs and signifiers subvert patriarchal systems within architecture and challenges the ways we both write about and speculate spatially. During this period, work by others such as Liz Diller, Liquid Inc. and muf challenged the boundaries of architecture due to their interdisciplinary approaches practicing between theory, art and architecture with speculative installation practices.[82]

Rendell questions what role does self-reflectivity have within architectural debate. Always slow to embrace current theories and practices in other disciplines, the situated-ness of the critic although commonly engaged in art, literature and cultural studies, has not been one many architectural writers and designers have taken on.[83] As acknowledged and supported by earlier feminist in the humanities and social sciences, one's positionality directly shapes who you are and how you see the world. As other disciplines have embraced and argued for this critical approach to research and creative practices, why would architecture not also begin to do the same? As feminist architects realized decades earlier, the boys' club of architecture is all about positionality although they would never publicly acknowledge or call it as such. But that is how the discipline has been operating for well over a century. Now women and people of color must call it out for what it is and through this, redefine the club and who can be members.

## SPACES OF POSSIBILITY

In *Framing Places: Mediating Power in Built Form*, architect Kim Dovey discusses the many ways built form reflects and reproduces power relations in the hopes of leading to more "imaginative, liberating and empowering placemaking practices."[84] Architecture is always determined by those with power and the capital to build. Our built environment "reflects the identities, differences and struggles of gender, class, race, culture and age … interests of the State in social order, and the private corporate interest in stimulating consumption."[85] Architecture cannot "claim autonomy from the politics of social change."[86] What we do is inherently a part of how people live their daily lives, for we design the spaces where this unfolds.

One of the critiques Dovey makes builds upon work by Thomas Markus arguing that architecture has traded more systemic power in planning and programming of spaces for aesthetics and form making. Architecture has become more about representation than about anything else and as a result "diminishes the engagement of architecture with issues of power … [and] serves to sustain the illusion that architecture can be practiced in a realm of autonomy from social power."[87] Architects and urban designers are imaginative agents. The power lies in the potential to "stimulate desire and to enlarge the public imagination [and] can be crucial to the discourses of power."[88] Dovey argues that being aware of how power is mediated through form enables us to "change the way it is practiced."[89] Although architecture acts as a structure for ordering social systems in space, it frames social actions, capacities to create change, or people's potential agency.[90] Here lies the real potential of architecture as an agent of social and political change. He concludes writing that if designers are critical within a certain moment of the process we should "keep alive the liberating spirit of design without the illusion of autonomy … places are programmed, designed and built by those with the power to do so. To practice in the light of this complicity is the primary liberating move."[91] Architects must use this awareness proactively and often.

Lisa Findley's book *Building Change Architecture, Politics and Cultural Agency* explores the current potentials within architecture to help produce and leverage architecture as an agent for social change. Because architecture is a cultural producer, architects are actively participating in constructing cultural agency and power all around us. "Architecture, like no other form of cultural production, can manifest renewed cultural agency by making it spatial, material, present and, in that sense, undeniable."[92] She advocates that architects need to use this cultural power opportunistically through "proactive cultural practice[s]."[93]

Although architecture has historically been associated with creating spatial representations of power, it does have the latent ability to work against the hegemony. Power, whether hegemonic or counter-hegemonic, must become spatialized. Findley cites Lefebvre's recognition that:

> [a] revolution that does not produce a new space has not realized its full potential; indeed it has failed in that it has not changed life itself, but has merely changed ideological superstructures, institutions or political apparatuses. A social transformation, to be truly revolutionary in character, must manifest a creative capacity in its effects on daily life, on language, on space ...[94]

What becomes spatial, built and occupied shapes those who move through and use space. Although architecture manifests power, it also and simultaneously reflects cultural agency. And here lies the opening for a potential challenge and change of space.

Findley mentions David Harvey's reference to the "insurgent architect" as a person who can be a proactive participant in reconfiguring the flows of cultural, political and economic systems of power. Although Harvey is not referring to the practitioner of architecture, she graphs his analogy onto architecture because there is such potential in thinking through the implications of his ideas and how they could pertain to socially engaged architectural practices. Harvey sees the figure of the architect as one having:

> centrality and positionality in all discussions of the processes of constructing and organizing spaces. The architect has been most deeply enmeshed throughout history in the production and pursuit of utopian ideals ... [t]he architect shapes space so as to give ... social utility as well as human and aesthetic/symbolic meanings. The architect shapes and preserves longterm social memories and strives to give material form to the longings and desire of individuals and collectives. The architect struggles to open spaces for new possibilities, for future forms of social life.[95]

Clearly the architect has potential for producing change. As spatial producers, we have the ability to reorganize and create differently people's every day environments. Whether it is at the scale of a clinic, a shelter, a hospital or even a sidewalk, this is where I find Findley's book most inspiring and relevant to the contested spaces being explored throughout this book. She concludes it is in the everyday where architecture's cultural and spatial agency exists and has power for change.

Possibility registers in a different way by Elizabeth Grosz where she asks:

> [h]ow to think architecture differently? How to think in architecture, or of architecture, without conforming to the standard assumptions, the doxa,

> the apparent naturalness, or rather the evolutionary fit assumed to hold between being and building? ... How to see dwelling as something other than the containment or protection of subjects? In short, how to think architecture beyond complementarity and binarization, beyond subjectivity and signification?[96]

She looks to Deleuze in seeking to provide not an answer to these questions but a response, a provocation. Understanding thought as an encounter from outside what we know, from our material reality and subjectivity, Grosz sees a potential in Deleuze's idea of "thought as difference."[97] For him, difference is a force, "a positive desire, which *makes* a difference, whether in the image form in the visual and cinematic arts, in the built form in architecture, or in concept form in philosophy." He wants thought to be reenergized and able to move beyond the forces restricting innovation and change - "to free thought from representation" and enable it to be transformative. One is to move beyond what confines and suppresses difference.[98]

If the hope for architecture is to not just rely on its given modes of production but to create something outside architecture's typical sets of responses, what enables this to happen? What other ways can architecture be conceived and produced? As Grosz writes, "[i]nsofar as architecture is seeking not so much "innovation," not simply "the latest fad," but to produce differently, to engender the new, to risk creating otherwise ... How to keep architecture open to its outside, how to force architecture to *think*?"[99] Thought may operate as an intrusion; a realigning of the known or something that produces a delay or moment of discontinuity. "Can [architecture] become something—many things—other than what it is and how it presently functions? If its present function is an effect of the crystallization of its history within, inside, its present, can its future be something else?"[100]

These are significant and difficult questions that this research is attempting to ask and work through. In other words, what can looking at the wide range of influences that both directly and indirectly shape spaces like abortion clinics, women's shelters and hospitals provide for the broader discipline of architecture and design? How does examining such spaces broaden and deepen the way people understand our built environment and what value is placed on such spaces? I am positioning this work somewhere between theory and practice. I am not necessarily interested in making these spaces "better" but of course that would be advantageous. I am more interested in discovering what the potential agency is within these spaces and how are people who use these spaces able to capitalize upon this potential and as a result alter, reorganize or subvert existing power structures and the spaces that reinforce them.

I aim to expose and make visual the complexities responsible for creating these contested landscapes. Building upon what architect Jos Boys has argued for in envisioning alternative possibilities for producing and consuming of space, the revealing of positionalities provides potential for thinking differently about economics and "meaning making" in space calling for the disruption between form and metaphor of particular social values in order for public debate to occur about what physical manifestations are relevant today.[101]

Although I am trained as an architect, this research locates itself between several different disciplines including architecture, geography, women's studies and law. This work could not be done otherwise and I would like to argue it gains more relevancy as a result of its interdisciplinary position. Working interdisciplinarily, Rendell writes is both ethical and political. This type of work requires one to step outside the comfort of what one knows into the possibility of "the emergence of new and often uncertain forms of knowledge." This new knowledge helps to reconfigure what we value as knowledge and critique what is knowledge and how it is produced.[102] In this way, I hope to use real world situations and spaces in order to posit speculations about the relationships between space, the powers that define it and gaps I can find between and among them for productive alteration. As Kenworthy Teather has suggested, individuals can change social structures through adapting their own personal practices because they are mutually constructed.[103] I see this as a productive area of potential for these contested spaces. Through the reconfiguring, re-occupying and intervening within state power, relationships can change and be lived differently.

**NOTES**

1 Colomina 1992.
2 Colomina 1992: Introduction.
3 Colomina 1992: Introduction.
4 For further discussion of this please see Despina Stratigakos's recent essay "Why Architects Need Feminism" in the online journal Places 2012.
5 Grosz 1992: 243–44.
6 Grosz 1992: 242.
7 Grosz 1992: 245–46.
8 Grosz 1992: 247.
9 Grosz 1992: 248.
10 Grosz 1992: 250.
11 Duncan 1996: Introduction, 1.
12 Duncan 1996: Introduction, 3, 4–5.
13 Taylor 1998: 129–30.
14 McDowell 1999: 4.
15 Teather 1999: 2.
16 McDowell 1999: 24.
17 Duncan 1996: Introduction, 5.
18 McDowell 1999: 29.
19 Longhurst 2001: 23.

20  Longhurst 2001: 25.
21  Longhurst 2001: 26.
22  Longhurst 1998: 20.
23  McDowell 1999: 34–36.
24  McDowell 1999: 49–50.
25  Young 1990: 160.
26  Young 1990: 163–64.
27  Young 1990: 166–67.
28  Young 1990: 168–69.
29  Longhurst 1998: 28–29.
30  Longhurst 1999: 78, 85.
31  Longhurst 2008: 124.
32  McDowell 1999: 175.
33  McDowell 1999: 174–75.
34  Duncan 1996: 2–3.
35  Fraser 1990: 73.
36  McDowell 1996: 40–41.
37  Duncan 1996: 142–43.
38  Brown and Erkarslan 2009: 295.
39  Blunt and Dowling 2006: 2, 22.
40  McDowell 1999: 71.
41  McDowell 1999: 73.
42  McDowell 1999: 75.
43  McDowell 1999: 78.
44  Johnston and Longhurst 2010: 29–30.
45  Hall 1992: 61–62.
46  Blunt and Dowling 2006: 15.
47  Johnston and Longhurst 2010: 42–43.
48  Duncan 1996: 131.
49  Duncan 1996: 131.
50  WomensLaw.org (updated June 21, 2012).
51  Centers for Disease Control 2010.
52  Brown and Erkarslan 2009: 295.
53  Pain 1999: 133.
54  Pain 1999: 126, 128, 133–34.

55  Pain 1999: 135.
56  Pain 1999: 131, 135.
57  Duncan 1996: 133.
58  Fraser 1990: 73.
59  Fraser 1990: 73.
60  Fraser 1990: 74.
61  Duncan 1996: 133.
62  Duncan 1996: 133–34.
63  Duncan 1996: 127.
64  Duncan 1996: 141.
65  Duncan 1996: 141–42.
66  McDowell 1999: 181.
67  Boys 1998: 203.
68  Rendell 2011: 18.
69  Rendell 2000: 230.
70  Weisman 1992: 1.
71  World's Columbian Exposition of 1893.
72  The Women's Building "Brief History."
73  Dwyer and Thorne 2007: 41.
74  Dwyer and Thorne 2007: 44–46.
75  Dwyer and Thorne 2007: 51–52.
76  Matrix Feminist Design Co-Operative (n.d.).
77  Weisman 2000: 1–5.
78  Hayden 2000: 507.
79  Hayden 2000: 507–509, 516.
80  Rendell 2011: 18–19.
81  Rendell 2011: 17–19.
82  Rendell 2011: 19–20.
83  Rendell 2011: 34.
84  Dovey 2008: 7.
85  Dovey 2008: 1–2.
86  Dovey 2008: 2.
87  Dovey 2008: 31.
88  Dovey 2008: 15.
89  Dovey 2008: 16.

90   Dovey 2008: 19.
91   Dovey 2008: 220.
92   Findley 2005: xiii.
93   Findley 2005: xiii.
94   Findley 2005: 30.
95   Findley 2005: 34.
96   Grosz 2001: 59.
97   Grosz 2001: 61.
98   Grosz 2001: 62–64.
99   Grosz 2001: 64.
100  Grosz 2001: 70–71.
101  Boys 1998: 216–17.
102  Rendell 2011: 21–3.
103  Teather 1999: 10.

# 3

## Legal Frameworks Understood Spatially

### GENERAL HISTORY AND CONTEXT OF ABORTION: UNITED STATES

In many parts of the world, abortion is fraught with religious and political influences. The US is no exception. Our current position is not so surprising given what one finds when examining the history of abortion in this country. This history "demonstrates the long legacy of a highly uneven geography of rights."[1] What is shocking, however, is when compared to all other industrialized Western countries, our teenage pregnancy and STD rates are among some of the highest and accessing age-appropriate sex education and abortion is among the lowest. To better understand our current situation, it is important to briefly highlight the broader history of abortion.

Beginning in antiquity, the Stoics believed that abortion should be allowed up to the moment of birth. The Pythagoreans, however, opposed abortion on the basis of their belief that the soul was infused into the body at the moment of conception.[2] Reflecting Pythagorean view, the Hippocratic Oath included the pledge: "I will not give to a woman an abortive remedy."[3,4] Early Roman law was silent on the issue, and abortion and infanticide was commonly practiced among the Roman upper classes. The rise of Christianity during the reign of Severus (A.D. 193–211) brought the first abortion prohibitions. Medieval theologians distinguished between the *embryo informatus* (prior to the endowment of a soul) and *embryo formatus* (after endowment with a soul).[5]

English Common Law, which became the basis of the United States' initial abortion policies, allowed the procedure up to quickening (the first time a woman feels the fetus move within her body).[6] Placing the soul's entry into the fetus at the time of quickening, approximately at four months, thirteenth-century Catholic theologian St. Thomas Aquinas designated the pregnant woman the expert in verifying her own pregnancy. Prior to quickening, she could not be declared pregnant. In colonial and early national America, this law was followed from the eighteenth through the mid nineteenth century. Colonial home medical guides

## USA Timeline

| 1870 | 1880 | 1890 | 1890 | 1900 | 1940 | 1950 | 1960 | 1970 | 1980 |

- 1865 — CIVIL WAR
- 1ST VICTORY OF ABORTION REFORM W/PASSAGE OF LIBERALIZING LEGISLATION IN COLORADO
- 1967 — 49 STATES AND D.C. CLASSIFIED ABORTION AS A FELONY
- 1968 — ABORTION STATUTES WERE CHALLENGED IN MANY STATES ON GROUNDS OF VAGUENESS, VIOLATION OF FUNDAMENTAL RIGHT OF PRIVACY, AND DENIAL OF EQUAL PRTOETION
- 1972 1973 — ROE VS. WADE

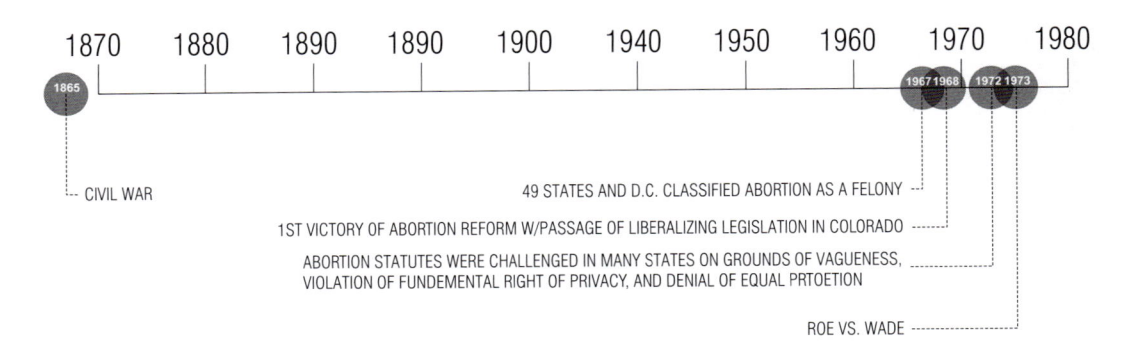

Fig. 3.1 US abortion timeline 1870–1970

included recipes for "bringing on the menses" with herbs either grown or found locally. These homemade remedies became commercially available by the mid eighteenth century. The first statutes restricting abortion appeared in the 1820s and 1830s as poison-control laws aimed at doctors and potion sellers.[7]

Prior to the Civil War, abortion practices remained largely unrestricted. But by the time of the war, many states had begun to revise their statutes in order to prohibit abortion at all stages of gestation, with exceptions for therapeutic abortions.[8] This legislative change resulted from the struggle between doctors ("regulars") and midwives and other abortion practitioners (irregulars"). Founded in 1847, the American Medical Association (AMA) enabled the exclusively male physicians' group to professionalize and exclude competitors. The doctors hoped to enhance their status by gaining authority over a realm that was not until this time either a medical domain or a moral issue. As with deliveries, doctors wanted to become the sole practitioners of abortion. Between 1850 and 1860 the AMA campaigned to limit the "irregulars" from practicing abortion in an effort to establish the belief that the medical profession was the only sanctioned body to perform such procedures. This campaign resulted in the 1860 law prohibiting abortion after quickening. In the 1870s, more restrictive abortion laws were passed, coinciding with major concerns about women leaving their traditional societal roles. These restrictions were followed in the 1920s with another wave of anti-abortion legislation, effectively making abortion illegal at all stages of pregnancy.[9] By the twentieth century, most state legislation prohibited abortion except when doctors deemed it permissible in special cases.[10]

In 1959, the American Law Institute (ALI) advocated legalizing abortion for reasons that would include the mental or physical health of the mother, pregnancy due to rape or incest and fetal deformity.[11] However, by 1967, 49 states and Washington D.C. had classified abortion as a felony. It is important to recognize even at this time each state legislature determined the legality of abortion. During that same year, Colorado became the first state to reform its abortion legislation.[12] On April 25, 1967 Governor John A. Love signed the first law to loosen state control

Fig. 3.2  *Roe v. Wade*

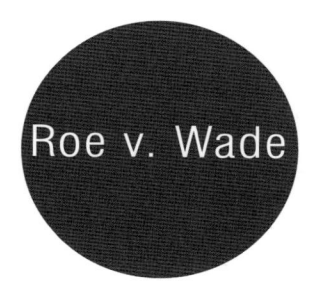

*Roe v. Wade*

Court stated woman's right to abortion fell within the right to privacy protected by 14th amendment; gave a woman total autonomy over the pregnancy during 1st trimester and states may not make abortions *unreasonably* difficult to obtain by prescribing elaborate procedural barriers

over abortion allowing the procedure in cases of rape, incest, or the permanent mental or physical disability of either the child or mother. California, Oregon and North Carolina passed similar laws within the year. On April 11, 1970 Governor Nelson A. Rockefeller signed a bill repealing New York State's 1830 law, which had banned abortion after quickening except to save a woman's life, while extending abortion rights up to the twenty-fourth week of pregnancy. Alaska, Hawaii and Washington soon passed similar laws. By the end of 1972, 13 states had laws as proposed by the ALI and four states allowed abortion on demand. However, only 31 states allowed abortion to save a woman's life.

On January 22, 1973, the Supreme Court handed down its landmark decision *Roe v. Wade* granting the right to abortion to all women.[13] The Court determined that the Constitution protects a woman's decision whether or not to terminate her pregnancy. In the companion case *Doe v. Bolton*, the Court held that a state may not unduly burden a woman's fundamental right to abortion by prohibiting or substantially limiting access to the means of effectuating her decision by *prescribing elaborate procedural guidelines* (italics are mine; to be discussed in more detail in Chapter 5). Writing the majority opinion, Justice Blackmun stated that the constitutional basis for the decisions rested upon the conclusion that the Fourteenth Amendment's concept of personal liberty and the right to personal privacy embraced a woman's decision whether to have an abortion. The cases referenced in the decisions "make clear that the right has some extensions to activities related to marriage, procreation, contraception, family relationship, and child rearing and education."[14] In Doe, the Court struck down state requirements that abortions be performed in licensed hospitals, be approved beforehand by a hospital committee, and two physicians concur in the abortion decision. The decision would not, however, apply to denominational hospitals and their employees. This continues to have repercussions today as witnessed in the debate over contraception coverage, mandated healthcare and Catholic hospitals refusal to provide reproductive healthcare on religious grounds.

Only four years after *Roe v. Wade* in 1977, the Supreme Court introduced a trilogy of restrictions limiting public funding of non-therapeutic or elective abortions. The Court held that states have neither a statutory nor a constitutional obligation to cover the expense of or allow access to public facilities for abortions. But they could cover these expenses if they chose to do so.[15] In addition, Congress passed the Hyde Amendment, specifying which abortion services are covered

Fig. 3.3 Hyde Amendment

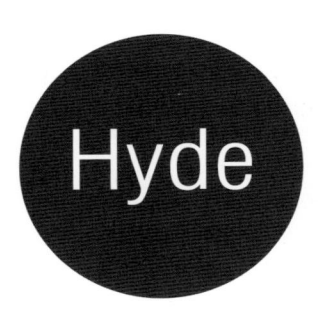

### Hyde Amendment HR2264

Permanent law a near ban on coverage of abortion services in a domestic health program

Federal funds are prohibited from being used to pay for abortion except when pregnancy results from rape, incest, or necessary to save a woman's life

under federal Medicaid. Although current coverage includes cases of rape, incest, life endangerment, and damage to a woman's physical health, Congress has rewritten the provisions a number of times. In 1979 the exception for physical health was excluded and in 1981, the exceptions of rape and incest were also excluded.[16]

This begins to raise several critical concerns around how space is beginning to be defined within abortion access. After Hyde, the space of state-funded abortion becomes a more highly regulated space compared with clinics and other spaces outside government purview. The legalized and theoretically protective space of abortion now begins to come under attack. Space that is privately owned and operated becomes more easily accessible both spatially and economically. Federally operated space is now legislated and regulated. The government has begun to insert itself more fully into the literal space of abortion.

**LEGAL = SPATIAL**

> *Congress shall make no law respecting an establishment of religion, or prohibiting the free exercise thereof; or abridging the freedom of speech, or of the press; or the right of the people peaceably to assemble, and to petition the Government for a redress of grievances. (First Amendment to the United States Constitution)*

> *The right of the people to be secure in their persons, houses, papers, and effects, against unreasonable searches and seizures, shall not be violated, and no Warrants shall issue, but upon probable cause, supported by Oath or affirmation, and particularly describing the place to be searched, and the persons or things to be seized. (Fourth Amendment to the United States Constitution)*

How do we understand the spatial implications of this complex historical legacy? In the most basic terms, there can be a court-determined line drawn on the ground that one side cannot cross. And although as we shall see, the distance dictated by the courts is important in real and physical terms, how do we begin to understand the larger issues around the spatial games being played out in this debate? Space becomes a metaphor for issues such as clinic access; the right to choose one's reproductive fate; different state attitudes toward abortion; discrimination against women of lower economic means; discrimination on the basis of race and ethnicity; and, ultimately, the inability to have full authority over one's decisions and one's body.

There have been a series of court rulings that have determined physical boundaries around both clinics and the people entering and exiting such spaces. Through these rulings, a series of definitions have emerged that codify the spatial relationships about abortion and public space as they pertain to the First Amendment. These terms and where they come from will be discussed later in this chapter.

**Bubbles and Abortion**

One would think such an unlikely pairing would not have anything to do with one another. However, over the past almost three decades a legal relationship has developed between bubbles and abortion clinics in this country. As legislated distances dictated by the courts, bubble laws protect people, clinics, and clinic sites from protestors attempting to prevent access into reproductive healthcare facilities providing abortions.

As the geographer Don Mitchell has mentioned, the choice of the word "bubble" to describe these sorts of laws is "in and of itself interesting." Denoting spaces of protection and impregnable to trespass, bubble laws are supposed to evoke zones of safety.[17] However, the first image that comes to mind are the bottles of bubbles and their plastic wands I use to get when I was a child. I remember the streams of bubbles that my brother and I would make. I recall their translucency, how they reflected the light with a somewhat pinkish-lavender sheen and how fragile the bubbles were, only lasting a few seconds at most. You could never run and catch them; they would pop before you could get to them. Yet, for abortion protection, the term synonymous with zones of safety where others cannot infringe into is the bubble. And as time continues to demonstrate, this bubble zone is easily manipulated and trespassed against, not ensuring real protection for women who brave the crowds to enter the many contested healthcare facilities across this country. So in reality, the bubble is not an apt analogy at all but rather one connoting abortion's still precarious position within contemporary society.

Legislated distances vary from state to state with most states having no bubble laws enacted. Currently there are three states with legislated zones of protection around a person and the buildings they are entering. In Colorado there is an 8-foot zone within 100 feet of clinics' doors; in Massachusetts there is a 35-foot zone around entrances and walkways of clinics; and in Montana there is an 8-foot zone within 36 feet of clinic doors.[18]

One of the courts primary concerns with bubble laws is the law's relationship to the First Amendment and what degree the law restricts one's right to freedom of speech and freedom to *peaceably* assemble. (Italic is mine, for it seems that many anti-abortion protesters do not adhere to the amendment's concept of *peaceably*). When the courts considered the three abortion cases discussed later in this chapter, one of the most discussed issues is whether restrictions violate or unduly restrict the First Amendment's right to free speech, "whether the challenged provisions of the injunction burden no more speech than necessary to serve a significant government interest."[19]

Another important application regarding the exercise of free speech is whether the speech being considered is "so intrusive that the unwilling audience cannot avoid it. Indeed, "[i]t may not be the content of the speech, as much as the deliberate 'verbal or visual assault,' that justifies proscription."[20] Further debating what the limits of speech are, the Court also references *Boos v. Barry*, 485 U.S. 322, "[a]s a general matter, we have indicated that in public debate our own citizens must tolerate insulting, and even outrageous, speech in order to provide adequate breathing space to the freedoms protected by the First Amendment."[21]

When considering free speech and abortion, the question has to be asked: how much is too much? At what point does the right to physical access become an equal to or greater issue than ensuring the right for someone to *peaceably* assemble and express their freedom of speech? And, what does *peaceably* really mean? Concerned with public safety, the courts must ensure the protection of abortion procedures, ensuring a woman's constitutional right of inter-state travel to have an abortion and that this right [is] not 'sacrificed in the interest of defendants' First Amendment rights.'"[22]

Bubble laws work by law enforcement. In cities with intense and repetitious levels of clinic protests including loud levels of noise and obstruction, there would typically need to be police officers or federal marshals present to maintain legislated distances. In some cases, there would be lines drawn on sidewalks and streets informing protestors and those entering and exiting clinics where these zones are precisely located. For example in Buffalo during the 1990s the NBC nightly news reported on how a "yellow line in front of a clinic on Main Street … ha[d] become a permanent fixture … By court order, protestors [could] not cross it."[23]

The specific cases highlighted below are ones that have become legal precedent and are typically referenced in abortion cases where limits of the First Amendment are being debated. Through these rulings, a series of definitions emerged determining physical boundaries around clinics and those entering and exiting such spaces regulating spatial relationships as they pertain to the First Amendment.

**The First Bubble Law: Boulder, Colorado**

Reacting to aggressive and confrontational tactics by anti-abortion protestors that had often impeded access, the Boulder City Council passed the first bubble law in 1986.[24] Originally referred to as a "Buffer Zone Ordinance," this ordinance protected those entering abortion clinics and doctor's offices from severe harassment from anti-abortion protestors. The ordinance stipulated within 100 feet from a clinic or office a demonstrator could not approach someone closer than 8 feet without explicit permission creating a bubble of protection around someone entering or exiting a building.[25] Senator Mike Feeley and State Representative Diana DeGette determined the 8-foot dimension through testing distances in a small hearing room in the basement of the Colorado Capitol in Denver. They walked around the room asking:

> [c]an you hear me now? ... How about now? When they found what seemed like the right distance—a comfortable distance, but close enough to hear each other at a normal tone of voice—someone left and came back with a tape measure. They were eight feet apart ... As they figured out how big the bubble should be, DeGette said, she looked not only at how far apart two people could hold a conversation, but also how close they should be for the woman to accept a pamphlet. "It's about two arms' lengths away," DeGette said. "If a protestor holds up a leaflet, I can lift my hand and take the leaflet."[26]

The Colorado legislature acknowledged that "the exercise of a person's right to protest or counsel against certain medical procedures must be balanced against another person's right to obtain medical counseling and treatment in an unobstructed manner."[27] A violation of this law would be a class three misdemeanor with punishment ranging from a $50 fine to six months' imprisonment and a $750 fine.[28] This eventually led the state of Colorado to pass the City Council ordinance into law protecting access to all health care clinics in 1993.[29]

**Hill v. Colorado (2000)**

The Supreme Court upheld the 1993 Colorado measure protecting those seeking abortion from harassment taking a "prophylactic approach." The Colorado law makes it unlawful for any person within 100 feet of a health care facility's entrance to "knowingly approach" within 8 feet of another person, without that person's consent, in order to pass "a leaflet or handbill to, displa[y] a sign to, or engag[e] in oral protest, education, or counseling with [that] person."[30]

**Madsen v. Women's Health Center (1994)**

Beginning in 1992, an abortion clinic in Melbourne, Florida received continued threats of picketing and protesting. The state court enjoined protesters from blocking or interfering with public access and from physically abusing those entering or leaving the clinic. When access was still being impeded six months later, the clinic sought to broaden the injunction because these activities were having detrimental physical effects on patients. (Injunctions do not address the general public but refer only to particular parties and their past violation(s) or, a party's imminent future violations.) For example, such activities were producing higher anxiety and hypertension levels in patients requiring increased levels of sedation, other protests were discouraging some potential patients from entering clinics, while some clinic employees' domestic lives were disrupted by protests outside their own homes.

The state court issued an amended injunction including the creation of a 36-foot buffer zone around clinic entrances and driveways and the private property to

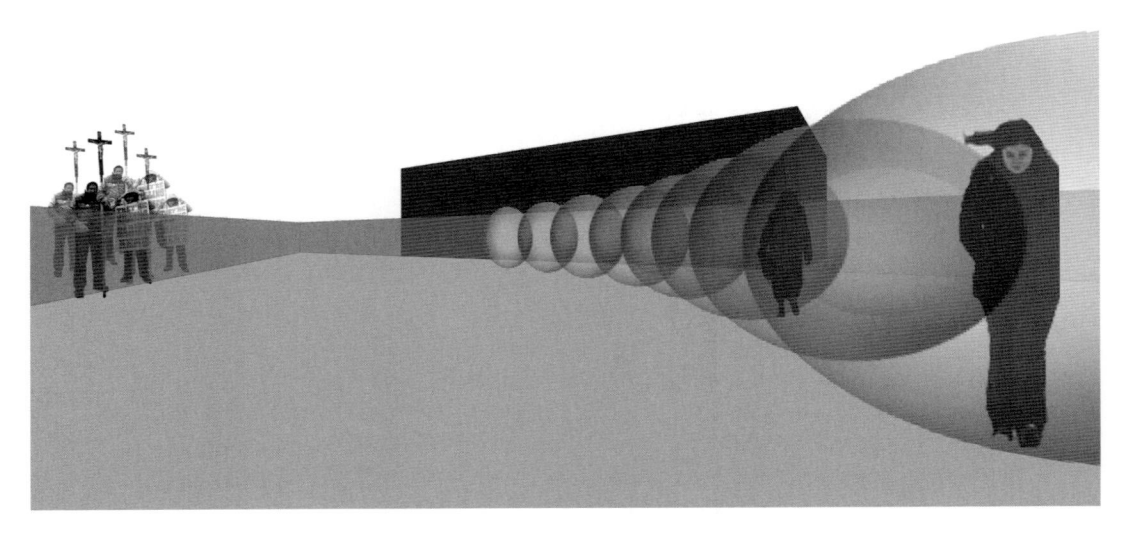

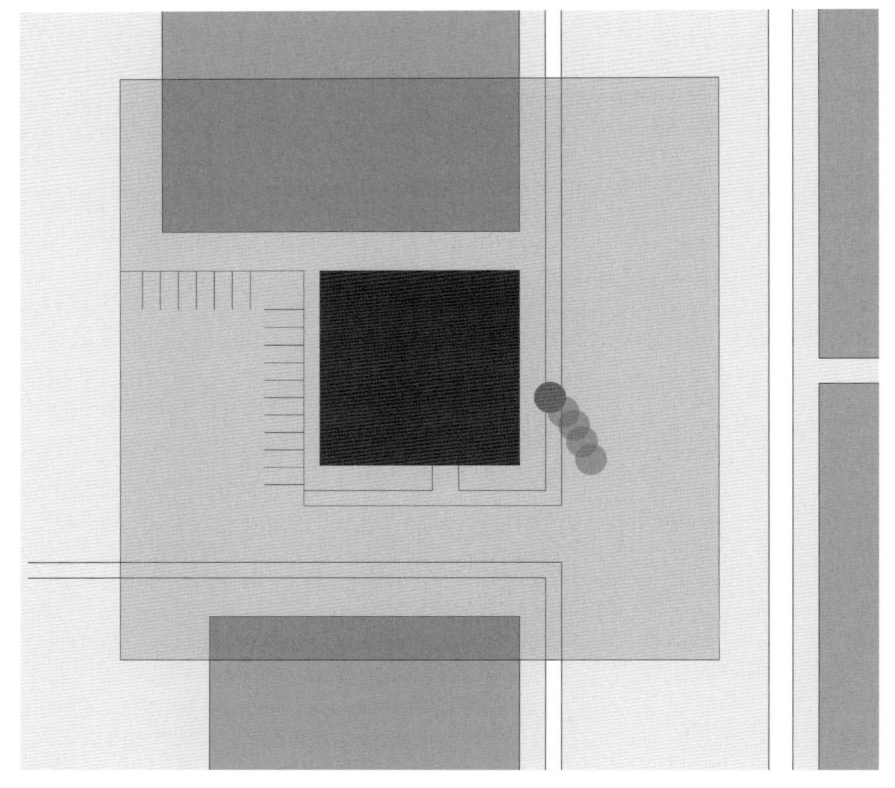

Fig. 3.4 *Hill v. Colorado.* Plan and perspective diagrams illustrating legislated spaces

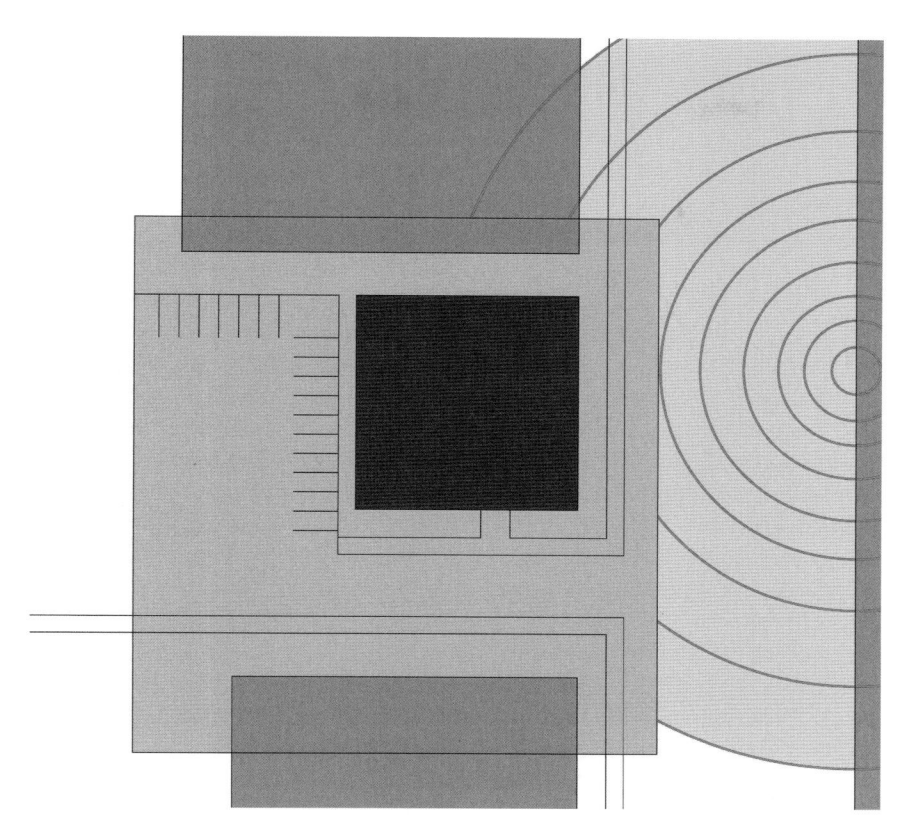

Fig. 3.5 *Madsen v. Women's Health Center*. Plan diagram illustrating legislated space and noise restrictions

the north and west of the clinic; restricting excessive noise-making within earshot during 7:30 a.m. until noon Mondays through Saturdays during surgical procedures and recovery periods (including singing, chanting, whistling, shouting, yelling, bull-horn use, auto horns, sound amplification equipment); restricting the use of "images observable" by patients inside the clinic; prohibiting protestors within a 300-foot zone around the clinic from approaching patients and potential patients who do not agree to talk; and creating a 300-foot buffer zone around residences of clinic staff. The Florida Supreme Court upheld the injunction.

The United States Supreme Court upheld part of the Florida state court decision protecting both the patients and the employees at the Women's Health Center. The Court recognized that "[t]he First Amendment does not demand that patients at a medical facility undertake Herculean efforts to escape the cacophony of political protests."[31] The Supreme Court agreed with the lower court and upheld noise restrictions from 7:30 a.m. until noon, Mondays through Saturdays, during surgical procedures and recovery periods, prohibiting singing, chanting, whistling, shouting, yelling, use of bull-horns, auto horns, sound amplification equipment, or other sounds within earshot of the patients inside the clinic and upheld the 36-foot buffer zone around the clinic entrances and driveway. Public areas are defined as surrounding health care facilities where demonstrations or access are restricted or sharply limited; they can cover the public entrances so doorways and driveways

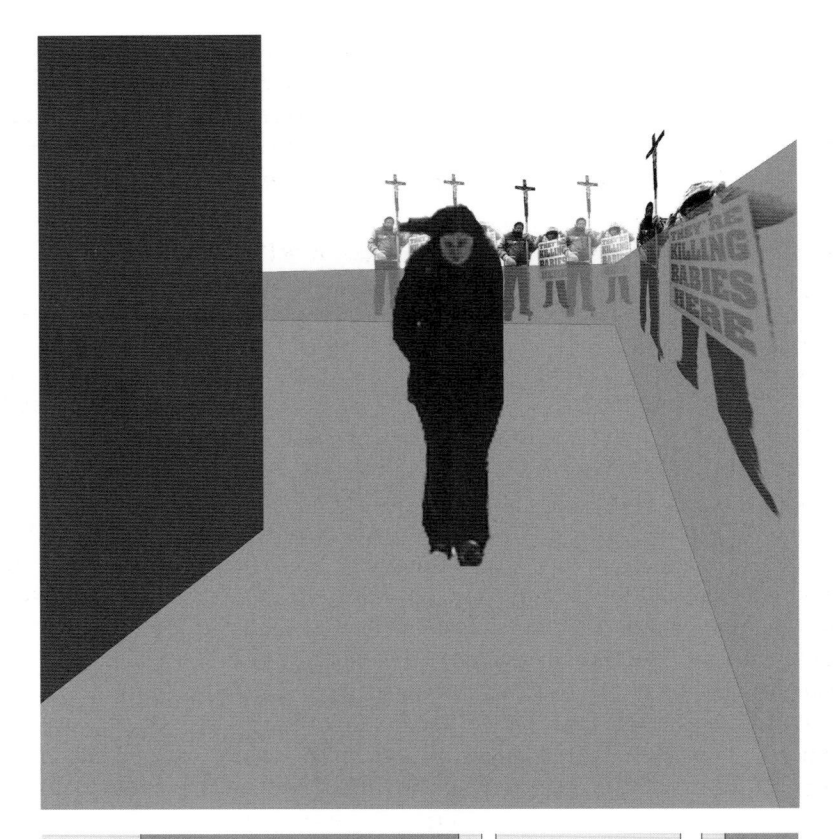

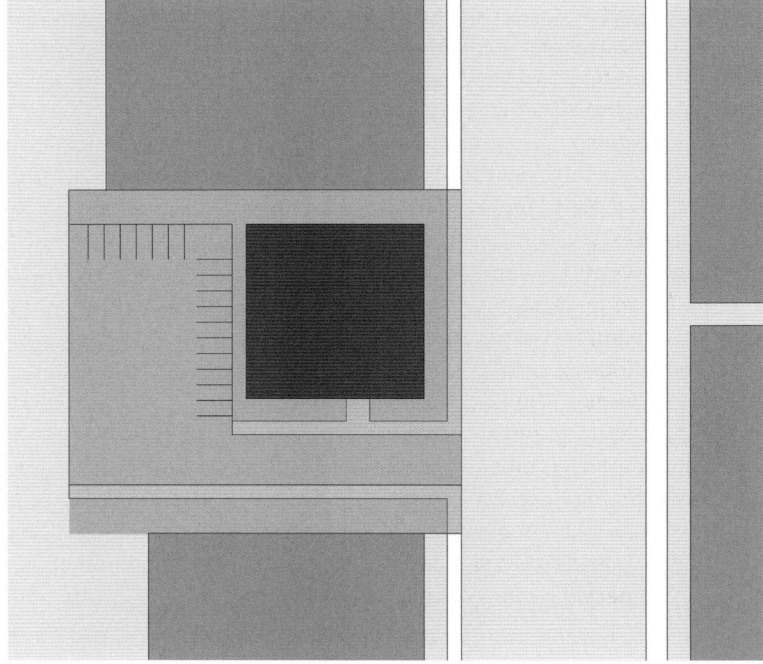

Fig. 3.6 *Schenck v. Pro-Choice Network of Western New York*. Plan and perspective diagrams illustrating legislated spaces

cannot be blocked; they also can limit what people can do around these areas.[32] However, the Court struck down as unconstitutional the 36-foot buffer zone as applied to the private property to the north and west of the clinic, the "images observable" provision, the 300-foot no-approach zone around the clinic, and the 300-foot buffer zone around the residences of employees.[33]

### Schenck v. Pro-Choice Network of Western New York (1997)

In 1990, doctors and clinics with Pro-Choice Network of Western New York in upstate New York around the Rochester and Buffalo areas filed a complaint in the District Court seeking to enjoin petitioners from blocking and other illegal conduct at their clinics. Prior to filing the complaint, these clinics experienced numerous large scale blockades where protestors engaged in activities such as kneeling, sitting and lying in clinic parking lot driveways and doorways, blocking or hindering car access onto the property and people access into the clinics. Smaller groups of protestors continually tried to stop or disrupt clinic operations through activities such as trespassing onto clinic parking lots and into clinic buildings, crowding around cars, surrounding, grabbing, pushing, shoving, yelling and spitting at women and their escorts entering clinics. "Sidewalk counselors," those approaching patients along public sidewalks in order to "counsel," used similar methods trying to persuade women entering the clinics not to have abortions.

A temporary restraining order (TRO) was issued by the District Court preventing demonstrations within 15 feet of any person or vehicle seeking ingress or egress of such facilities creating a "floating buffer zone" around a person with an exception that two "sidewalk counselors" were allowed to have "a conversation of a nonthreatening nature" with people entering or exiting the clinic. If a counselee indicated she did not want sidewalk counseling, the counselor must "cease and desist" from doing so. Protests were quieter and smaller for the first month following the TRO but after that, their prior intensity levels resumed. A preliminary injunction was issued 17 months later. In addition to the "floating buffer zone" previously included in the TRO, the new injunction included preventing demonstrations within 15 feet of clinic doorways and entrances, parking lot and driveway entrances, and clinic driveways creating a "fixed buffer zone." In addition, to address the sidewalk counselors the injunction required once the "cease and desist" request was invoked, the counselors must retreat 15 feet from the person they were counseling and remain outside the boundaries of the buffer zones.

The Supreme Court upheld part of the New York State court decision protecting those seeking abortion. The Court concurred with the lower court and upheld a ban on demonstrating within a 15-foot fixed zone around doorways and doorway entrances, parking lot entrances, driveways and driveway entrance of the clinic facilities. However, the Supreme Court struck down the ban on demonstrations within 15 feet of any person or vehicle seeking access to or leaving such facilities. They deemed the second part violated the First Amendment and burdened more speech than was necessary to serve relevant governmental interests.[34] The Courts

Fig. 3.7 Key spatial terms

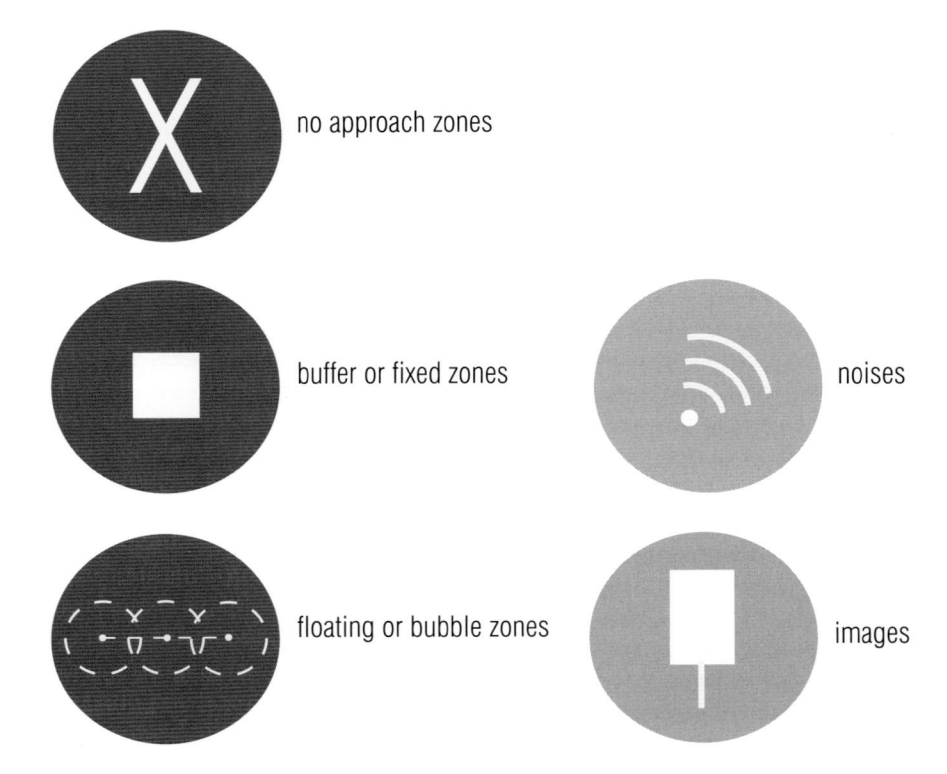

no approach zones

buffer or fixed zones

noises

floating or bubble zones

images

have stated they are concerned with public safety, ensuring the safety of abortion procedures, ensuring a woman's constitutional rights of inter-state travel to have an abortion and that this right should not be "sacrificed in the interest of defendants' First Amendment rights."[35]

All three cases affect direct mobility around and into the space of clinics for patients, employees and protestors. What immerged from these rulings were a series of key spatial terms impacting the actual space around these reproductive health clinics. These include *no-approach zones*: areas where no one can come within a legislated distance of a person when she is within a certain distance from a reproductive health care facility; this zone requires the assent of the person to come closer than the no-approach zone permits; *buffer zones*: defined public areas surrounding health care facilities where demonstrations or access are restricted or sharply limited; they can cover public entrances so doorways and driveways cannot be blocked; they also can limit what people are allowed to do around these areas;[36] *floating zones*: or a "bubble zone," these zones are similar to the no-approach zones but "float" with someone as they move to and from a reproductive health care facility, as if she were in a bubble;[37] *noise and image zones*: areas where severe noise is prohibited because it causes undue stress upon an abortion clinic patient and areas where there will be no use of "images observable" by patients inside the clinic.[38]

Fig. 3.8  FACE law

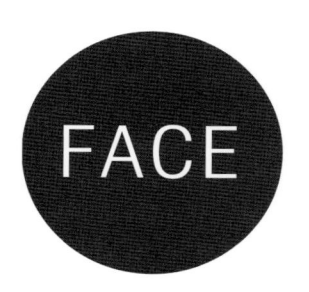

**Freedom of Access to Clinic Entrance Act [1994]**

This act is to protect and promote the public safety and health and activities affecting interstate commerce by establishing Federal criminal penalities and civil remedies for certain violent, threatening, obstructive and destructive conduct that is intended to injure, intimidate, or interfere with persons seeking to obtain or provide reproductive health services.

It also provides protection to churches and other places of worship, and to their congregants.

Another important federal law passed in 1994 by President Clinton is the Freedom of Access to Clinics Act (FACE), which protects anyone exercising free choice in obtaining reproductive health services and exercising First Amendment religious freedoms. The Act makes it unlawful for a person to use force, threat of force, or physical obstruction intentionally in order to injure or intimidate a person who is obtaining or providing reproductive health services or exercising the right of religious freedom at a place of worship. FACE also makes it unlawful to intentionally damage or destroy property of a facility providing reproductive health services or a place of worship.[39]

These court rulings and federal laws produce a complex set of spatial relationships. At first, they would appear to resolve the geographic and spatial aspect of the abortion controversy by literally drawing a line on the ground equaling the dimensions ordered by the Court. Indeed, there are many examples where yellow lines have been drawn on sidewalks, doing just that. In the abstract, such demarcation is exactly what the courts have asked for. But in practice, implementation of these laws does not work this way. Imagine the conflict, fear, anger and hostility that make filing a lawsuit mandatory. The spaces where these struggles occur are fraught with complex dynamics that laws often cannot completely control. Sometimes the architecture aids one side over the other; sometimes it does not. When I say architecture, I am referring to a myriad set of spatial relationships such as the literal building, where the clinic is sited on the property; access to the building, the space one passes through to enter the clinic; where windows are located; and what can be seen from and into the clinic. I am also referring to other environmental factors, including the invisible lines mandated by court rulings; the U.S. marshals required to enforce these laws; layers of different state legislation imposing increased abortion restrictions; the lack of public transportation throughout the United States; and the lack of federal funding for women's healthcare.

**Spatial Complexities**

One of the criticisms of bubble laws comes from Dr. Warren Hern, one of the few late-term abortion providers left in the United States and director of the Boulder Abortion Clinic. He has observed at first hand how difficult this law is to enforce.

Patients become terrified by the harassment at such a close range and have no real way of invoking the bubble law for their protection. Police are not regularly present to witness violations and when they are, they must first issue a warning. He believes this law is more symbolic than anything and offers no real protection from anti-abortion harassment. He states the law assumes those involved in protesting actually respect the law, the Constitution and the rights of others. However, from his experience he has witnessed protestors outside his clinic are people who have utter disregard and contempt for the law and for those women seeking care. He argues for a more effective law, similar to the protection mandated around polling places, where political activity must remain 100 feet or more from the building, as he says, a constitutional compromise. Eight feet, as dictated by Colorado state law, is still close enough were protestors can successfully terrorize people coming to health facilities.[40]

After eight feet, you can still try and speak to someone—it does not prevent protest from happening but protects the woman going into the clinic. Some clinics have noted patients undergo an extreme level of emotional distress as a result of protestors standing beside a patient. "[A]nti-abortion leaders have been known to boast that when they 'demonstrate' outside of clinics, medical complications increase."[41] Both Young and Fraser believe public space is a space that everyone has access to; however, when it comes to the abortion debate, access becomes a slippery slope. There must be an acknowledgement that there is a difference between contestation and domination. The laws allow anti-abortion protestors to intimidate patients, employees and doctors to such a degree where for decades abortion clinics have closed all across the country. Not only with fewer clinics, but also many of the remaining clinics still in operation continue to receive protestors interested in dominating, overpowering and preventing a woman's ability to access abortion. Through the gradual closure of clinics, the possibility of access to any clinic becomes further diminished and will eventually lead to no choice in some states. When only one abortion clinic remains in a state, like it does in South Dakota, Mississippi, North Dakota, Wyoming and Arkansas, is this choice? In theory, we want the right to voice our dissent but who is accountable when this dissent, often unlawful and unregulated, prevents access and choice from still being possible?

I believe most people would agree that these laws are difficult to implement. But this difficulty works to the advantage of those protesting outside clinics. For example, in *Schenck v. Pro-Choice of Western New York*, the floating buffer zone was struck down because the Court believed these floating zones would be difficult to enforce. If protesters who thought they were keeping pace with the targeted individual from a distance of 15 feet actually strayed to within 14 or 13 feet of the individual for a certain period of time, then they would be in violation of the injunction.[42] As a result there is no floating zone of protection for people accessing abortion in western New York.

I have been following postings by abortion escorts for women obtaining abortions in Louisville, Kentucky on *Everysaturdaymorning Blog*. People post weekly about their experiences helping women and their families' access reproductive healthcare. I have noticed over time how often the protestors intimidate and disrespect both a woman and her family's personal space as she is trying to make her way to the clinic. Because patients must park in a lot that is not adjacent to the clinic, there is time and space for protestors to try and engage her as she is escorted to the clinic. There have been many posts where the patient's friends or family come to near blows with protestors because they feel continually under verbal assault as their personal space is constantly being violated. A recent post mentioned a young woman who had covered her head with a towel so she could have some privacy walking from the car to the clinic.[43]

When it comes to the point where clinics are measuring noise levels outside their buildings on an often-daily basis as a way to try and convenience local police to uphold noise ordinances, what good is the insurance that speech will not be too intrusive? It already has been and continues to be. From archival research at the Sallie Bingham Center for Women's History and Culture, it became apparent there was a gap between Attorney General Janet Reno's request for clinic protection and the support of local police to carry out the attorney general's decrees. Some police blatantly did not follow some of her orders. The coordination and support between federal and state law enforcement was not well implemented resulting in a lack of clinic protection across the US.

## GENERAL HISTORY AND CONTEXT OF ABORTION: CANADA

Birth control laws of Canada during the late nineteenth century were similar in nature to those of both Britain and the United States. The selling, advertising or distributing of contraceptives or abortifacients was illegal and if a woman was found to have obtained her own abortion, she could be incarcerated for up to seven years.[44] The 1892 Criminal Code of Canada Section 251 defined when a child becomes a human being as "has completely proceeded, in a living state, from the body of its mother, whether it has breathed or not, whether it has an independent circulation or not, and whether the navel string is severed or not. The killing of such child is homicide when it dies in consequence of injuries received before, during or after birth." The code stipulates that if the death was necessary to preserve the life of the mother then that person is not guilty of any offense.[45]

This law was in affect making abortion illegal in Canada until 1969 when under Prime Minister Pierre Trudeau, the Criminal Code was reformed through Bill C-150. The reform included decriminalizing contraception, homosexual acts between consulting adults and legalizing abortion under certain circumstances.[46] This resulted in a formal process a woman was required to navigate to procure an abortion and therefore institutionalizing the medical establishments control over access. A woman was now completely dependent upon an arduous and time-consuming set of procedures and regulations. Requiring a referral from her doctor, she would then have to go before an accredited hospital based Therapeutic Abortion Committee (TAC) comprising three or more doctors, none of whom could be her own personal doctor, for the committee to deem that the abortion was medically necessary to preserve her "health."[47] "Health" was quite a broad and interpretive measure to be used in determining whether a woman needed an abortion or not. This was practiced

Fig. 3.9 Canada abortion timeline 1800s–1988

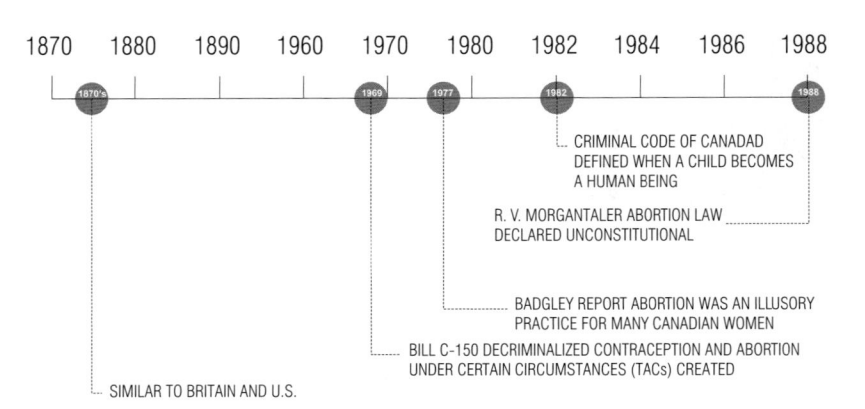

Canada Timeline

1870　1880　1890　1960　1970　1980　1982　1984　1986　1988

- 1870's — SIMILAR TO BRITAIN AND U.S.
- 1969 — BILL C-150 DECRIMINALIZED CONTRACEPTION AND ABORTION UNDER CERTAIN CIRCUMSTANCES (TACs) CREATED
- 1977 — BADGLEY REPORT ABORTION WAS AN ILLUSORY PRACTICE FOR MANY CANADIAN WOMEN
- 1982 — CRIMINAL CODE OF CANADAD DEFINED WHEN A CHILD BECOMES A HUMAN BEING
- 1988 — R. V. MORGANTALER ABORTION LAW DECLARED UNCONSTITUTIONAL

with shocking inconsistency throughout the country. Hospitals were not required to form TACs so few did and those that were created were mostly located in urban areas. There was no appeal process created so if a woman was not in agreement with the TAC decision she had absolutely no recourse available.[48]

In 1977 the *Report of the Committee on the Operation of the Abortion Law*, informally referred to as the *Badgley Report* after the committee chair sociologist Robin Badgley, found that "the procedure provided in the Criminal Code for obtaining therapeutic abortion is in practice illusory for many Canadian women."[49] Although deaths from abortions had decreased since the 1969 abortion law, TACs were only established in 20.1 percent of hospitals throughout the country creating vast differences in women's abortion access.[50] Clearly the 1969 law reform was not working. Parliament had established a system whereby women were at the mercy of a committee of doctors that under no clearly defined terms, ruled whether a woman was in need of an abortion or not.

Synonymous with Canadian abortion reform is Dr. Henry Morgantaler. A well-known doctor throughout Canada, he has passionately fought for women's reproductive rights for decades. A Holocaust survivor, he emigrated from Poland to Montreal in 1950 where he established a family medical practice. After the 1969 reform, he began to perform abortions full time in his Montreal clinic where in open opposition to the Criminal Code, he bypassed TAC requirements.[51] His was the first abortion clinic in Canada. He believed that only the woman should make the decision whether to continue with her pregnancy and that no woman should be forced by the state or anyone else to carry a pregnancy to term.[52] Raided in 1970, Dr. Morgantaler was charged but continued to provide abortions. Finally in 1975 he began to serve an 18-month jail sentence after his appeal had been rejected. A re-trial was ordered in 1976 after serving 10 months in jail and he was acquitted 9 months later.[53] In 1983 he opened clinics in Winnipeg and Toronto.[54] The Toronto clinic was raided and in the next five years, his legal case worked its way to the Canadian Supreme Court.

Finally in 1988 Dr. Morgantaler's case provides the opportunity for the Supreme Court of Canada to declare the abortion law unconstitutional. Violating Section 7 of the Charter of Rights and Freedoms, the Court ruled that the law infringes upon

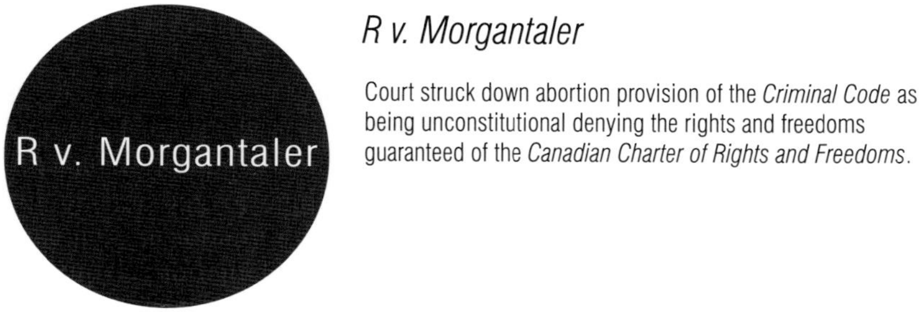

## R v. Morgantaler

Court struck down abortion provision of the *Criminal Code* as being unconstitutional denying the rights and freedoms guaranteed of the *Canadian Charter of Rights and Freedoms*.

Fig. 3.10   *R v. Morgantaler*

a woman's right to "life, liberty and security of person." Chief Justice Brian Dickson writes: "[f]orcing a woman, by threat of criminal sanction, to carry a fetus to term unless she meets certain criteria unrelated to her own priorities and aspirations, is a profound interference with a woman's body and thus a violation of her security of the person."[55] This was a milestone. However, although now legal, there were no federal laws forcing unwilling doctors or hospitals to perform abortions.[56] So in a similar situation to the US, although abortion is legal on paper, if there are so few places to go to actually exercise your right, is it really a right?

Following the 1988 Supreme Court decision, Canada's abortion law has gone through a series of both expansions and contractions. A few will be highlighted. In 1989 the Supreme Court rules that a man "has no legal right to veto a woman's abortion decision." Also during that same year, the Supreme Court refuses to hear a case arguing for fetus rights. In 1991 the Supreme Court rules that unless a child is fully born alive, she does not have legal rights. Unlike in the United States where fetal rights have become a current anti-abortion focus at both state and federal levels, in Canada this idea was legally declared moot. In 1992 the Ontario New Democratic Party (NDP) government creates an injunction against protestors outside hospitals and abortion clinics, thereby limiting free speech. In 1994 the Ontario NDP grants an interim injunction prohibiting protestors from coming closer than 500 feet from abortion providers' homes and 30 to 60 feet from abortion clinic entrances. There have been a number of provincial laws (Nova Scotia in 1989 and New Brunswick in 1994) banning abortions outside hospitals but these were followed in 1995 by both federal and provincial rulings in both provinces requiring private abortion clinics to be allowed. In 1995 Dr. Morgantaler wins his challenge to the Prince Edward Island policy only funding "medically necessary" abortions. As a result, abortion is ruled a basic health service and must be included in the provincial government's health funding. In 1995 British Columbia's NDP government creates a bubble zone around abortion clinics but then this is greatly restricted in 1996. The year 1999 sees two important rulings. The first allows nurses the right to decline assisting in providing abortion services in a northern Toronto hospital in Ontario. The second is the approval by Health Canada for a morning-after pill to be available to the Canadian public. In 2000, British Columbia allows morning-after pills to be sold without a prescription and Quebec follows in 2001. Due to workload problems, the last hospital in New Brunswick performing abortions announced in 2006 it would be suspending this medical service. Despite federal requirements that all provinces must pay for abortions performed in clinics, New Brunswick remains the only province refusing to do so.[57]

Canada — Number of Hospitals Providing Abortions

YUKON
1 (50%)

NORTHWEST TERRITORIES
2 (67%)

NUNAVUT
1 (100%)

BRITISH COLUMBIA
26 (29%)

ALBERTA
6 (6%)

SASKATCHEWAN
4 (6%)

MANITOBA
2 (4%)

ONTARIO
33 (17%)

QUEBEC
31 (24%)

NEWFOUNDLAND & LABRADOR
3 (31%)

PRINCE EDWARD ISLAND
0 (0%)

NOVA SCOTIA
4 (13%)

NEW BRUNSWICK
1 (4%)

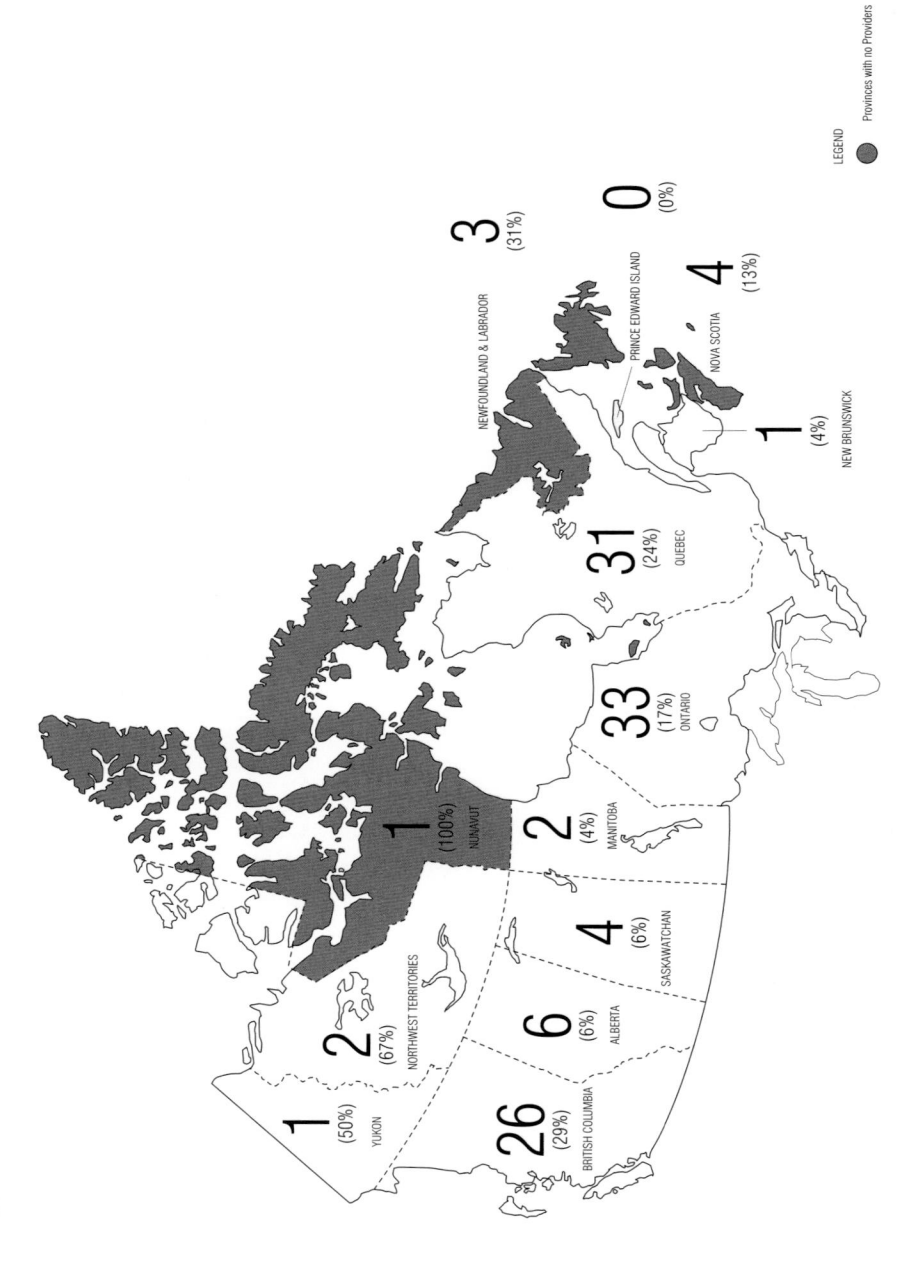

LEGEND
● Provinces with no Providers

Fig. 3.11a   Abortion in Canada

This map and the diagrams below illustrate where in the country a woman can access hospital and clinic abortions and what provinces have no providers. The provincial abortion funding policies have been explained demonstrating another mechanism for restricting abortion access.

| PROVINCE/TERRITORY | | PROVINCIAL ABORTION FUNDING POLICY |
|---|---|---|
| BRITISH COLUMBIA | C$ | FULL FUNDING FOR HOSPITAL AND CLINIC ABORTIONS |
| ALBERTA | C$ | FULL FUNDING FOR HOSPITAL AND CLINIC ABORTIONS<br>QUOTA IMPOSED ON NUMBER OF PROC. FUNDED AT CALGARY CLINIC<br>OUT-OF-PROVINCE WOMEN MUST PAY A FACILITY FEE |
| SASKATCHEWAN | C$ | FULL FUNDING FOR HOSPITALS ONLY<br>THE SASKATCHEWAN GOVERNMENT HAS BEEN STRONGLY OPPOSED TO CLINICS OPENING IN THEIR PROVINCE |
| MANITOBA | C$ | FULL FUNDING FOR HOSPITALS AND WINNIPEG CLINIC (SINCE 2004 ONLY)<br>FUNDING FOR ABORTION CLINICS RESULTING FROM A LAWSUIT THAT FOUND THAT THE GOVERNMENT'S HOSPITAL ONLY FUNDING POLICY CONTRAVENED WOMEN'S RIGHT TO ACCESS TIMELY SERVICES UNDER THE CANADA HEALTH ACT |
| ONTARIO | %C$ | FULL FUNDING FOR HOSPITAL AND CLINIC ABORTIONS<br>NORTHERN HEALTH TRAVEL GRANTS AVAILABLE WITH REFERRAL FOR NORTHERN WOMEN WHO MUST TRAVEL SOUTH<br>25% OF ALL ABORTIONS ARE PERFORMED IN TORONTO BASED CLINICS<br>66% OF ALL ABORTIONS TAKE PLACE IN SOUTHERN ONTARIO |
| QUEBEC | %C$ | FULL FUNDING FOR ABORTIONS IN HOSPITALS AND COMMUNITY HEALTH CENTERS (CLSC)<br>PARTIAL FUNDING FOR CLINIC ABORTIONS, WOMEN PAY REMAINDER (APPROXIMATELY $200)<br>APPROX. 70% OF ABORTION SERVICES IN QUEBEC ARE CONCENTRATED IN THE MONTREAL AREA<br>PRIVATE CLINICS PERFORM APPROXIMATELY 50% OF ABORTIONS IN THE CITY OF MONTREAL |
| NEW BRUNSWICK | C$ | FULL FUNDING FOR HOSPITAL ABORTIONS WHEN PROCEURE IS APPROVED BY TWO DOCTORS<br>NO FUNDING FOR CLINIC ABORTIONS<br>DR HENRY MORGENTALER IS CURRENTLY CHALLENGING THE PROVINCES FUNDING POLICY IN COURT<br>NB IS THE ONLY PROVINCE TO REQ. TWO PHYSICIANS TO APPROVE A WOMEN'S ABORTION REQ. |
| NOVA SCOTIA | %C$ | FULL FUNDING FOR HOSPITAL ABORTIONS<br>PARTIAL CLINIC FUNDING, WOMEN PAYS THE REMAINDER |
| PRINCE EDWARD ISLAND | C$ | APPROXIMATELY 30% OF HALIFAX CLINIC PATIENTS ARE FROM PEI<br>THE PROVINCE PAYS FOR ABORTIONS IN ONE HALIFAX HOSPITAL ONLY IF THE DEPARTMENT OF HEALTH AND SOCIAL SERVICES APPROVES THE PROCEDURE AS "MEDICALLY NECESSARY"<br>AS OF 2005, ONLY ONE HALIFAX HOSPITAL WILL ACCEPT REFERRALS FOR PEI WOMEN NEEDING AN ABORTION. HER PEI DOCTOR MUST REFER HER THERE AND APPLY TO THE PROVINCE TO HAVE THE PROCEDURE COVERED |
| NEW FOUND./LABRADOR | C$ | FULL FUNDING FOR HOSPITAL AND CLINIC ABORTIONS |
| YUKON TERRITORY | C$ | FULL FUNDING FOR HOSPITAL ABORTIONS<br>PARTIAL FUNDING FOR TRAVEL FOR WOMEN LIVING OUTSIDE WHITE HORSE<br>THE YUKON GOVERNMENT HAS A RECIPROCAL BILLING AGREEMENT WITH BC, ALLOWING WOMEN TO ACCESS FUNDED HOSPITAL ABORTION SERVICES IN BC<br>PARTIAL FUNDING IS PROVIDED FOR CLINIC ABORTIONS IN ALBERTA AND BC |
| NORTHWEST TERRITORIES | C$ | FULL FUNDING FOR HOSPITAL ABORTIONS<br>PARTIAL FUNDING FOR TRAVEL |
| NUNAVUT TERRITORY | C$ | FULL FUNDING FOR HOSPITAL ABORTIONS AND TRAVEL<br>WOMEN ARE FLOWN FROM NUNAVUT TO OTTOWA IF OVER 13 WEEKS |

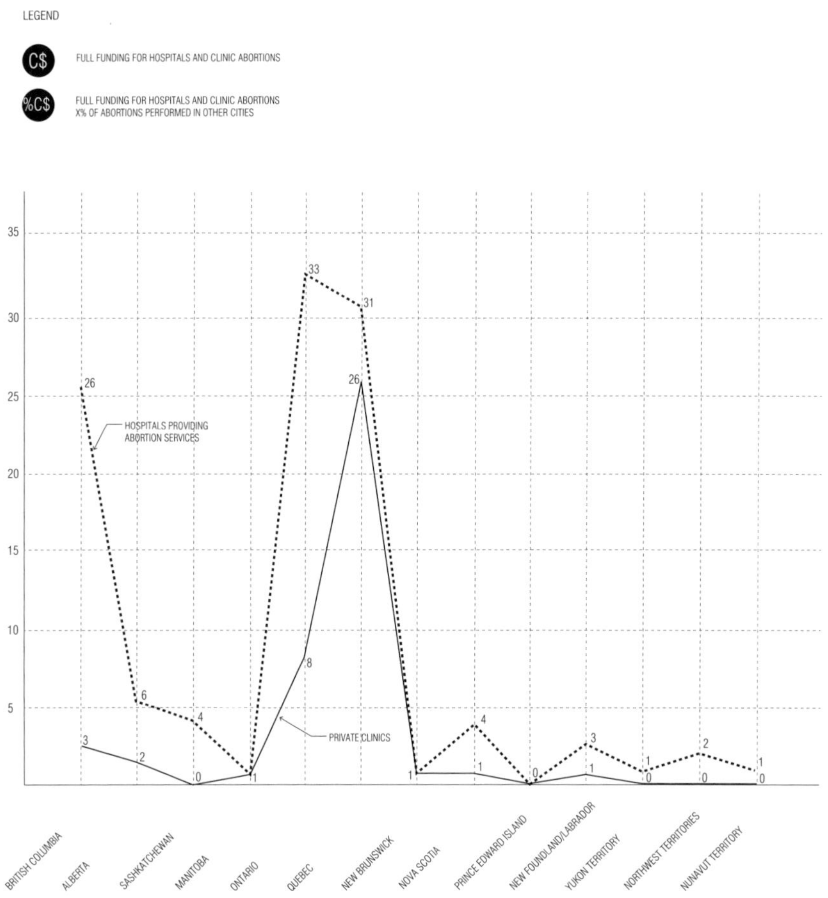


Fig. 3.11b Abortion in Canada

## GENERAL HISTORY AND CONTEXT OF ABORTION: MEXICO

It is necessary to contextualize abortion in Mexico in relation to dramatic changes in Mexican demographics, the rise of women's rights and the evolution of Mexican law reform. These are interdependent issues that have been affected over various periods in Mexico's history. Several will be highlighted in order to have a better understanding of abortion law in Mexico today and how the last 150 years have significantly influenced Mexican legal policy.

When Mexico regained its independence from Spain in the early 1800s, one of the first significant reforms the Mexican Reform Laws of 1859 focused on was the separation of Church and state. This law prevented elected or appointed officials from using their personal or religious beliefs to influence public policy.[58] During the next century Mexico fought the Catholic Church's influence in all aspects of Mexican life. One result of the Mexican Revolution was to outlaw the Church all together. The Constitution of 1917 denied churches legal status, members were not allowed to own property, religious clergy could not wear their habits in public and diplomatic ties to the Vatican were severed. However, in 1939 the Catholic Church re-established its powerful presence and influence on all aspects of Mexican life once again.[59] It is common knowledge that the Catholic Church still remains an ever-present political force to be reckoned with.

The 1968 student movement was instrumental in beginning to alter power structures in Mexico. Comprising diverse groups including urban and rural workers, artists, intellectuals and radicalized Christian sectors, the movement sought a more diverse political arena and the elimination of restrictive political and social controls by the state. By the early 1970s, women started organizing and women's groups began to be created. *Voluntary Motherhood* became a publicly discussed topic serving as an umbrella for issues of women's control over their own reproductivity. Arguing for legalization of contraception and abortion, these groups also strongly advocated that women's legal equality would not possibly be created without a woman's ability to *voluntarily* become a mother.[60]

The Mexican Constitution was amended in 1973 granting women equality before the law including the legalization of contraception. Women "were given the right to decide 'in a free, informed, and responsible manner about the number and spacing of their children'...."[61] These new laws provided a mechanism for women to receive contraception without the consent of their husbands or partners. Abortion was not included at this time in hopes of not jeopardizing the state's relationship to the Catholic Church. Categorized as "planned parenthood," these new laws were in part created to help reduce the rapidly increasing Mexican population that had been taking place by the mid 1970s.[62]

For the first time in Mexican history the state-led Interdisciplinary Abortion Group (Grupo Interdisciplinario del Aborto, GIA), publicly debated and discussed the decriminalization of abortion in 1976.[63] It comprised attorneys, demographers, economists, physicians psychologists, anthropologists, philosophers and various religious representation including a Catholic priest, a Protestant pastor and a Jewish rabbi. GIA recommended the complete abolishment of criminal abortion

## Mexico Timeline

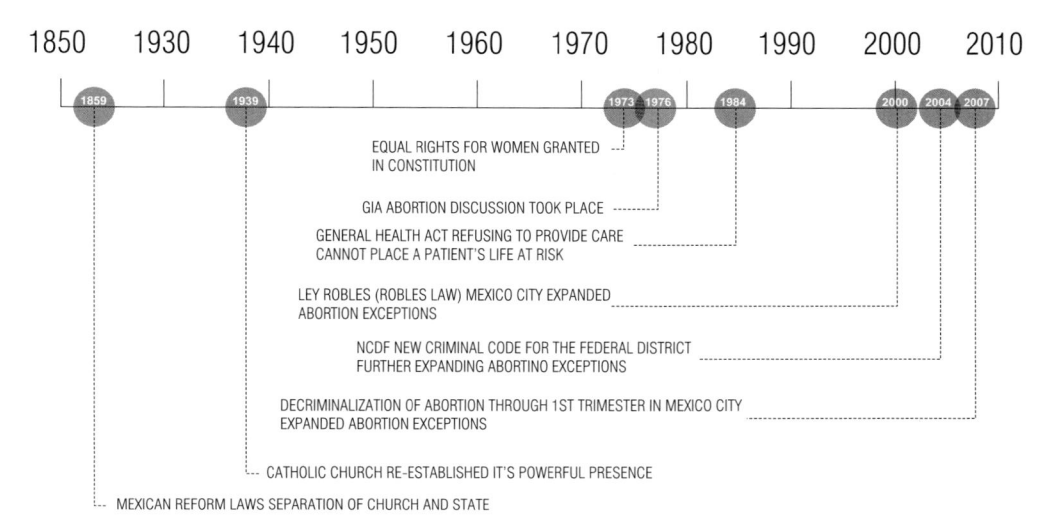

```
1850    1930    1940    1950    1960    1970    1980    1990    2000    2010
 |1859    |1939                           |1973 1976  |1984            |2000 2004 2007
```

- EQUAL RIGHTS FOR WOMEN GRANTED IN CONSTITUTION
- GIA ABORTION DISCUSSION TOOK PLACE
- GENERAL HEALTH ACT REFUSING TO PROVIDE CARE CANNOT PLACE A PATIENT'S LIFE AT RISK
- LEY ROBLES (ROBLES LAW) MEXICO CITY EXPANDED ABORTION EXCEPTIONS
- NCDF NEW CRIMINAL CODE FOR THE FEDERAL DISTRICT FURTHER EXPANDING ABORTINO EXCEPTIONS
- DECRIMINALIZATION OF ABORTION THROUGH 1ST TRIMESTER IN MEXICO CITY EXPANDED ABORTION EXCEPTIONS
- CATHOLIC CHURCH RE-ESTABLISHED IT'S POWERFUL PRESENCE
- MEXICAN REFORM LAWS SEPARATION OF CHURCH AND STATE

Fig. 3.12 Mexico abortion time line 1850–2007

sanctions and for the procedure to be included in general health coverage. These recommendations were never published nor followed.[64]

The General Health Act in 1984 held providers culpable for refusing care when a patient's life is at risk. Described as an aggravated offense, providers could be either fined or imprisoned if discovered to deny services when a person's life is in jeopardy. Although not explicitly referring to conscientious objection, abortion providers are clearly indicted in this Act.[65] In 1990 the Mexican state of Chiapas loosened its abortion restrictions by passing a law expanding abortion rights. As a result either a couple or a single woman would be able to request an abortion for reasons regarding family planning concerns or economic situations.[66] In 1992 the federal Law on Religious Associations and Public Culture further instituted one's religious beliefs could not prevent one from following the rule of law. One caveat with this law is Mexican state laws override this federal law.[67] The Platform for Action of the UN Women's Conference in 1995 further condemned "forced motherhood as a violation of women's human rights."[68] Mexico is still in violation of this UN platform but depending upon where in the country you live, a woman has less or more freedom to abortion. Sound familiar?

### Mexico City (Federal District)

The liberalizing of the Federal District's abortion laws has only happened during the past 12 years yet offers several important issues to consider when comparing how quickly positive change has been legislated. Mexico City has the most liberal abortion laws throughout Mexico. It is interesting to compare Mexico City's history to the continued restricting of abortion access in the United States. The Federal District's Penal Code of 1931 stated abortion was legal in cases of rape, to save the

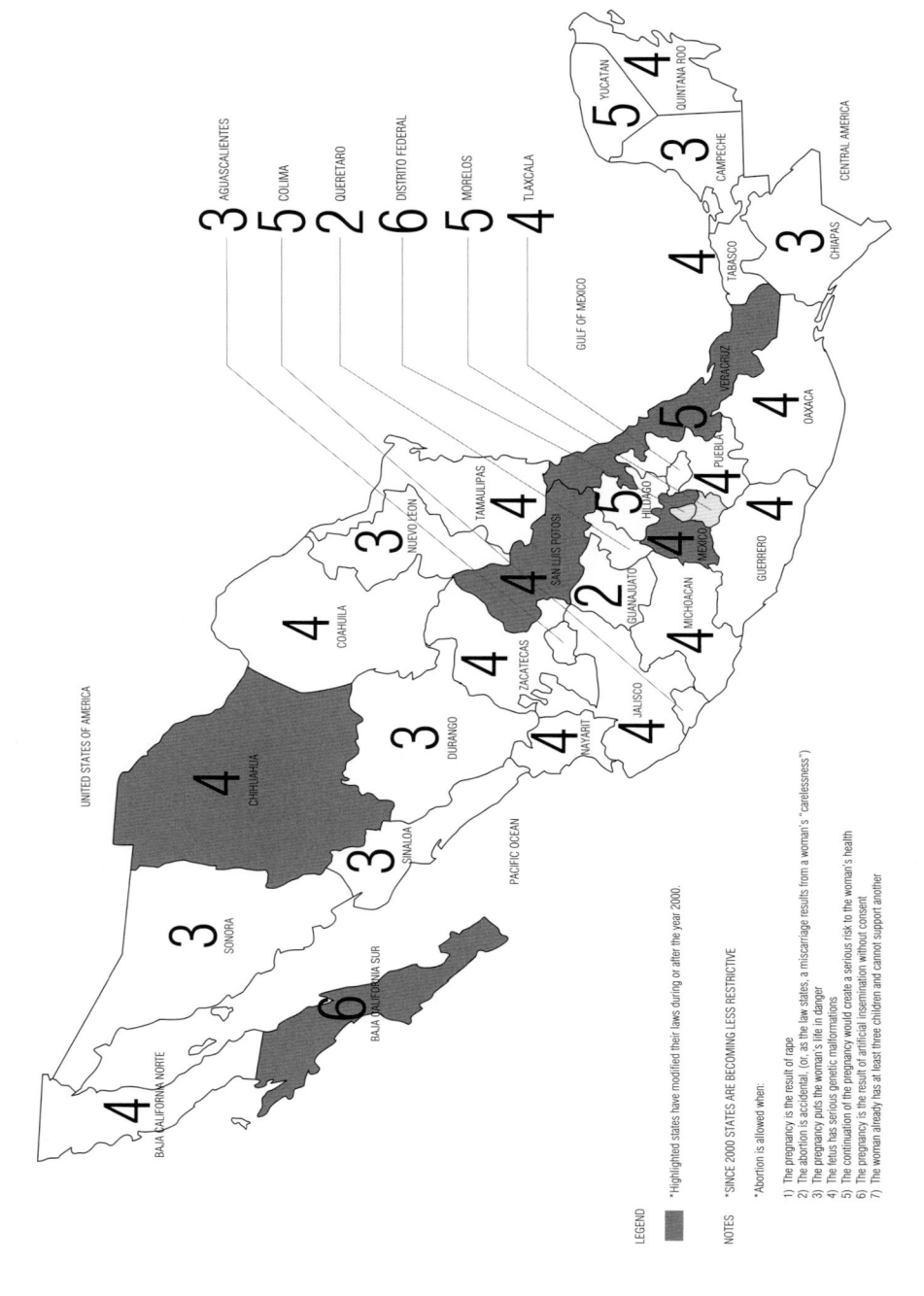

Fig. 3.13a  Abortion in Mexico

This map and the diagrams below illustrate which states have more liberal policies in Mexico. These are further discussed in Chapter 5.

| STATES_SINCE 2000 STATES ARE BECOMING LESS RESTRICTIVE | | | | | | |
|---|---|---|---|---|---|---|
| AGUASCALIENTES | RAPE | ! | X | | | |
| BAJA CALIFORNIA NORTE | RAPE (A) | ! | X | | | OTHER (B) |
| BAJA CALIFORNIA SUR | RAPE | ! | X | ● | HEALTH | OTHER (B) |
| CAMPECHE | RAPE | ! | X | | | |
| COAHUILA | RAPE (A) | ! | X | ● | | |
| COLIMA | RAPE (A) | ! | X | ● | | OTHER (B) |
| CHIAPAS | RAPE (A) | | X | ● | | |
| CHIHUAHUA | RAPE (A) | ! | ✱ | | | OTHER (B) |
| DISTRITO FEDERAL | RAPE | ! | ✱ | ● | HEALTH | OTHER (B) (D) |
| DURANGO | RAPE | ! | X | | | |
| GUANAJUATO | RAPE | ! | | | | |
| GUERRERO | RAPE | ! | | ● | | OTHER (B) |
| HILDAGO | RAPE (A) | ! | ✱ | | HEALTH | OTHER (B) |
| JALISCO | RAPE | ! | X | | HEALTH | |
| MEXICO | RAPE | | X | ● | | |
| MICHOACAN | RAPE | ! | X | | HEALTH | |
| MORELOS | RAPE | ! | X | ● | | OTHER (B) |
| NAYARIT | RAPE | ! | X | | HEALTH | |
| NUEVO LEON | RAPE | | X | | HEALTH | |
| OAXACA | RAPE (A) | ! | X | ● | | |
| PUEBLA | RAPE | ! | X | ● | | |
| QUERETARO | RAPE | ! | | | | |
| QUINTANA ROO | RAPE (A) | ! | X | ● | | |
| SAN LUIS POTOSI | RAPE | ! | X | | | OTHER (B) |
| SINALOA | RAPE | ! | X | | | |
| SONORA | RAPE | ! | X | | | |
| TABASCO | RAPE | ▲ | X | | | OTHER (B) |
| TAMAULIPAS | RAPE | ! | X | | HEALTH | |
| TLAXCALA | RAPE | ! | X | | HEALTH | |
| VERACRUZ | RAPE (A) | ! | X | ● | | OTHER (B) |
| YUCATAN | RAPE | ! | X | ● | | OTHER (C) |
| ZACATECAS | RAPE | ! | X | | HEALTH | |
| TOTAL | 32 | 30 | 29 | 13 | 11 | 12 |

LEGEND

- RAPE Rape
- ! Abortion due to an accident
- X Risk to the woman's life
- Fetal Impairment
- HEALTH Risk to the woman's health
- OTHER Other Causes
- ● The indication is included in the state's penal code.
- ✱ The state's penal code makes no explicit mention of "Risk to the woman's life", but it is included under "Risk to the woman's health".
- ▲ Based on an integrated interpretation of Article 14 (exclusions for criminal responsibility) and Article 61 (which mentions accidental abortion) of the Penal Code of the state of Tabasco, abortion without wilful intervention by the woman or the doctor is not penalized.
- *Highlighted states have modified their laws during or after the year 2000.

NOTES

(A) In these cases, the laws mention time periods during which the termination of pregnancy can take place. Some codes signal "within three months, counted from the day of the rape" while others state "within 90 days of gestation" or during the "first three months" of pregnancy

(B) Artificial insemination without the woman's consent.

(C) Socio-economic reasons (for women with 3+ children).

(D) Abortion not penalized up to 12 weeks of gestation.

Fig. 3.13b Abortion in Mexico

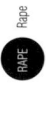

life of the mother or when abortion occurs due to an accident.[69] This was the oldest criminal code in the republic,[70] and defined abortion as "the death of the product of conception at any moment during pregnancy."[71]

From 2000 onwards, there have been a series of legislative reforms rewriting abortion policy in Mexico City. I would like to highlight the three most significant reforms. The first is commonly referred to as the Ley Robles or Robles Law, named after the interim mayor of Mexico City, Rosario Robles. The law expands the possible exceptions to accessing abortion and slowly begins to move abortion away from the procedure being one of a moral offense. The law includes an exception to a woman being artificially inseminated against her will, changing the language from "product of conception" to one concerned with the threat to a woman's health, an exception regarding "genetic or congenital conditions affecting the fetus "which may result in physical or mental damage ... [that could] put the product of conception's survival at risk.""[72] Also noted are the replacement of "mother" with "woman" and the added stipulation of a 24-hour time limit for a rape or insemination survivor to be authorized for an abortion once rape and pregnancy were confirmed.

The second change occurred in the 2004 reform. Focusing on the issue of a woman's consent, this new legislation increased imprisonment from three to six years to between five and eight years if an abortion had been performed without the consent of the woman. The language around abortion was also altered so that if abortion was performed under the permitted circumstances there was no longer any criminal responsibility assigned, officially decriminalizing abortion. In addition two articles were added in a sister reform to the Health Law of Mexico City. The first article included the obligation of city-run public health institutions to perform abortions for free in cases allowed by Mexico City law, provide information about abortion alternatives and established a five-day time limit for the procedure once a woman had submitted a petition for the legal abortion. The second article established the right for conscientious objection for health providers but provided an exception if the woman's life was in danger. If a doctor decided to refuse to perform an abortion, the provider was obligated to provide a referral for another doctor who would agree to perform the abortion.[73]

In 2007, the third change fully decriminalized abortion during the first trimester. It should also be noted that the Legislative Assembly redefined the crime of abortion as "the interruption of a pregnancy after the 12th week." Pregnancy was also defined "as the process of human reproduction starting with implantation of the embryo in the wall of the uterus ..." allowing for emergency contraception to be used because it is beyond the definition of pregnancy and abortion.[74] Sister reform further stipulated that all women are entitled to free legal abortions in city hospitals. One of the most important aspects of this ruling is that it provides the right AND the mechanism to access abortion. An additional article was added to Mexico City's Health Law requiring public health policies to prioritize sexual and reproductive health. The article stipulates:

> 'permanent, intensive and integral' education and training campaigns promoting sexual health, reproductive rights, and responsible "maternity and paternity," family planning, and contraception services aimed at

*reducing the number of abortions through the prevention of unplanned and unwanted pregnancies, reducing reproductive risk, avoiding the propagation of sexually transmitted diseases, and helping the exercise of sexual rights taking into account a gender perspective, and respect for sexual diversity in accordance with the characteristics of the multiple population groups, especially girls and boys, adolescents and youths.*[75]

The first year after abortion was made legal in Mexico City, the 12 hospitals where the procedure was offered developed complications and in particular, many of the doctors who were performing abortions became conscientious objectors. This resulted in a major strain of available resources due to a reduction of doctors to provide the service. Additionally, more space was needed and due to the numbers of women now seeking access, there was tremendous overload for those doctors providing abortions. Health care providers and women were both noting the hostile environment.

To help mitigate these situations, in May 2008 the Mexico City Ministry of Health opened the first facility to specifically provide abortion care, the Beatriz Velasco de Aleman (BVA). Two years later, the second public health facility, Santa Catarina, was opened to provide further access to abortion services. As has been noted in 2011, most legal abortions accessed through the public health system occur in these two facilities.[76]

There has been a trickle down affecting other more progressive Mexican states as a result of the liberalizing of Mexico City abortion legislation, especially in the case of rape.[77] However, what this has also produced for women living in states with far stricter abortion laws is a great deal of inter-state and cross-border traffic by women seeking abortions. Women will travel great distances to access safe care. One study documented women who traveled up to seven days crossing the border to find safe abortion care with the full intention of returning to Mexico afterwards.[78]

There are those critics who ask if the courts have any right to be making these decisions. University of Toronto Faculty of Law Professor and Director of the Reproductive and Sexual Health Law Rebecca Cook points out that the Supreme Court in the United States, Canada, Mexico and Portugal are all deciding abortion laws but questions what are their proper roles in the legalities of abortion.[79] Philosopher and Princeton University Professor Peter Singer argues that abortion should not be a criminal offense or a constitutional issue. Abortion is a political issue and should be decided by a democratically elected body, not by an unelected body such as a Supreme Court. He cites both Australia and New Zealand where there is no constitutional right to abortion yet abortion is covered by public health care and much better protected than in the United States.[80]

Although the United States passed the earliest legislation (1973) compared to either Canada (1969 requiring TAC approval and 1988 without) or Mexico City (2007), depending upon where in the country one lives their policies have become more and more restrictive and as a result are drastically reducing a woman's ability to access abortion. Canada's law is the most liberal in the Western world; abortion is entirely decriminalized with no restrictions for the full nine months of pregnancy and can be paid for by the national health care system.[81] Although Mexico is one of the more restrictive countries in the world for abortion access, Mexico City offers an interesting recent history in how laws have become far more liberalized. Due to both the election of more liberal politicians and a strong women's movement, abortion policy was drastically rewritten. The legislation moved from one of public morality to one of women's health and autonomy. This shift is important because it eliminated the possibility of fetal life as a legal question placing emphasis on the wellbeing of a woman's physical body, no longer focusing on the question of moral agency. In addition what is even more instrumental is that the law requires the means to procure an abortion making her decision possible with "permanent, intensive and integral education and training campaigns promoting sexual health, reproductive rights, and responsible 'maternity and paternity.'"[82] This is absolutely critical because the law institutionalizes education as integral to the larger concerns around abortion and age-appropriate sex education has proven instrumental in reducing unwanted pregnancies. The US has so much to learn from such policies.

## NOTES

1. Weinbar 2007: 13.
2. Rubin 1994: 3.
3. Rubin 1994: 4.
4. NOVA (n.d.).
5. Rubin 1994: 3.
6. Rubin 1994: 4.
7. Gajdušek 2004.
8. Lewis and Shimabukuro 2002.
9. Hames 1993: 54.
10. Simonds 1996: 27–8.
11. National Right to Life (n.d.).
12. Lewis and Shimabukuro 2002.
13. National Right to Life (n.d.).
14. Lewis and Shimabukuro 2002.
15. Lewis and Shimabukuro 2002.
16. National Abortion Federation (NAF) (c).
17. Mitchell 2005: 78.
18. Guttmacher Institute 2009.
19. *Schenck v. Pro Choice Network of Western New York* (1997): [***LEdHR2D] [2D] footnote 9.
20. *Erznoznik v. Jacksonville* (1975) as cited in *Hill v. Colorado* (2000): [***LEdHR3A] [3A].

21 *Hill v. Colorado* (2000): II A; *Schenck v. Pro Choice Network of Western New York* (1997): [***LEdHR17] [17] [***LEdHR18A] [18A].
22 *Hill v. Colorado* (2000).
23 Boettcher 1992.
24 National Abortion Federation (NAF) (a).
25 Hern 2000.
26 Soraghan 2000: A-09.
27 Chen 2003: 50.
28 Chen 2003: 50 and see footnote 101.
29 Hern 2000.
30 FindLAw for Legal Professionals (a).
31 *Madsen v. Women's Health Center* (1994): 772–3.
32 The Feminist Majority Foundation and NOW Legal Defense and Education Fund 1996: 5.
33 *Madsen v. Women's Health Center* (1994): 773–5.
34 *Schenck v. Pro Choice Network of Western New York* (1997).
35 *Schenck v. Pro Choice Network of Western New York* (1997).
36 The Feminist Majority Foundation and NOW 1996: 5.
37 Mitchell 2005:78.
38 *Madsen v. Women's Health Center* (1994).
39 United States Department of Justice Civil Rights Division (n.d.).
40 Hern 2000.
41 Choices West 1995.
42 *Schenck v. Pro Choice Network of Western New York* (1997): footnote 9.
43 *Everysaturdaymorning Blog* 2012.
44 Sethna 2011: 90.
45 Tremeear 1908: Part VI, 190. See also CBCnews Canada 2009.
46 Sethna and Hewitt 2009: 464.
47 Sethna 2011: 95.
48 Sethna 2009: 470.
49 Sethna 2011: 101.
50 Sethna 2011: 101.
51 Sethna 2011: 95–6.
52 CBC Digital Archives 1969–1989.
53 CBCnews Canada 2009.
54 Sethna and Doull 2007: 642.

55   CBCnews Canada 2009.
56   CBC Digital Archives: 1969–1989.
57   CBC Digital Archives: 1969–1989.
58   Sánchez-Fuentes et al. 2008: 352.
59   Lamas 1997: 61.
60   Ortiz-Ortega and Barquet 2010: 113, 116.
61   Ortiz-Ortega et al. 1998: 154.
62   Ortiz-Ortega et al. 1998: 154.
63   Ortiz-Ortega and Barquet 2010: 115.
64   Lamas 1997: 58.
65   Casas 2009: 81.
66   Lamas 1997: 60.
67   Casas 2009: 81.
68   Billings et al. 2002: 87–8.
69   Billings et al. 2002: 88.
70   Lamas 1997: 65.
71   Madrazo 2009: 266.
72   Madrazo 2009: 266–7.
73   Madrazo 2009: 267–8.
74   Madrazo 2009: 268.
75   Madrazo 2009: 266–8.
76   Van Dijk et al. 2011: 168.
77   Sánchez-Fuentes et al. 2008: 348.
78   Grossman et al. 2005: 236.
79   Cook 2010.
80   Singer 2010.
81   AbortionInCanada.ca (b) and Kishen and Stedman 2010: 571.
82   Madrazo 2009: 267–68.

# 4

## Case Studies and Spatial Awareness

While doing research for this project, I became aware of many individuals and organizations that actively work or worked to legalize abortion often at great expense to themselves. These people went to extreme measures to create ways to provide reproductive care, challenging spatial and legal constraints. Some included in this chapter provide provocative examples of unusual types and uses of space while many examples demonstrate the ingenuity and extent people have been pushed in order to provide reproductive healthcare and safe housing for survivors of domestic violence. In most cases, this type of thinking takes place before abortion was legal in the United States and where it is still illegal in most parts of Mexico. From domestic spaces, motels, offices, to pharmacies and even bodies of water, geography takes on a different meaning once it is co-opted for women's reproductive healthcare. These case studies offer insights into the politics of space and how challenging the norms around the abortion debate can create progressive and successful alternatives. Examples are activist in nature and collaborate with local communities providing care to a diversity of women that is sometimes out in the open and visible but oftentimes invisible to the public. Similarly the case studies for women's shelters challenge the more common practice centered on secrecy of location and actively seek to engage their local communities as partners in protecting and working towards less violence in the home.

Another component of the case studies is to outright challenge the often naïve and simplistic depictions by the popular media and entertainment industry of abortion and domestic violence. Films like *Juno* and *Knocked Up* as well as MTV's "16 and Pregnant" and "Teen Mom" either glorify the pregnant teenager or young woman by skirting around the complex social, economic and political issues these women encounter. As media critic Jennifer L. Pozner acknowledges, "[f]or two seasons of "16 and Pregnant" and "Teen Mom," we have never seen any pregnant teen seriously consider abortion."[1] Popular cultural rarely includes any realistic depiction of the internal deliberation and struggle weighing a young woman's options and decision she makes. Apparently the industry feels no responsibility to produce critical or thought provoking work on this subject matter as a means to create productive public dialogue. Let's just ignore and pretend abortion is a non-issue. There are a few exceptions worth mentioning. Most recently in US domestic television programming abortion has been addressed front and center in a surprisingly frank discussion by three teenagers about their choices to have an abortion on MTV's "No Easy Decision."[2] The episode begins by shadowing one young teenage mother as she and her boyfriend consider their options regarding an unplanned pregnancy painfully deciding to have an abortion due to their economic situation. Episodes of "Gray's Anatomy" and "Friday Night Lights" also dealt with abortion where after a female surgeon uses several episodes to consider whether to get an abortion or not finally decides that is the right choice for her[3] and after much contemplation a tenth-grade teenager in Texas finally determines to get an abortion.[4] Foreign films such as the British film *Vera Drake* (2004) and the Romanian film *4 months, 3 weeks and 2 days* (2007) focus on an older mother's experience aiding women seeking abortions until the local police find out and in the latter, the agonizing process and experience of a college student going through an illegal abortion with the help of her friend.

## ABORTION

### Army of Three or The Three Crusaders: California

In the 1960s the Army of Three included Patricia Maginnis, a medical technician, Rowena Gurner, a Bay area activist, and Lana Clarke Phelan, a Long Beach, California secretary and housewife, hoped to eliminate abortion laws altogether.[5] They conspired to do this through eventually getting arrested and having the California law against abortion declared unconstitutional. This proved far more difficult than they imagined. Under the San Francisco Municipal Ordinance 188 it was unlawful to distribute leaflets on information about birth control, venereal disease or abortion. Eventually after many attempts, Pat was arrested around 1968 for pamphleting and her case resulted in the local ordinance being declared unconstitutional. Aiming to overturn the state law, this local victory was not enough. Realizing they needed to be arrested for breaking state abortion laws that included aiding others in obtaining abortions or undergoing an abortion, the Army of Three created "classes in abortion" in order to hopefully be arrested again.[6] Successful about a year later, they were arrested in San Mateo County. Although their case was not settled until after *Roe v. Wade* legalized abortion, the Army of Three were successful in having California's state abortion law finally declared unconstitutional.[7]

Divided into four parts, the "abortion class" was comprehensive in scope. Ensuring all who attended would leave with a broad understanding, the class included information from the legislative consequences to the physical realities of self-induced abortion. Part one included a history of abortion legislation for that particular state where classes were taking place and required all in attendance to write letters to their representatives demanding the repeal of that state's abortion law. Part two discussed contraception, the use of certain contraceptive devices and the process of going to Mexico to receive an abortion. Part three presented the sterile technique and part four taught how to self-induce an abortion.[8]

The specific type of space used by the Army of Three was never a priority rather it was the delivery of class content that was the driving motivation. The location was merely a place where the abortion classes could be held. However, it is interesting to note that locations included apartments and houses in cities and towns throughout the United States and even Rowena Gurner's own home in Palo Alto, California.[9] These domestic environments became the backdrop and space for abortion activism. It is not surprising that the realm typically associated with the feminine became the space of illegal activist action, education and empowerment. What has been considered the place of exploitation and confinement became the space of defiance and liberation.[10]

Their activist work transitioned into an underground feminist health agency, Association to Repeal Abortion Laws (ARAL), and maintaining an abortion referral list ("The List") for women seeking access across the border. ARAL's primary role was monitoring and insuring the listed abortion providers were safe for those women seeking their services. ARAL demanded "excellent medical care, humane treatment, low prices, and, when the specialists failed, refunds for incomplete abortions."[11] Sending a list of requirements the potential providers must fulfill prior to be included on The List, ARAL functioned as licensers and regulators on behalf of these women.[12]

**Feminist Women's Health Center: California**

In 1967 an abortion reform bill had been passed in California yet legal abortions were still difficult to procure. If a hospital's Therapeutic Abortion Committee (TAC) could not be convinced to grant permission to a woman seeking an abortion, she would have to find one illegally. The National Organization of Women (NOW) referred women to illegal clinics and had begun to consider the idea of opening their own illegal clinic. Carol Downer, a mother of six, became involved with the local Los Angeles NOW chapter in part due to her own abortion experience. Studying under Lana Clarke Phelan from the Army of Three, Carol became educated about abortion and what was happening in the burgeoning abortion debate.[13]

She had an epiphany of sorts due to witnessing the insertion of an intrauterine device (IUD) at an illegal abortion clinic. Realizing the more a woman knows about her body the more power she has over the control of her body:

> [t]he only way that they can keep abortion illegal is to keep us in total ignorance of our bodies ... once you ... realize that abortion is so simple and so easy to do that any woman who has knitted and sewn and made pottery or done any of the multitude of things that women constantly do-we realized that we could do this.[14]

This led to the organization of a "Self-Help Clinic" located within Everywoman's Bookstore in Venice Beach on April 7, 1971.[15] During that meeting, Carol brought the women into a small office area and after clearing off the desk she proceeded to perform a cervical examination on herself. She also explained how abortions could be performed with the use of suction and a flexible straw-like device called the cannula that she had witnessed at an illegal abortion clinic in Los Angeles.[16]

Teaming up with Lorraine Rothman, a mother of four and a public school teacher who was present that day, Downer and Rothman went on to create the Del-Em, commonly referred to as the "menstrual extraction" device. With help from friends, this allowed a woman to extract the contents of her uterus at the time of her period. The women categorized the procedure as part of other similar "home-maintenance routines" such as self-catheterization and at-home bladder instillations. As described in a 1971 issue of *The Spokeswoman*, "if one can extract one's period when it is on schedule, one can also extract it when it is late. And what policeman or court could ever impinge on such an exercise?"[17]

During the August 1971 NOW national conference, organizers prevented Downer and Rothman from presenting their menstrual extraction technique on the assertion that the idea was "too shocking." So instead, using their hotel room as their classroom, Carol and Lorraine demonstrated to a packed room of women for two days.[18] This then led to a national tour providing information, self-examination and menstrual extraction demonstrations in addition to selling the two-dollar plastic speculums needed for the examinations.

Menstrual extraction and self-help classes were part of a much broader set of concerns around a woman's autonomy and having control over her own body. Not only focused on reproductive control but also the ability to have access to other much needed social services, the women's movement was arguing for the necessity of support such as maternity and childcare. Because abortion was illegal and of immediate concern, abortion provided the mechanism to raise public attention and debate around these topics and garner wider public assistance for the larger demands women were seeking.[19] Not unlike the Army of Three, Downer and Rothman's activism centered upon education as the central mechanism for change. Incremental in scale, these two women were able to greatly impact abortion accessibility through redefining the terms and location of female healthcare. If you can extract your period within the privacy and safety of your own home with a group of other supportive women, you are able to take control over your own reproductive cycle. As a result of more women becoming educated about their own sexuality as well as through these discussions occurring openly and in public, women themselves were redefining women's reproductive healthcare and the space where this healthcare could take place.[20]

### Jane: Chicago

Another important case study was a group in Chicago officially known as The Abortion Counseling Service of Women's Liberation, but more informally referred to as "Jane." Organized in 1969, the group's initial focus was on screening abortionist in an effort to ascertain which providers were knowledgeable and dependable. Abortion was illegal in Illinois in the late 1960s except in order to save a mother's

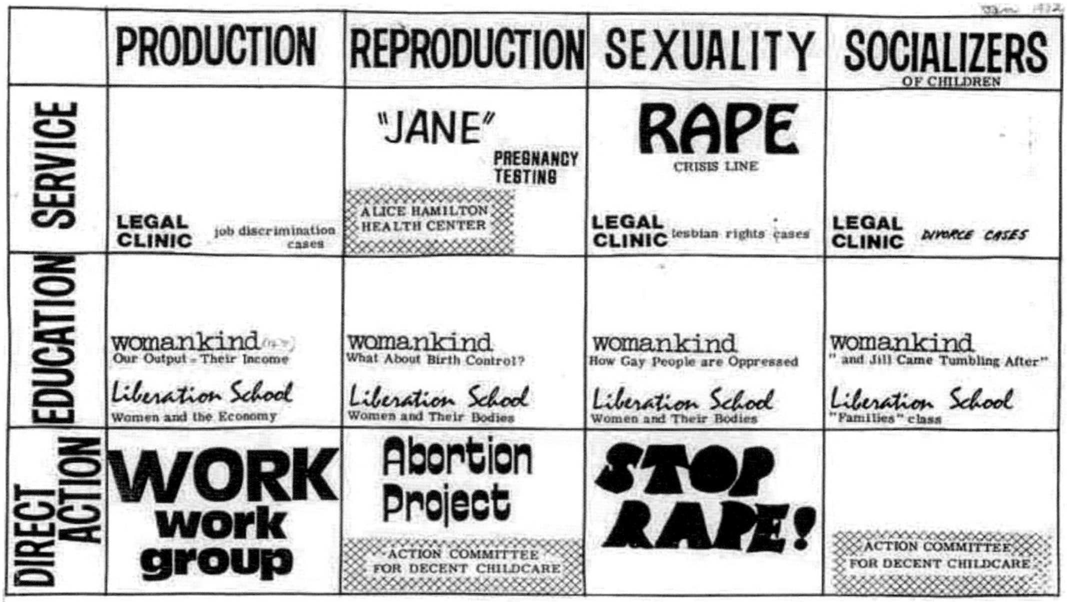

|  | PRODUCTION | REPRODUCTION | SEXUALITY | SOCIALIZERS OF CHILDREN |
|---|---|---|---|---|
| SERVICE | LEGAL CLINIC — job discrimination cases | "JANE" PREGNANCY TESTING — ALICE HAMILTON HEALTH CENTER | RAPE CRISIS LINE — LEGAL CLINIC lesbian rights cases | LEGAL CLINIC DIVORCE CASES |
| EDUCATION | womankind — Our Output – Their Income — Liberation School — Women and the Economy | womankind — What About Birth Control? — Liberation School — Women and Their Bodies | womankind — How Gay People are Oppressed — Liberation School — Women and Their Bodies | womankind — " and Jill Came Tumbling After" — Liberation School — "Families" class |
| DIRECT ACTION | WORK work group | Abortion Project — ACTION COMMITTEE FOR DECENT CHILDCARE | STOP RAPE! | ACTION COMMITTEE FOR DECENT CHILDCARE |

Fig. 4.1 Event Matrix. A chart of most of the activities of the CWLU in 1972 Source/Credit: CWLU Herstory Project

life and the decision to have an abortion, similar to many other states at the time, was in the hands of a hospital board.[21] In their original informational pamphlet they state "Women should have the right to control their own bodies and lives. Only a woman who is pregnant can determine whether she has enough resources—economic, physical and emotional—at a given time to bear and rear a child."[22]

Women often found hospital emergency rooms unsupportive. If abortion was thought to be the reason she was being admitted, hospital staff were known to withhold medical care, even wait to examine a woman in labor until after the police were called. Other staff had been known to refrain from providing medication unless the woman was willing to disclose her personal story, and still others would flatly deny any medical care at all.[23] There were repeated stories that if a woman was either Black, Hispanic or on welfare with a history of previous pregnancies, hospitals would attempt to perform a complete hysterectomy often using the excuse that the procedure was necessary to save her life and solicited the woman's permission while she was heavily in labor.[24] Many abortionists were part of a corrupt system that involved either paying for police protection or paying the Mafia to remain in business.[25]

Jane soon realized that as long as women were dependent upon illegal practitioners, they would remain vulnerable. If these men could provide illegal abortions, some who were not even real doctors, then why could they not do the same? Over the next several years, a few women within the group learned to perform abortions and Jane became a fully self-reliant abortion service. Part of a growing movement of women's liberation, Jane was "committed to the creation of alternative institutions … controlled and designed by women to meet women's needs."[26] The success of their work depended upon their anonymity and because

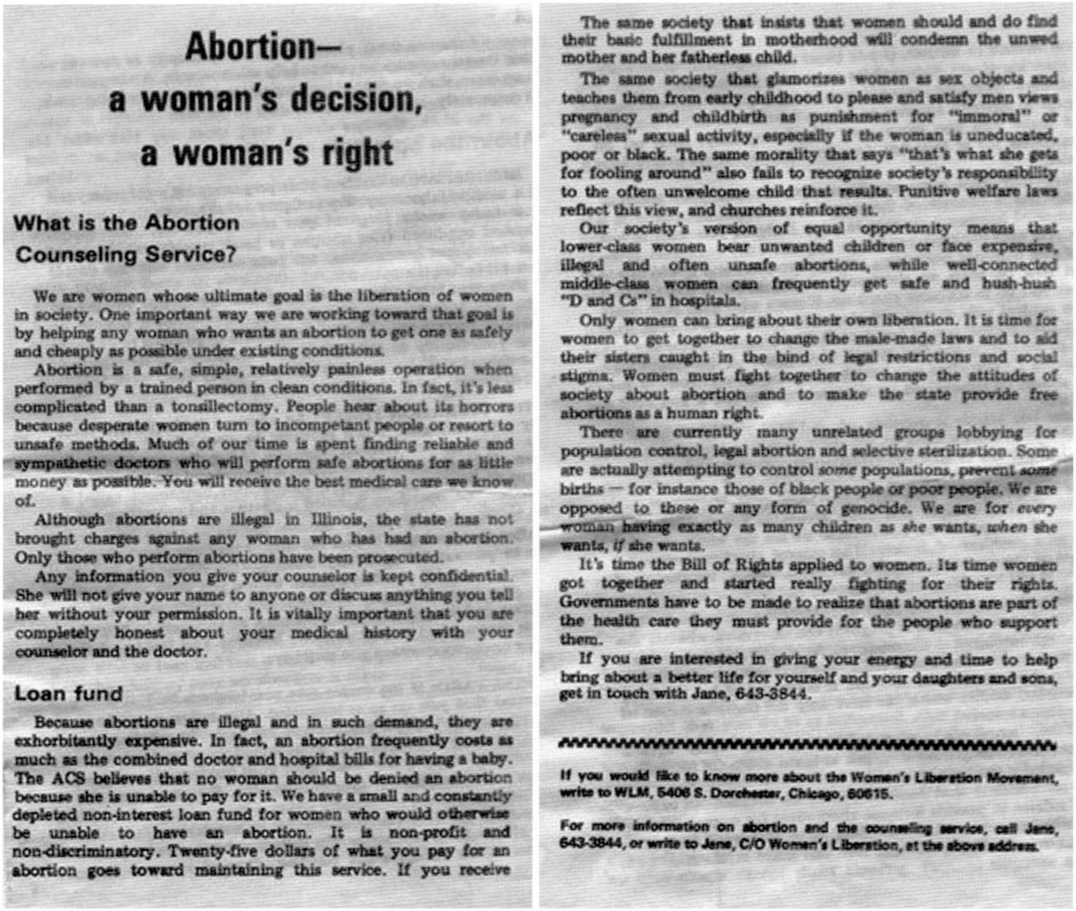

## Abortion—
## a woman's decision,
## a woman's right

### What is the Abortion Counseling Service?

We are women whose ultimate goal is the liberation of women in society. One important way we are working toward that goal is by helping any woman who wants an abortion to get one as safely and cheaply as possible under existing conditions.

Abortion is a safe, simple, relatively painless operation when performed by a trained person in clean conditions. In fact, it's less complicated than a tonsillectomy. People hear about its horrors because desperate women turn to incompetent people or resort to unsafe methods. Much of our time is spent finding reliable and sympathetic doctors who will perform safe abortions for as little money as possible. You will receive the best medical care we know of.

Although abortions are illegal in Illinois, the state has not brought charges against any woman who has had an abortion. Only those who perform abortions have been prosecuted.

Any information you give your counselor is kept confidential. She will not give your name to anyone or discuss anything you tell her without your permission. It is vitally important that you are completely honest about your medical history with your counselor and the doctor.

### Loan fund

Because abortions are illegal and in such demand, they are exhorbitantly expensive. In fact, an abortion frequently costs as much as the combined doctor and hospital bills for having a baby. The ACS believes that no woman should be denied an abortion because she is unable to pay for it. We have a small and constantly depleted non-interest loan fund for women who would otherwise be unable to have an abortion. It is non-profit and non-discriminatory. Twenty-five dollars of what you pay for an abortion goes toward maintaining this service. If you receive

The same society that insists that women should and do find their basic fulfillment in motherhood will condemn the unwed mother and her fatherless child.

The same society that glamorizes women as sex objects and teaches them from early childhood to please and satisfy men views pregnancy and childbirth as punishment for "immoral" or "careless" sexual activity, especially if the woman is uneducated, poor or black. The same morality that says "that's what she gets for fooling around" also fails to recognize society's responsibility to the often unwelcome child that results. Punitive welfare laws reflect this view, and churches reinforce it.

Our society's version of equal opportunity means that lower-class women bear unwanted children or face expensive, illegal and often unsafe abortions, while well-connected middle-class women can frequently get safe and hush-hush "D and Cs" in hospitals.

Only women can bring about their own liberation. It is time for women to get together to change the male-made laws and to aid their sisters caught in the bind of legal restrictions and social stigma. Women must fight together to change the attitudes of society about abortion and to make the state provide free abortions as a human right.

There are currently many unrelated groups lobbying for population control, legal abortion and selective sterilization. Some are actually attempting to control *some* populations, prevent *some* births — for instance those of black people or poor people. We are opposed to these or any form of genocide. We are for *every* woman having exactly as many children as *she* wants, *when* she wants, *if* she wants.

It's time the Bill of Rights applied to women. Its time women got together and started really fighting for their rights. Governments have to be made to realize that abortions are part of the health care they must provide for the people who support them.

If you are interested in giving your energy and time to help bring about a better life for yourself and your daughters and sons, get in touch with Jane, 643-3844.

∿∿∿∿∿∿∿∿∿∿∿∿∿∿∿∿∿∿∿∿∿∿∿∿∿∿∿∿∿∿∿∿

If you would like to know more about the Women's Liberation Movement, write to WLM, 5406 S. Dorchester, Chicago, 60615.

For more information on abortion and the counseling service, call Jane, 643-3844, or write to Jane, C/O Women's Liberation, at the above address.

Fig. 4.2 Jane newspaper publicity Source/Credit: CWLU Herstory Project

abortion was illegal, they worked to keep everything confidential with as little documentation and record keeping as possible.[27] The group's structure aimed toward less hierarchy and more collaboration. In trying to deconstruct perceived differences of status within their organization, members rotated through different volunteer positions helping diffuse perceptions of power. Everyone was exposed to and participated in all levels of involvement with the patients. This strategy also helped protect the volunteers from being labeled as the "abortionist," "the nurse," the "money collector," and so on, and this proved useful once arrested when no one person could ultimately be held accountable.[28] Through these various mechanisms, Jane strove to ensure the safety of all involved: both the women receiving abortions and the members of Jane aiding these women.

The code name Jane was agreed upon because the name was so inconspicuous. No one was named Jane within the group and Jane immediately conjured the anonymous condition of woman in reference to such nicknames as "plain Jane, Jane Doe, or Dick and Jane." Using the name Jane also protected all involved and seemed to be more reassuring if a message from Jane was left for someone seeking an abortion.

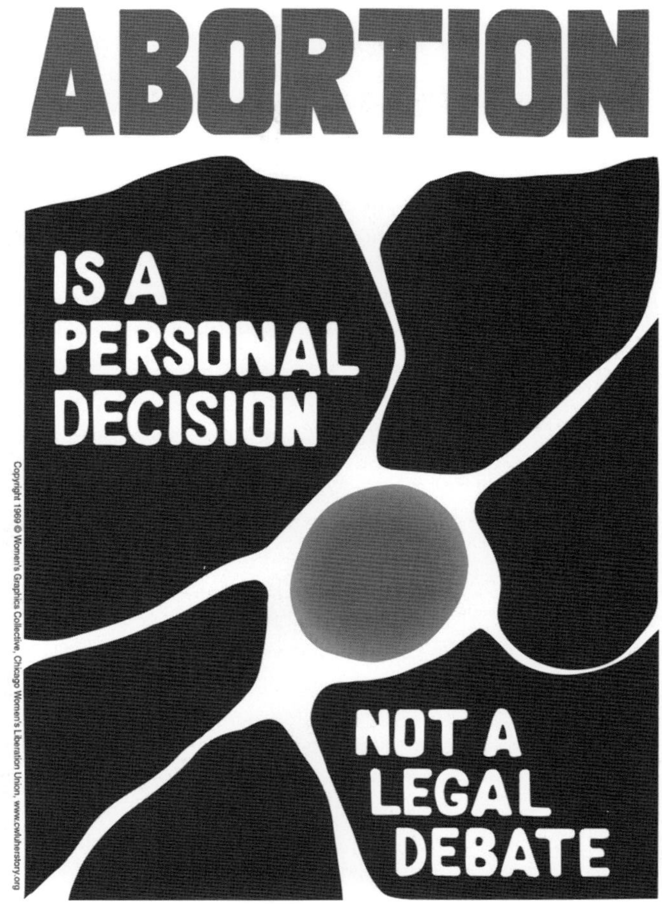

It provided anonymity and no one would know what the message would be in reference to.[29] Listed as "Jane Howe" in the phonebook, women found out about the service through various means: word of mouth, alternative newspapers, referrals from sympathetic doctors, and even from the police.[30]

The process evolved but essentially it worked this way: a woman seeking an abortion would call "Jane" and leave a message. These calls would be returned and each woman seeking an abortion would be assigned a counselor. As a prerequisite to being accepted for the service, counseling must occur prior to the scheduling of her abortion. During the counseling session, a price would be agreed upon. Over the four years Jane existed and once they no longer depended upon a "doctor" for regular appointments but were performing abortions themselves, the price dropped to $100 for an abortion from an average of $300. No woman was ever turned away because she did not have the money as long as she could pay something.[31] Once the counseling session had occurred, the date and time of the abortion was set. The night preceding the abortion, women received telephone calls with the address of what was known as the "Front." The actual abortion occurred at another location known as "the Place." A driver shuttled women back and forth between the two different sites. Both the "Front" and the "Place" were always located in domestic spaces; either generously provided by friends of Jane members or eventually rented by the group. The Front provided protection and a literal spatial division from unexpected visitors and police raids. This scenario was created as a result of near arrests. The group realized if they had one space serving as a buffer to the actual space where abortions were performed, they would provide themselves a little time to help the women leave before the police could arrive.[32]

The service became aware they were constantly under surveillance. From members being watched and followed, harassing of former patients, tapping of phones, to being greeted by name or by "Jane" on the street or in stores by police, there was always looming concern and fear for all involved. Jane realized that at some point they would probably be arrested and eventually during their third year

Fig. 4.3 Abortion is a personal decision
Source/Credit: Chicago Women's Graphics Collective

in operation there was a surprise siege.[33] They were acquitted after abortion was legalized in January 1973.[34]

Jane members estimate that during their four-year history they performed over 11,000 abortions.[35] These women risked their lives in order to provide safe health care to women seeking help. They did so by rethinking how health care could be provided and where this could happen. Space plays a major role in how Jane functioned, from creating varying zones of protection from intruders, to maintaining anonymity of location in order to safeguard the vital work Jane was providing for their Chicago community. Domestic space became the space of choice, liberation, security and safety from the law. By co-opting domesticity as a place of power and subterfuge, Jane used a series of spatial relationships to protect the services they were providing to women of all walks of life.

**Clergy Consultation Service on Abortion: New York**

In the spring of 1967 a group of clergy first met to consider what they could do on a larger scale to help women seeking abortions in New York City. Individually several of the clergy were already referring women for abortions but realized they were ignorant about the procedure itself. The first step required they educate themselves in order to be able to better counsel women seeking help. They brought in doctors to discuss the procedure and what a woman would experience, even using a life-size model to help illustrate. Legal consultation from the New York Civil Liberties Union (NYCLU) described their potential legal risk advising if the clergy functioned somewhat conservatively in regard to the law they may actually be able to do something without being prosecuted. This advice included only referring women to out-of-state licensed gynecologists making it more difficult to prosecute due to multiple jurisdictions, never assume or admit they were breaking the law because as clergy they "were bound to follow a higher moral law" and that all of their activities should be done as publicly and openly as possible.[36]

Howard Moody, an American Baptist minister at Judson Memorial Church,[37] agreed to become the group spokesperson and subsequently many of the activities became housed there. The Clergy Consultation Service (CCS) decided to have as little formal organization as possible with no officers and no bank account linked to the CSS. They did have an answering machine at the Judson Church and ministers and rabbis counseled out of their individually affiliated offices. This decentralization diffused culpability and could be argued as a part of their larger pastoral and rabbinical responsibilities.[38]

The public announcement on May 22, 1967 in the *New York Times* clearly stated their purpose was "not to provide abortions, but to offer compassion and to increase freedom of women with problem pregnancies" listing all participating 21 ministers and rabbis.[39] The CCS's statement of purpose included the recognition that:

> Therefore believing as clergymen that there are higher laws and moral obligations transcending legal codes, we believe that it is our pastoral responsibility and religious duty to give aid and assistance to all women with problem pregnancies. To that end we are establishing a Clergymen's

*Consultation Service on Abortion which will include referral to the best available medical advice and aid to women in need.*[40]

This was quite a radical stance in the late 1960s when even publicly uttering the word "abortion" was considered taboo.[41] They discovered the medical establishment was not interested in this area of health care and in fact was part of the problem by ignoring women in need. Additionally at this time in 1967 it was illegal to aid or abet a woman attaining an abortion and one could be fined $1,000 and up to one year in prison.[42]

A woman would leave a message on the CCS answering machine. Her call would be returned and a counseling session would be scheduled with a clergyman. She was required to bring a doctor's note stating she had received a pelvic exam with the precise length of her pregnancy. This was a prerequisite for a doctor referral and was instituted due to a near-death experience of one young woman who was further along than thought at the time of her abortion. The referred doctors underwent a three-to-four week trial period with thorough follow-up reports by the women who had accessed an abortion from them. Once a doctor received consistently positive reports, he would be officially added to the list.[43]

During the summer of 1968, the New York CCS began to consider the idea of a national CCS. Although not a part of their intention when they began over a year earlier, it was realized there was a clear need to establish a national network to better facilitate the referral systems. Created in November 1968, the National CCS was also housed in Judson Church but still with no real formal structure. Each local entity had autonomy and was self-governing. All CCSs agreed to three requirements: one, no participating clergy would ever charge a counseling or referral fee; two, all clergy must provide person-to-person counseling; and three, there would be no counselors referring to non-approved resources.[44]

After a year in service, the CCS realized they were only serving white middle-class women who could afford the $500–600 abortion fee plus travel expenses. They had helped almost no poor women or women of color. Deciding something must change to better serve a more diverse group of women combined with the New York State legislature's inability to change abortion law, the CCS decided to open an abortion facility that would directly violate the law and "to expose the hypocrisy of a law which allowed "therapeutic" abortions for the rich but denied them to the poor."[45] One consideration eventually not supported was an abortion ship just outside the three-mile limit that would fly under a foreign flag. But in December 1969 a prospectus for a Reproductive Crisis Facility was drafted. It included three key provisions. First, this would be a pilot project for abortion prior to 10 weeks in an ambulatory outpatient office; second, the facility would assist women's problem pregnancies with counseling, medical assistance and contraceptive education, examinations and psychiatric consultation (required by New York state); and third, women would be provided with safe, humane and inexpensive treatment regardless of their ability to pay. The facility would be created as a non-profit.

All felt the location should be near Judson Church since the NY CCS would be operating under its direction yet they were finding it difficult to rent a space for less than one year. In the end, Judson Church agreed to allow the "abortorium" facility to be housed on the second floor of the church owned brownstone located directly behind the church.[46] The following month New York State legislature passed the Cooke/Leichter Abortion Reform bill legalizing abortion up to 24 weeks. Within days an out-of-town doctor approached CCS about the possibility of opening a clinic. They agreed to work with this doctor and therefore the clinic was never housed on church property. NY CCS was directly involved in creating what they hoped would become the model clinic with its low fee structure and referral service.[47]

The CCS provides an interesting example for many reasons. Probably the most obvious is how a religious group worked both illegally yet positively in public for women's reproductive rights. One is hard pressed to find such a diverse group of religious affiliates standing up for a woman's bodily autonomy today. Second, the ability of such a group thinking quite creatively and openly challenging legal structures demonstrates a resolve worth remembering and being inspired by. Third and probably the most significant in terms of the politics of space is the direct engagement of religious space as spaces of subversion and empowerment. Each of the clergy used their own offices for abortion counseling and although the clinic was never housed on the church's building property, it was approved to be located there. Judson Church was committed to social and political engagement to affect structural change using their religious space to do so.

### Overground Railroad

On July 4, 1989 the day after *Webster v. Reproductive Health Services* decision was announced allowing states to pass restrictions on abortion rights,[48] women at the annual Quaker meeting in Pennsylvania were angered into action. Building upon the Quaker's historical work with the Underground Railroad transporting southern slaves to freedom in the north, the Overground Railroad was seen as a way to ensure women access to safe abortions in states where it was legal.[49] Volunteers provide a woman seeking an abortion "information, transportation, housing, an escort to a clinic, or money for transportation and other costs." The all-volunteer group works on a first name basis maintaining confidentiality to protect all involved.[50] Not officially connected to the Religious Society of Friends, the Overground Railroad created a network of volunteers willing and able to escort women across state lines for reproductive healthcare.[51] The volunteers would provide a network of "safe houses" similar to those created during the Underground Railroad used to house fugitive slaves. Women would receive free accommodations as they make their way from a contested state to a different state with more liberal abortion policies.[52]

### Women on Waves: Netherlands

A contemporary case study is Women on Waves, a non-profit organization founded by Dr. Rebecca Gomperts in the Netherlands in 1999. Their website declares:

> Every 8 minutes somewhere in the world a woman dies needless as a result of illegal, unsafe abortion. In response to this violation of women's human rights and medical need, Women on Waves sails to countries where abortion is

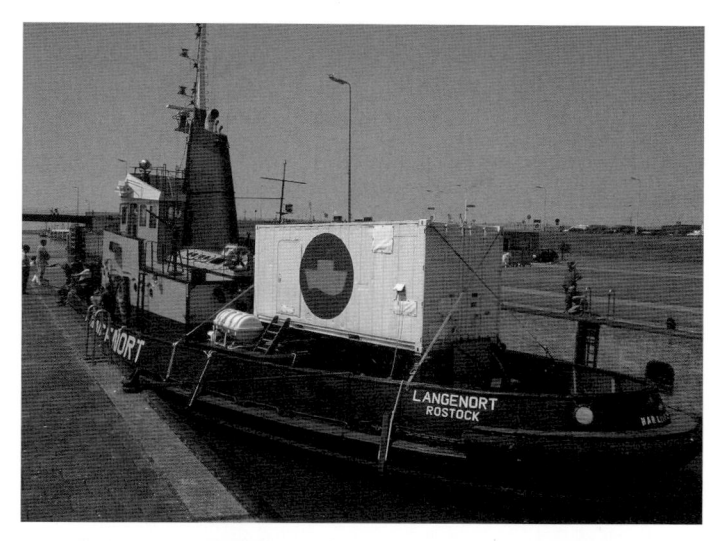

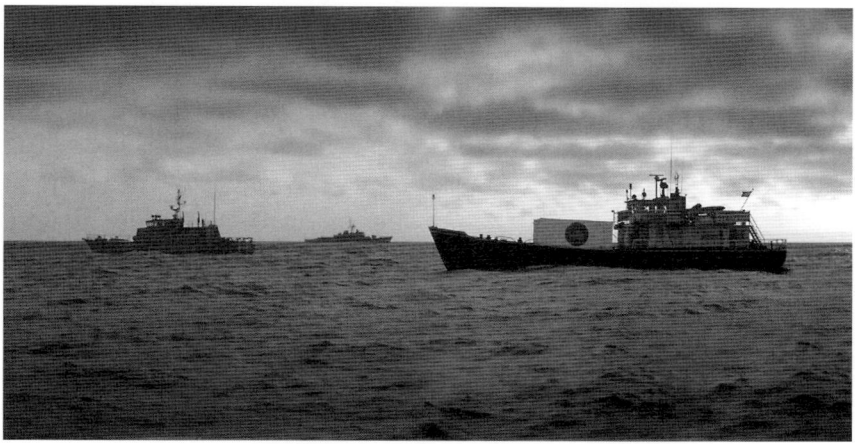

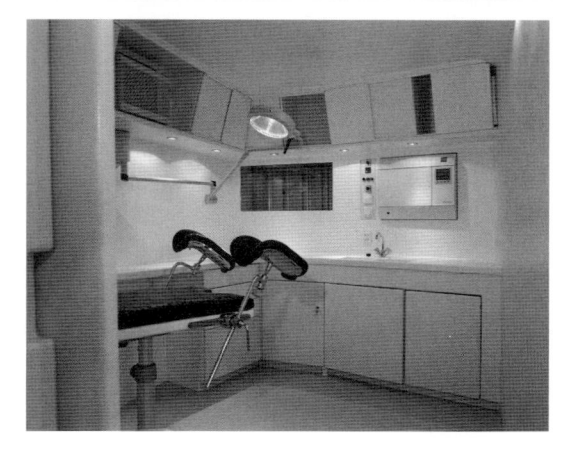

Figs 4.4 and 4.5 and 4.6   Women on Waves. Exterior and interior views of the abortion boat
Sources: Fig. 4.4: Women on Waves; Figs 4.5 and 4.6: Atelier Van Lieshout

*illegal. This is done at the invitation of local women's organizations. With the use of a ship, early medical abortions can be provided safely, professionally and legally. Women on Waves aims to prevent unsafe abortions and empower women to exercise their human rights to physical and mental autonomy, by combining free healthcare services and sexual education with advocacy.*

Operating a mobile reproductive health clinic created from a shipping container that can be secured onto a ship, Women on Waves sails to countries where abortion is illegal.[53] Docked 12 miles out in international waters beyond a nation's legal border, Women on Waves waits while boats are ferried from the visited country out to board their ship. Because Dutch law governs Women on Waves in international waters, reproductive health care and abortion can be provided to women once on board.[54] Women on Waves have traveled to Ireland (2001), Poland (2003), Portugal (2004), Spain (2008) and Morocco (2012), in addition to establishing abortion hotlines in Ecuador (2008), Argentina and Chile (2009), Peru and Pakistan (2010), Venezuela and Indonesia (2011) and Kenya (2012).[55]

As the Women on Waves website states, after becoming an abortion doctor, Gomperts worked with Greenpeace and sailed on the Rainbow Warrior as its doctor. While in South America, she came in contact with many women who lacked access to reproductive healthcare including safe and legal abortions. This experience became a motivating factor for Women on Waves. Additionally another influence on this project can be traced back to her undergraduate education in visual arts. Through this exposure as an art student, Gomperts understands the importance of aesthetics, design and branding as a way to garner public support. All three are integral to the project's success. The abortion boat is designed by Atelier Van Lieshout, a Dutch firm operating within the disciplines of architecture, art and design.[56] Dr. Gomperts has even called the ship "an art work in itself."[57]

On board, a fully functioning medical staff is available for patients. Services such as legal and medical workshops, sex education, contraception, ultrasounds and counseling are provided once no longer docked. The abortion pill can be dispensed once in international waters.[58] As Carrie Lambert-Beatty, a Harvard University Associate Professor and Director of Graduate Studies for Film and Visual Studies, has eloquently written, this project is an innovative and controversial instance of feminist activism. Using the radical idea that the power "of one nation-state over the bodies of its women could be evaded by a short boat trip registered to another " is both "outrageous in its simplicity as well as its implications … using international waters as a refuge for women's rights."[59] Pushing the boundaries of the geopolitical, Women on Waves occupies a legal space where a woman can seek assistance, information and reproductive health care outside her own country where such information is difficult to find and abortion is criminalized. Connected with neoliberal policies, this project exploits the idea of free trade zones and International waters and exists because it plays against hegemony's own system through legal loopholes of globalization. Creating a different interpretation of sovereignty, Women on Waves occupies this newly interpreted space.[60]

Many of these case studies create different approaches toward accessing women's healthcare confronting spatial politics in the process. In particular Jane reclaims the domestic, a privatized realm as a space of empowerment and control over a woman's body. In contrast, Women on Waves create a spectacle on a national and global scale while administering reproductive healthcare to women. These two approaches implicate assumptions about women's physical relationships to private and public space through politicizing the private as an empowered place of access and bringing a most intimate and private decision out into the public realm for media coverage and publicity.

## Dr. George Tiller

Probably the most well-recognized doctor for abortion care in the United States is the late Dr. George Tiller of Wichita, Kansas. He was one of the most outspoken proponents for abortion access and one of the few publicly acknowledged doctors in the country who would perform late-term abortions for women with serious health problems or fetal anomalies. Throughout his time as an abortion doctor, he and his practice had been under siege by anti-abortion protestors. In hopes of closing his practice anti-abortion protestors had bombed and blockaded his clinic an untold number of times. He had previously been shot and had been legally prosecuted numerous times. There was even a website maintained by anti-abortion people providing all the building and site security information. From this website it was clear that the clinic was under heavy surveillance. Killed by Scott Roeder, an anti-abortion zealot,[61] Dr. Tiller was serving as an usher handing out church bulletins in his church foyer on May 31, 2009 when he was fatally shot.[62]

Dr. Tiller was deeply concerned with a woman's abortion experience. So much so that he reconsidered what role space could play in helping to begin the mourning and healing process for those who had to make difficult decisions to end a pregnancy due to major health complications. One of the most moving spaces I have read about in the design and use of abortion clinics is described by Carole Joffe in her book *Dispatches from the Abortion War The Costs of Fanaticism to Doctors, Patients, and the Rest of Us*. She writes about being deeply affected by images of a private space created specifically for parents and their spiritual practices. Often these grieving parents wanted a room where they could seek counseling by a chaplain or a room to use for religious observances or their own spiritual practice. Called the Quiet Room, it provided a space of solace and comfort during this difficult and emotional experience.

Joffe mentions abortion practices that have set aside spaces for meditation and others that include religious materials. She has heard of women who have even brought their own clergy with them to an initial clinic visit.[63] During my time conducting interviews with abortion providers, I often noticed clinics clearly caring about the design of their spaces and how their spaces could create a more positive experience for their patients. One clinic I visited has a space referred to as the Sanctuary Room. Decorated in soothing colors with big soft sofas and ambient light, the space creates a peaceful and soothing environment in addition to the larger semi-public waiting area women occupy prior to their procedures. In the Sanctuary Room, a woman could choose to be quiet, play music softly or read.[64]

The clinic created this space to be one that would support their patients' desire for further privacy and solitude that is separate from the common areas shared by other patients and clinic employees.

**The Abortion Caravan: Canada**

The Vancouver Women's Caucus (VWC) emerged during the turbulent 1960s as part of the larger movement radically rethinking society's power structures that continued to create oppression for women and people of color. Protesting the newly passed 1969 abortion law, the VWC decided to travel from Vancouver to the Canadian capital in Ottawa scheduled to arrive on Mother's Day.[65]

The caravan carried a coat-hanger-filled coffin calling attention to the untold number of women's deaths from illegal abortions. Hoping to have the abortion law repealed, the VWC staged this public event to put pressure on the Canadian Parliament to take further action. Driving 300 miles a day, the caravan would reach out to the public in each stopover with guerilla theater, food and public meetings. Once arriving in Ottawa, the women demanded to meet with Prime Minister Trudeau. Unable to do so, they left the coat-hanger-filled coffin at the main entrance to his residence. Two days later, women's liberation groups joined the caravaners in protesting at the House of Commons. About 25 women peacefully entered the public galleries of the House with forged passes. Once inside, the women locked themselves to their seats with bicycle chains they had smuggled in. At the predetermined time, the women all denounced the new abortion law resulting in the first ever shutting down of the House. Weeks later the VWC members met with Trudeau to discuss the abortion law. He was unsympathetic telling them "Canadian women seeking abortions could always travel to the United States."[66]

**Dr. Henry Morgantaler**

As discussed in Chapter 3, the most well-known abortionist throughout all of Canada is Dr. Henry Morgantaler. He passionately believes that a woman has the right to end her pregnancy without risking her own life. He has been arrested many times, served time in jail[67] and was instrumental in seeing Canada's abortion law overturned on 28 January 1988. In *R. v. Morgantaler* the Supreme Court struck down the abortion law declaring the law did not follow the *Charter of Rights and Freedoms* violating a woman's security of person.[68] Dr. Morgantaler has always believed abortion to be a basic human right and has spent his life fighting for this to happen in Canada. He was awarded the Order of Canada in 2008 for his services to women and leadership in civil liberties.[69]

Although two dramatically different examples, both the VWC and Dr. Morgantaler demonstrate how civic action can significantly influence political will. Both passionately committed to abortion rights, each capitalized upon media attention to gain publicity and support for repealing abortion laws. Morgantaler continues to fight for greater reproductive freedom throughout Canada today.

## Abortion Tourism: US and Mexico

Prior to abortion becoming legal in the United States, there was a constant flow of women crossing the border into Mexico seeking abortions. Although also not legal in Mexico, abortion was much easier to procure there than in the US at that time. This cross border traffic had been occurring since at least the early 1950s. It was so common that at one point during this time period, San Diego police would not allow women less than 18 years of age to cross without parental permission. The image of the female tourist was instrumental in a woman's ability to successfully subvert the law. Women were recommended to carry as little luggage as possible, wear make-up so as to appear conservative and buy a few souvenirs to be able to show the border agents.[70]

Not only did abortionists find this to be a lucrative opportunity, a supporting industry around abortion benefited from this trans-national three-day migration. Airline services, for one, were able to financially gain from the surge in international travel. Elizabeth Canfield, a Planned Parenthood counselor in Albuquerque, New Mexico who worked from 1968 to 1971 with Clergy Counseling Service for Problem Pregnancies in Los Angeles, referred many American women to abortionists in Mexican border cities. She remembers one travel agent "didn't want to know anything about what [women] were doing when we made reservations through her. One day she called me and said, 'You won't believe this, but we received an award for selling the most three-day weekends in Mexico.' Her boss kept asking how it was that so many of her clients wanted to go there. She was mortified!"[71]

Once abortion became legal in the US, the regular traffic of American women seeking abortions across the border into Mexico came to a halt.[72] Now the reverse is taking place for Mexican women who can afford both the time and money to cross into US border towns where they believe they will find safer abortions. American women are also seeking abortion-inducing drugs in Mexico because they are less expensive and can be bought over the counter in a pharmacy or on the black market. So although abortion tourism from the US into Mexico may not be as regular today as before *Roe v. Wade*, there is still much travel by women crossing from Mexico into the US seeking reproductive healthcare either medically or surgically.[73]

## MEXICO

### GIRE, Grupo de Información en Reproducción Elegida (Information Group on Reproductive Choice)

One of the most influential Mexican non-profit non-government organizations formed in 1992 provides and disseminates information on reproductive rights, specifically about abortion. Because information is inherently biased and the public is so misinformed, GIRE seeks to communicate information typically not included in public discourse focusing upon legal, bioethical and social perspectives. GIRE aims to "promote a rational discussion that addresses the issue of abortion without interference from dogma or prejudice."[74] In large part their work focuses on those who are making the decisions and creating and influencing policy: government officials, media outlets and opinion leaders. GIRE works to redirect public associations about abortion through expanding the discussion to include critical issues of public health and social justice. If Mexico is to become a truly democratic country, then women's health and access to health services must become a much greater priority. GIRE is concerned the more normative pro-abortion argument centered upon a woman's ownership of her body is not influential enough as one more directly connected to the broader democratic concerns Mexico continues to face. GIRE's core issue has become "who decides and according to what precepts are decisions made in a diverse society with democratic aspirations?"[75] Among GIRE's many achievements include the instrumental role GIRE played in the decriminalization of abortion in Mexico City in 2007, the creation of the largest single library of reproductive and sexual rights material in Mexico and the continued involvement promoting public debate on abortion and reproductive rights.[76]

### The Case of Paulina del Carmen Ramírez Jacinto

Probably the most referenced abortion case throughout all of Mexico that dramatically shifted the understanding of how abortion restrictions and conscientious objectors create major impediments to abortion access involves the case of Paulina del Carmen Ramirez Jacinto. As Rosario Taracena, communications specialist for GIRE has written, Paulina's case has influenced public opinion towards further supporting a woman's right to decide whether she has an abortion than any other event to date.[77]

In July 1999 13-year old Paulina was raped and stabbed by a thief who had broken into her family's house. Nineteen days later Paulina discovered she was pregnant. She and her mother went through the proper channels and procedures seeking a legally authorized abortion. Another 15 days later she received permission from the State Attorney's Office ordering the abortion to be performed at the Mexicali General Hospital in Baja California. She was not admitted into the hospital for another 41 days, placing her pregnancy much closer to the end of the first trimester. Over the course of a week while in the hospital she encountered various people trying to persuade her to change her mind; from visitors forcing her to watch a pro-life film, to the Attorney General personally taking her and her mother to visit a priest where they were told abortion is a sin and could result in excommunication from the church, to the hospital director misrepresenting the risks of abortion stating she could die or become sterile. In addition, the hospital director stated all the hospital gynecologists refused to perform the abortion due to conscientious objections.[78] After all of these tactics and delays, the abortion was never performed. Influenced and pressured by such faulty information, Paulina's mother signed a document resending their desire for an abortion just 16 days before the three-month limit for her legal abortion.

Due to the extensive and pervasive media attention Paulina's case received, the feminist organizations Alaíde Foppa and Diversa offered to intervene on behalf of her case. They filed a complaint to the Baja California Law Offices for Human Rights and Citizen Protection in late October 1999.[79] Upholding the complaint, the Commission recommended the following: compensation to Paulina and her family, a trust fund to be created for Paulina and her son and penal consequences for the responsible officials who prevented Paulina's abortion. The governor rejected all three and the case was then sent under appeal to the National Human Rights Commission where once again they ruled in Paulina's favor. More than a year later, the governor offered Paulina a vacant piece of land and some money, far less than was originally recommended.[80]

Due to the fact that Paulina's case drew an enormous amount of publicity and placed a face and name with the extreme prejudices women seeking abortion face, this event clearly demonstrated to the public the lack of social justice women could receive when seeking a legal abortion in Mexico. Although Paulina went through every appropriate legal channel available to her, she was still unable to access an abortion. As cultural critic Carlos Monsiváis has stated, "Paulina's case [was] 'the collective discovery of horror.'"[81]

**INTERVIEWS**

**Spatial Awareness—It's All in the Details**

Over the course of interviewing many providers across the US, I became aware of how small details produced dramatically positive effects. I would like to mention just a few. As all women will recognize who have had an annual gynecological exam, as you lie on the table staring up at a ceiling usually consisting of white ceiling tiles, you wonder what else could you be looking at other than a ceiling tile grid and fluorescent lights. This Midwest clinic had the insight that fluorescent lighting can be rather harsh creating a cold and impersonal environment. With a desire to help improve patient care, one of the clinic staff suggested changing the degree of lighting in the exam rooms to improve the environmental quality and possibly make a woman's experience better. The clinic installed fluorescent decorative light panel diffusers with floral imagery in the ceilings of each exam room. The rooms now have a light pinkish, lavender hue completely altering the room's atmosphere. Being slightly abstracted but yet recognizable as flowers, they are nice to look at while lying prostrate on the table.

One of health care's greatest travesties is in how awful their spaces can be. This is exemplified through their poor color choices. Apparently someone has unfortunately determined that health care colors should only be sea green, gray, purple and white. Varying little across types of medical practices, one finds these colors used in offices spaces of general practitioners, dentists, emergency rooms, cardiologists, oncologists, abortion providers, and so on. Color can be a simple yet powerful spatial device. Most clinics are unable to spend much money on interiors so paint color becomes an inexpensive and easy way to dramatically improve their spaces. In one particular clinic in the South, a new owner who had recently bought a practice decided the environment of the clinic must dramatically improve in order to convey how different the practice was going to be under new directorship. This owner completely altered the clinic's image through color. She had the waiting areas and hallways painted with a selection of bright yellows and lavenders. In addition, new oversized comfortable red furniture was placed in the waiting area. When entering this clinic, you would never imagine this was a medical facility much less an abortion clinic by the décor and uplifting energy of the space. Of the clinics I have been to, this one stands out above all others. Because of the place's vitality, I would argue that a patient's experience dramatically improves.

Another interesting use of materials, plants of all shapes and sizes, are located in another clinic's reception and waiting area. Upon entering one is instantly struck by the beautiful greenery just inside the door and the other plants on the receptionist's desk; all of which immediately lightens the room's feeling and one's mood. As you make your way into the waiting room you encounter even more plants in this space too. Such a small token, the plants provide a welcome change to the atmosphere of a medical facility. Invoking a connection to domesticity and gardening, the plants positively alter the spatial dynamic of this abortion clinic.

## WOMEN'S SHELTERS

There are several overlaps in concerns about location and security between abortion clinics and women's shelters. Like abortion clinics, two of the most important concerns surrounding women's shelters are location and security of the shelter. For decades it has been the practice to keep the location of shelters secret. One is never to give the address out to strangers or even family members under the premise that secrecy provides a more secured space and women and their children will be safer from their abusers.

Current debate appears to be shifting regarding issues of secrecy around shelters. Margaret Hobart, with the Washington State Coalition Against Domestic Violence, has noticed a lot has changed pertaining to information in the past 30 years. The idea of secrecy and what is required now to keep something secret is much more difficult if not nearly impossible due to the continuing evolution of technology. For example cell phones have GPS (global positioning systems) and are traceable in real-time. Mapping someone's latitude, longitude and movement with an accuracy of up to 15 meters is now easier than ever.[82] Everything you do with the phone including taking photos becomes traceable and locatable through geo-tagging. Many cars are also equipped with GPS so they can be mapped and traced as well. One program services director I spoke with mentioned that the National Network to End Domestic Violence (NNEDV) has created a tech support division to help shelters better understand and address just such concerns.[83] The NNEDV"s Safety Net Project web page "addresses how technology impacts the safety, privacy, accessibility and civil rights of victims." This includes information on technology safety planning for phone, computer, email, instant messaging, spyware, social networking and other related technologies and privacy related concerns.[84]

There is movement away from the idea that a shelter must remain secretive and instead many organizations now focus on making a shelter safer. For example in Pennsylvania they no longer require shelter locations to remain secretive. Dr. Hobart states that if the idea of making a place secret is exchanged with making it safe, this can result in shelter residents and their children feeling safer and more protected. There is a concern shelter spaces are considered to be more like prisons than housing. She cites a number of different approaches shelters have been able to use to accomplish truly functioning and secure spaces working *for* the residents without over burdening them. For example, security cameras and closed circuit systems located all around shelter buildings are far more ubiquitous these days, as are keyed entry systems with either hotel-like key cards or heat sensors. There can often be perimeter fences around more isolated shelters that remain locked at all times and are only open for the residents by either a security guard or a staff person.

Another way shelters have begun to re-think secrecy and security is through their locations and the way in which their program components are dispersed throughout a location. In some cases shelter programs have reconsidered the 'everything within one building model' scattering shelter apartments throughout a larger apartment complex. Their secrecy is in the idea the shelter does not advertise their location meanwhile the women and their children are not hidden away in some undisclosed building. Their anonymity works because "each resident has the ability to not open their door and use their phone. Same as you or me."[85]

There are several benefits to this spatial configuration. The individual families have far more privacy and space than being housed within one building that requires sharing many amenities like kitchens, dining rooms, play areas and bathrooms. The families are not forced to be a part of other families' moments of conflict and discipline. The families can have friends and other family members over helping maintain contact with their individual support networks. One of the disadvantages to the individually located apartments is the difficulty a woman has making contact with shelter staff as well as other shelter residents. The whole concept of communal space must be reconfigured within the staff office areas. When shelters are located within a larger apartment complex, the communal space's attraction is created through the needs women may have—be those through food, clothes, toys, and so on. The staff creates positive incentives to bring the women to the office and communal areas and this also facilitates promoting more contact among the shelter residents as a result.

Several shelters have an online presence showcasing their new buildings and renovated spaces, even calling for donations for the work they want to do. Although it is common to ask for contributions and donations, a few of these shelters documented the renovation processes and posted images of their recently upgraded and well-designed spaces. Dr. Hobart mentioned an interesting aspect to the programs that no longer proscribe to the secrecy model. The communities these programs are located in all have embraced them. Aware that they live by or near a women's shelter, residents invested in their communities are attentive and supportive of these programs. They look out for them—an informal neighborhood watch—and will call the police when they notice anything different or unusual about cars and people in the area. The shelter residents have noted they feel safer because their newfound community is aware of their presence and they know the shelter is going to be looked after.

Another interesting result of this change is one that demonstrates an ability to move from a conversation around secrecy to one of security. When the security is good, women feel safe. They are more able to embrace their community and begin the process of healing and moving beyond the traumatic events that have required they leave their homes and seek refuge elsewhere. One of the prices of secrecy Dr. Hobart believes is that secrecy keeps resources out and thus keeps the community at a distance. People cannot help if they do not know their neighbors need help. However, one caveat is that the position a program takes is inherently dependent upon the geography of place and the community the shelter serves.[86] Ultimately the shelter must understand these factors and work towards the best ways to accommodate and support the women and children of their communities.

## NOTES

1. Harris 2010.
2. Harris 2010.
3. Piazza 2011.
4. Bellafante 2010.
5. Chalker and Downer 1992: 104.
6. Baehr 1990: 15.
7. Baehr 1990: 17.
8. Baehr 1990: 15–16.
9. Baehr 1990: 15.
10. The Association for the Repeal of Abortion Laws, ARAL, eventually became the National Association for the Repeal of Abortion Laws, NARAL, and is now the National Abortion Rights Action League.
11. Reagan 2003: 354–5.
12. Reagan 2003: 363–4.
13. Baehr 1990: 21.
14. Baehr 1990: 21–2.
15. Chalker and Downer 1992: 114.
16. Baehr 1990: 22.
17. *The Spokeswoman* 1971: 1.
18. Chalker and Downer 1992: 113–18.
19. Baehr 1990: 23–5.

20  The Feminist Women's Health Center is still in operation with several other affiliates across the country. It is the first women's health clinic run by women for women. Please see www.fwhc.org for more information.
21  Kaplan 1995: x, 4.
22  CWLU herstory project (a).
23  CWLU herstory project (e).
24  CWLU herstory project (f).
25  CWLU herstory project (b).
26  Kaplan 1995: 72–3.
27  Kaplan 1995: xviii.
28  CWLU herstory project (d).
29  Kaplan 1995, 27.
30  Ter Hor 1999.
31  Kaplan 1995: 175.
32  Kaplan 1995: 92.
33  CWLU herstory project (g).
34  Chicago Women's Liberation Union (n.d.). this is part of CWLU herstory project so shouldn't it be referenced as the others? CWLU herstory project h?
35  Kaplan 1995: 280.
36  Carmen and Moody 1973: 23–6.
37  Religious Coalition for Reproductive Choice (n.d.).
38  Carmen and Moody 1973: 28–9.
39  Fiske 1967.
40  Carmen and Moody 1973: 31.
41  Carmen and Moody 1973: 27.
42  Carmen and Moody 1973: 36, 40.
43  Carmen and Moody 1973: 43, 49.
44  Carmen and Moody 1973: 51–2.
45  Carmen and Moody 1973: 62, 67.
46  Carmen and Moody 1973: 68–71.
47  Carmen and Moody 1973: 72–4.
48  *The Body Politic* 1993: 13.
49  Chalker and Downer 1992: 50.
50  *The Body Politic* 1993: 13.
51  *Los Angeles Times* 1992.

52  Salter 1992. Also found information about the network and how it would work in New York in Merle Hoffman Papers Box CH2 Duke University Sallie Bingham Center for Women's History and Culture.
53  Women on Waves 2011.
54  Lambert-Beatty 2008: 309–10.
55  Women on Waves 2012.
56  "Atelier Van Lieshout" (n.d.).
57  Verhagen 2001.
58  Lambert-Beatty 2008: 312.
59  Lambert-Beatty 2008: 313.
60  Lambert-Beatty 2008: 324.
61  Joffe 2009: 134.
62  Stumpe and Davey 2009.
63  Joffe 2009: 135.
64  Interview with author, July 2011.
65  Sethna and Hewitt 2009 for more detailed information on the Vancouver Women's Caucus and the Abortion Caravan.
66  Sethna 2011: 100.
67  CBCnews Canada 2008.
68  Sethna and Doull 2009: 163.
69  CBCnews Canada 2008.
70  Nathan 2000: 123.
71  Nathan 2000: 123.
72  Nathan 2000: 123.
73  Please see the following articles for more information on abortion tourism and cross-border medical access: Sethna 2011: 89-108, Monk et al. 2009: 799–806, Hoffman 2005, Tillman 2010, Ball 1967: 293–301, and Ojeda 2006: 53–69.
74  "What is GIRE?" Grupo de Información en Reproducción Elegida 2007.
75  Lamas 1997: 61.
76  "Our Objectives," Grupo de Información en Reproducción Elegida 2007.
77  Taracena 2002: 103.
78  Lamas and Bissell 2000: 12–14.
79  Lamas and Bissell 2000: 13.
80  Taracena 2002: 103–4.
81  Lamas and Bissell 2000: 20.
82  Rose India Technologies Pvt, Ltd 2008.
83  Interview with author December 2011.

84 National Network to End Domestic Violence (n.d.).
85 Hobart 2011.
86 Hobart 2011.

# 5

## Landscapes of Access: United States, Canada and Mexico

This chapter looks more closely at how differences of access are spatialized in the United States, Canada and Mexico. I am interested in understanding and making visual to what effect varying degrees of legislation impact the landscapes of reproductive healthcare access. As well, security has become a critical issue for abortion clinics, women's shelters and hospitals. This chapter will discuss different approaches toward security and how each of the three program types thinks about and employs security technologies.

### UNITED STATES

#### Statistics

Although *Roe v. Wade* (1973) remains legally intact, the states independently control and govern degrees of access. In 2005 87 percent of U.S. counties had no abortion provider, with 97 percent of counties in non-metropolitan areas having no provider.[1] As a result, approximately one in four women who have had an abortion were required to travel 50 or more miles for the procedure.[2] The availability of access is also dependent upon where in the country one lives. Extreme examples are demonstrated by Connecticut and Mississippi where 13 percent of counties in Connecticut and a maximum of 99 percent of counties in Mississippi are without providers.[3] As more restrictive legislation continues to be passed, certain groups find it increasingly difficult to exercise the legal right to abortion, as granted by federal law. Women below the federal poverty level now have over 40 percent of all abortions, with black and Hispanic women constituting the greatest percentage of the women having these abortions.[4]

Clinic violence is probably the single greatest factor for the decline in abortion providers. The National Abortion Federation has tracked clinic violence since 1977. The over 6,000 documented incidents of violence against clinics include

USA County With and Without Providers

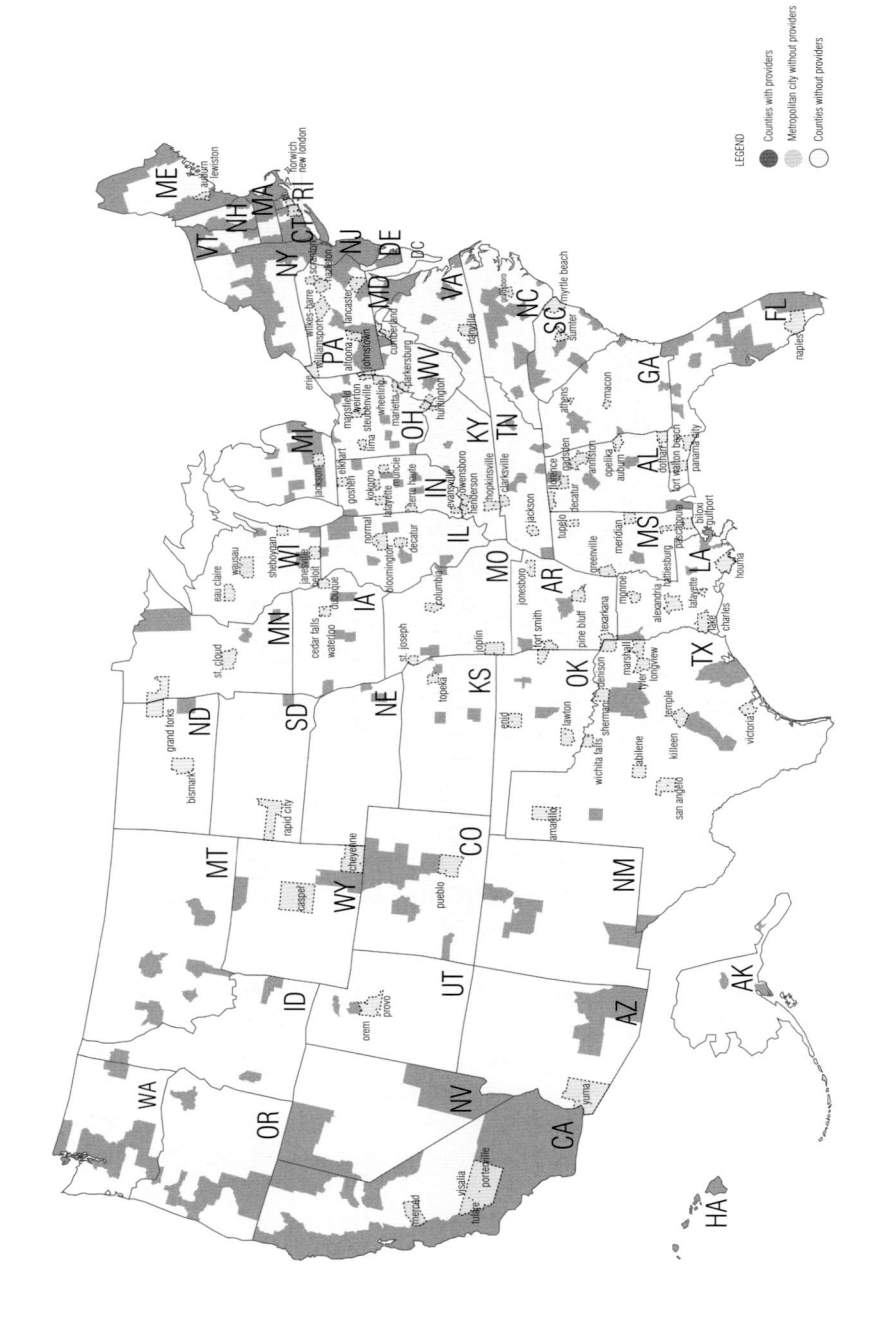

Fig. 5.1 USA county with and without providers

The diagram above illustrates counties with and without providers. The vast white areas of the map are counties with no providers. The light gray areas are metropolitan cities without providers and the darker gray areas are counties with providers. This clearly demonstrates the disparities between counties with providers (typically population densities and urban areas) versus areas of the country where there is a real dearth of providers.

8 murders, 17 attempted murders, 41 bombings, 175 incidents of arson, 170 burglaries and 523 stalkings. In addition there have been over 33,000 arrests for clinic blockages and over 170,000 incidents of clinic disturbances (including hate mail, Internet harassments, hoax devices, harassing calls, bomb threats and picketing.)[5]

The second most important factor in the decline in abortion providers stems from the exclusion of contraception and elective abortion content in preclinical education at medical schools in North America. A recent study found inclusion of such education varied widely by topic and region. Of the respondent schools, 33 percent did not include any discussion of elective abortion procedures. That schools in the South were less likely to address some topics of contraception and elective abortion than schools in other regions suggests how culture influences medical education. Exposure to these topics in preclinical curriculum is greatly lacking; when they *are* covered, more time is allotted to oral contraceptives than to elective abortion procedures. This imbalance yields medical students who are not fully prepared to discuss accurately a complete range of contraceptive options with their patients.[6] A long-time supporter and provider of comprehensive women's reproductive health, Dr. Takey Crist, opined:

> *the medical community—specifically ob/gyns—has allowed the provision of abortion services to become marginalized. If 80 percent of ob/gyns in this country provided abortions as part of their normal practice, physicians such as David Gunn (who was killed outside an abortion clinic) would not have had to travel to five different cities a week to provide services. By eliminating abortion training and making it, at best, elective, and at worst, unavailable, the ob/gyn community devalues the service early in a resident's training. At the very beginning residents are given the message that abortion are less than "normal" or "necessary" surgical procedures.*[7]

In recent correspondence with Medical Students for Choice (MSFC), it was mentioned that there are recommended "women's health competencies" issued by the Association of Professors of Obstetrics and Gynecology (APGO) but as of yet there are no formal detailed "requirements" concentrating on family planning. One issue helping to change curricula includes questions on the "shelf" and USMLE exams necessitating some reproductive healthcare knowledge. I was told this is a big step forward. I also inquired regarding general requirements for medical school education and MSFC responded by saying this is a difficult topic to answer because the range of knowledge considered ideal by many different constituencies is so immense that it could not be covered adequately in four years of education. Consequently, MSFC is fighting that perception every step of the way as they work to have basic family planning and abortion content introduced into required curricula.[8]

USA Providers by State

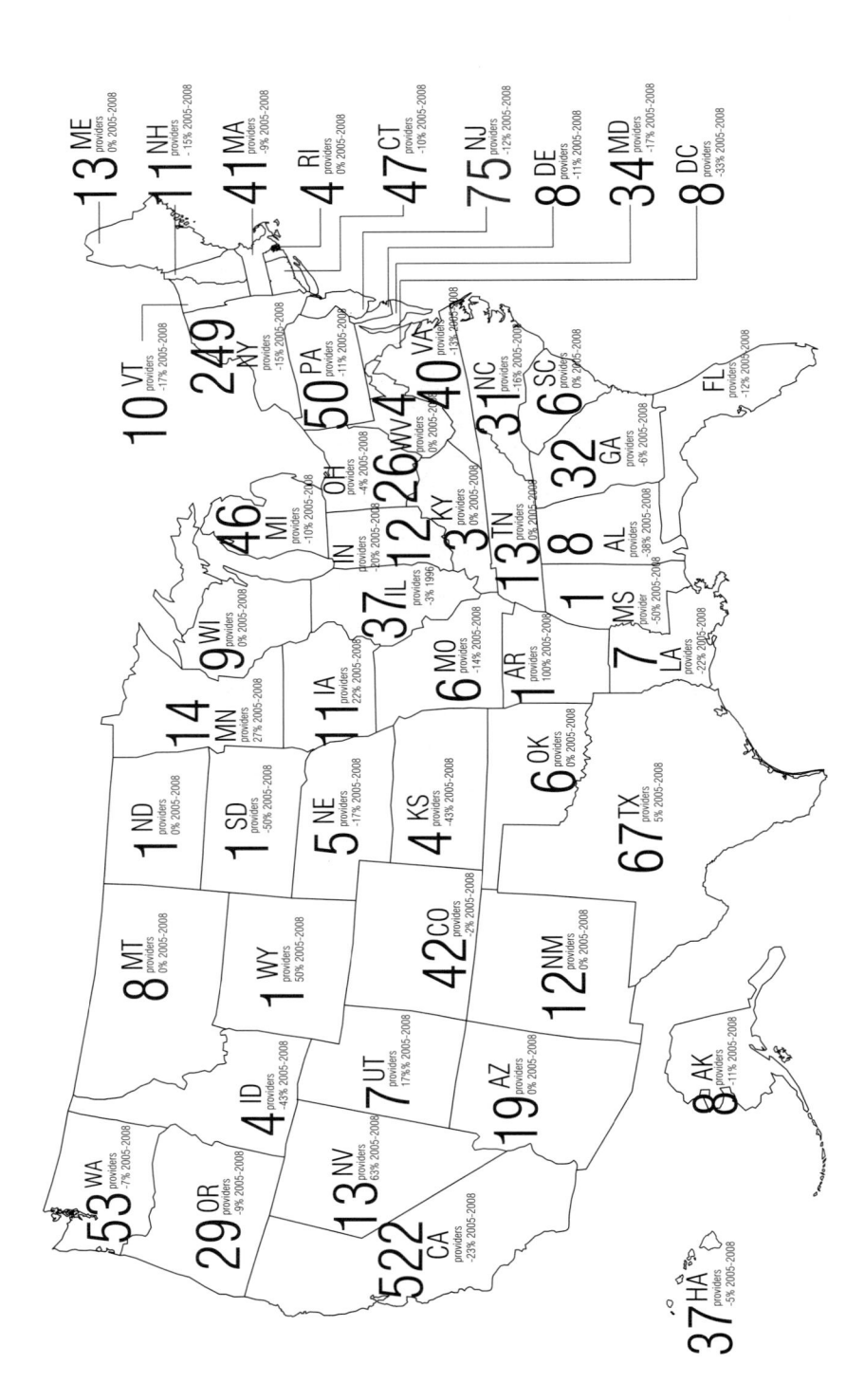

Fig. 5.2a  USA providers per state
This map and the diagram opposite provide the number of providers per state.

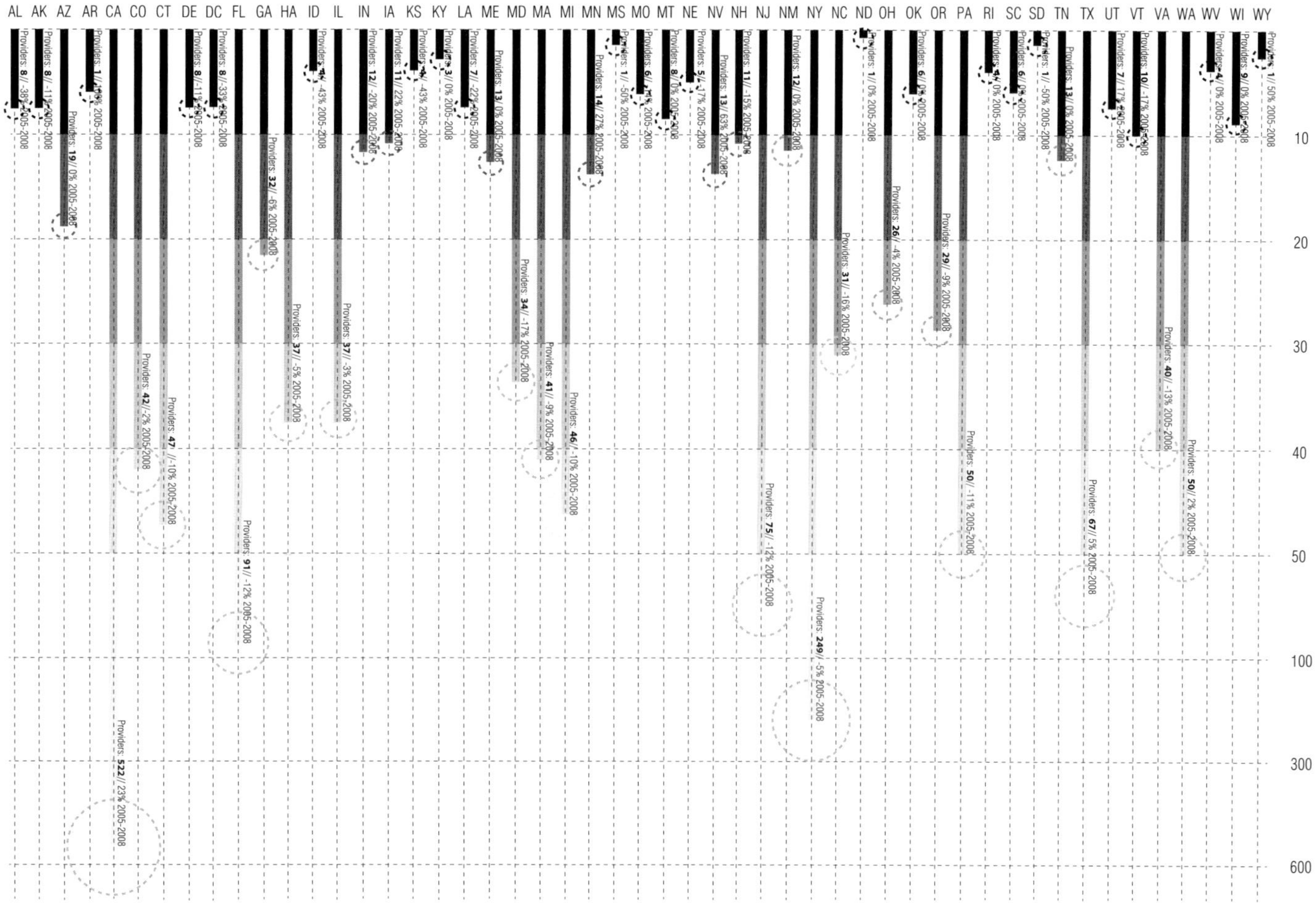

Fig. 5.2 b  USA providers per state

## Methodology

One important aspect of my research and working methodology was through conducting on-the-ground interviews with those who are the most familiar with the ongoing attack against abortion—the individual providers themselves. All of the people interviewed discussed the daily impact protestors have on both the patients who come to them seeking reproductive healthcare and the impact on their own profession and lives. The decision to go and interview people across the country came after several years of attempting to do research with a local Planned Parenthood (PP). Understanding PP's reticent to allow researchers into their facilities and speak with employees and patients, and after finally receiving a no to my research proposal seeking permission to conduct interviews and distribute questionnaires, I was forced to rethink my approach to the project and a way to proceed forward. This actually required me to recalibrate the scale at which this research should be conducted and with whom I should really be speaking. As a result, I first shifted my focus to the national level to better understand how political and governmental actions affect and greatly influence abortion policy. Second, I then examined the most restrictive states through a series of themes. These include poverty levels for single mothers with children under five years of age, the number of restrictions each state has passed, the number and location of abortion clinics, the number and location of hospitals, the number and location of pharmacies and whether they stock and sell the morning-after pill, and then compared this data to other social and cultural forces like the number of religious institutions, Native American reservations and gambling establishments. These cross-comparisons were done to make evident larger social and cultural conditions and how these possibly influence larger political and social forces connected to a particular state or region's identity. I quickly learned that state restrictions well exceeded my expectations, given the fact that antiquated laws still remain on the books. For example, in Colorado, Illinois, Louisiana, Kentucky, North Dakota, Pennsylvania, Rhode Island and South Carolina there is still an unconstitutional law mandating husband notice and/or consent before married women may obtain an abortion. In addition to the antiquated laws, I was surprised to see some of the more moderately restrictive states have some level of family planning and emergency contraception support. Regarding poverty, what I found was not that different from what I expected. Where state poverty levels are highest so are the number of reproductive healthcare restrictions.

The data included provides a way to examine the larger issues around spatial access. These factors impact real space, real buildings and ways people choose to navigate around them. Integral to this research is interpreting how legislation and court rulings affect on-the-ground access and usage of abortion facilities and how thinking through these spatial issues can help to reconfigure and redefine the abortion debate. Space matters. Space is at stake. Control over geography is being legislated by those who want to eliminate a woman's right for reproductive choice. We must reclaim this real space and not allow further violation of these rights to continue.

Over the past several years I have conducted interviews with independent abortion providers and abortion networks around the country in both states that have the most highly restrictive abortion legislation and in those where there is far more accessibility. The actual configuration and layout of the clinics was less the focus but more how clinics circumnavigated the myriad security concerns and legislative restrictions—ways they are creatively maneuvering this shaky terrain. Every interview left me with a mixed set of emotions: a deep sense of awe, respect and inspiration for all of these exceptional and fearless individuals who risk their lives almost daily to continue to provide abortions. In addition I felt their anger, frustration and real concern about the state of abortion in the United States today and although legal, depending on where in the country they are located, it is not always accessible. I believe this research demonstrates further how deeply divided this country is on issues pertaining to basic human rights which women's reproductive healthcare is a part and how inequalities continue to deepen affecting those who have the weakest voice and least representation.

Over the course of interviewing providers, repeated subjects emerged that clinics across the country would often mention. The results of the interviews discussed below will address these broader topics and will then go into more specific detail where alarming differences were brought to my attention. Out of respect to all of the providers who agreed to be interviewed I have not included any names or exact locations and only mention the region where they are located in order to protect both their privacy and safety. The interviews will be discussed by region.

Another important component of my methodology involves the translation of various data into diagrams. These diagrams seek to clearly illustrate what I have found and propose alternatives to change it. The exploratory mappings that have emerged seek to visually represent a wide range of issues around abortion access as well as examining the most highly restrictive states with the fewest number of providers. When researching these particular states, information sought typically included documenting all the current state restrictions, all religious institutions in the state, any cultural landmarks or events that are state-specific, calling every pharmacy in the state to determine whether they stocked and sold the morning-after pill, sometimes called Plan B® or emergency contraception (EC), determining if and where abortion clinics were located, determining how someone without a car could access these places including bus and train fares, distances and fees required to use this type of transportation.

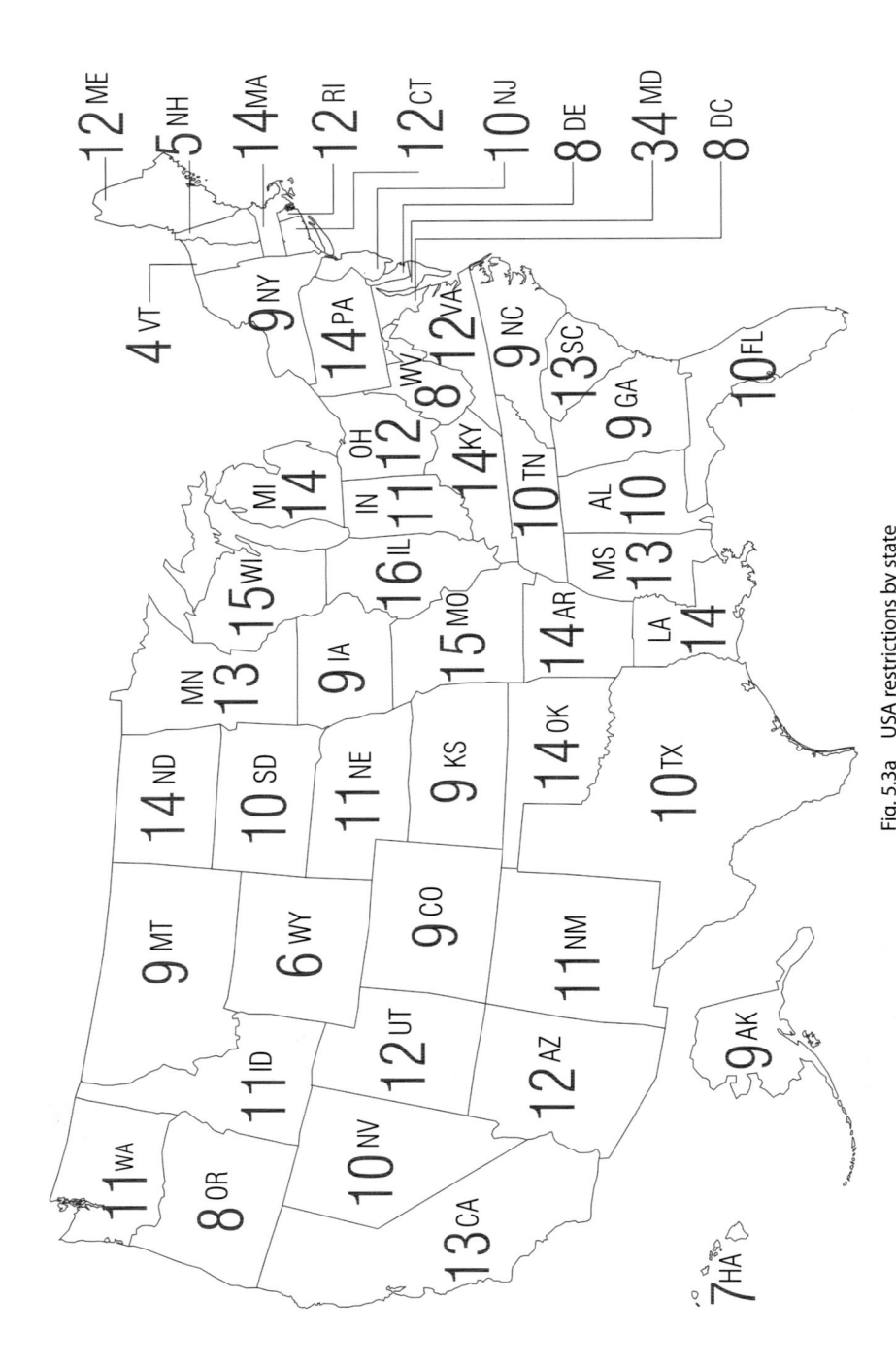

Fig. 5.3a  USA restrictions by state

These two diagrams focus on the number of restrictions by state. The diagram above provides the total number of restrictions in each state and the diagram opposite, through the use of icons, individually lists each restriction with an index further explaining each icon. The graphic icons were created to make more legible the restrictions of each state.

USA — Number of Restrictions

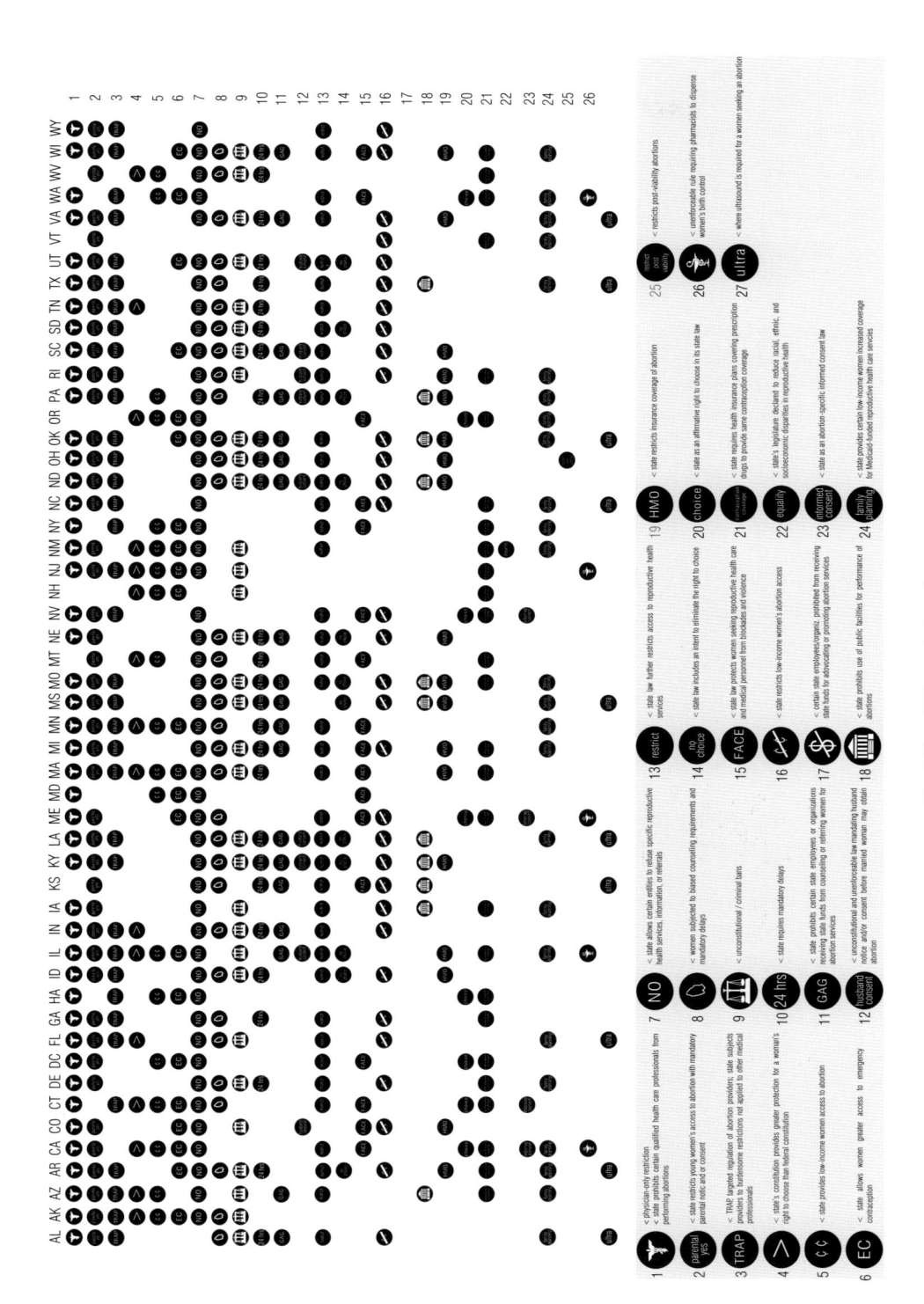

Fig. 5.3b  USA restrictions by state

## Interviews

How did they get here? What brought these individuals to provide reproductive healthcare? Several directors mentioned their own personal abortion experience influencing their career choice to ensure others did not suffer as a result of having an abortion, while some doctors felt there needed to be more female abortion doctors practicing and decided early on while in medical school and still others came into the profession as part time work eventually working their way up into directing and owning their own clinic. One director said that she made the decision a long time ago "[t]hat this is a cause worth dying for … [I'll] fight to the very end, to the very end." "If women can't make this decision, we can't make any decisions."[9] Another provider mentioned that she knows she is helping others through a crisis situation, "I am respecting other people's choices."[10] Another provider has witnessed how women have come to expect difficulties in receiving reproductive healthcare. In one particular southern clinic if women were really over weight, one doctor would refuse to perform their abortions. The women's feelings were not hurt; they expected to be treated like this. "It tells you about health care there." This clinic owner is invested in making the experience the most positive one possible. "As a woman, that is how I feel. I have been there. It was not positive. And that is what this is all about."

## US REGIONS

### South

As a region, the south is the most restrictive area of the United States when it comes to abortion access. The providers I interviewed here have all experienced inordinate degrees of harassment, protesting and the continued passing of more restrictive state abortion legislation. Some have received bomb threats while several clinics have been bombed. Every provider I interviewed in the south is the target of regular protests and most experience this almost daily. All commented that clinic procedure days are the most intense and highly attended days of protest, especially Saturdays when there are greater numbers of protestors present. The clinics have grown to expect this and have developed various mechanisms to try and handle the onslaught of more people outside their clinic, the increased noise levels and the unreliable monitoring by police. Patients are always informed of these high-protest traffic days and often if possible decide to schedule their abortion on a different day.

Clearly each clinic is legally required to adhere to state codes for abortion clinics and spatial flow must enable a smoothly operating clinic, even more important during higher patient volume days. Certain states have far stricter code requirements than others. These requirements are enforced through regular clinic inspections by the Health Department. Clinics can be warned, fined or even temporarily closed and put on probation depending upon the degree of violation found. One clinic owner in the south told me about two occurrences that reflect a cavalier and often times seemingly unlawful attitude by local authorities. The first was a recent issue with the state health department. Showing up almost weekly to

CASE STUDIES AND SPATIAL AWARENESS 105

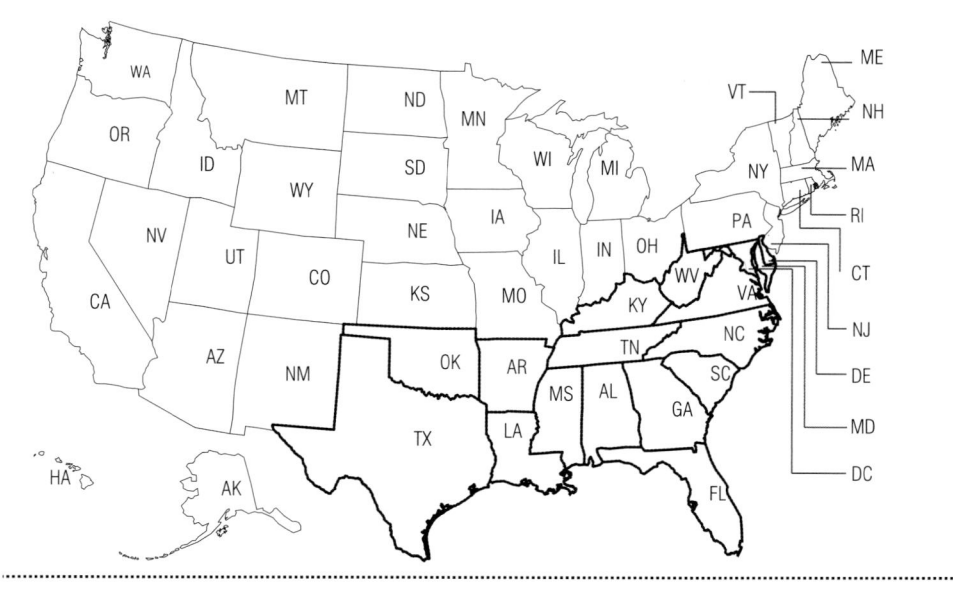

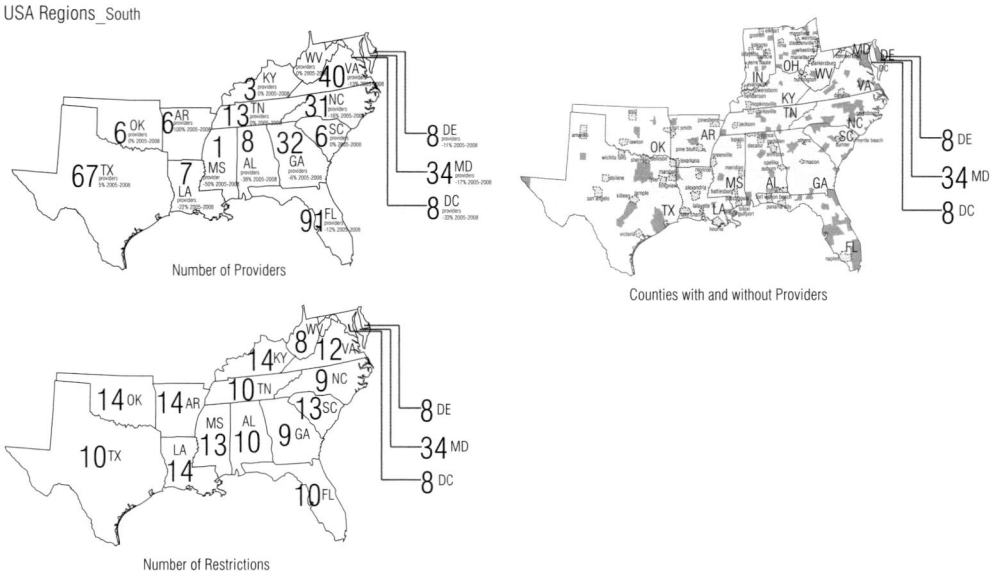

**Fig. 5.4 Southern region synopsis**
This map excerpt provides an overview of the states officially included as part of the south defined by the US Census Bureau. Included are the number of abortion providers and number of state restrictions.

inspect her clinic, they began to ask for the doctors' schedules. Her response was "[t]here's nothing in the rules that say you need a schedule … [I'm] not going to do it … You're putting my doctors at risk."[11] This has yet to be resolved. The second involved the health department copying clinic information without redacting during their inspections. The clinic owner observed that the health department would come and copy whatever they wanted and take it out of the clinic with patient names still legible. She lets them do this now because of two experiences several years ago. The experience of one of her colleagues who owns and runs a clinic in a neighboring city requested a hearing rather than being placed on probation. The clinic was closed for a month because "it took this long for a hearing to be scheduled." When it was time for the owner's hearing, she was informed that she could not bring her attorney or have any legal representation.

Her own experience was similar. She had the option of either being placed on probation or requesting a hearing. She wanted a hearing, however the state attorney said he "would be happy to give [her] a hearing but I don't know how long it will take." He asked her how long could she afford to be closed waiting for her hearing? Both clinic owners knew what the state was doing was illegal, but it was done. The message was loud and clear. Either you play by this state's rules or the state will make it that much more difficult to operate your clinic and you will be closed while you fight your case.[12]

Another significant logistical concern described to me focused on the lack of parking near one of the clinics I visited. Prior to arriving the owner informed me to not park along the residential street adjacent to this clinic because I could be ticketed or even towed. Although parking is allowed along all the other side streets in this neighborhood of this southern city, it is not allowed along the clinic's street. One of the neighbors, president of a local community organization, bought every house on the clinic block and was able to eliminate all on street parking along the entire street. The clinic owner has tried to rent parking spaces from nearby businesses but none will agree because they are fearful of retaliation against their own customers by the anti-abortion protestors. Although the clinic has its own lot adjacent to the building, the need for overflow parking does occur and the lack of street parking has made it much more difficult for clinic patients to find parking nearby.

From these descriptions in the southern states I visited, it is clear abortion clinics are being discriminated against by state governments, local business owners and community partners. One clinic owner said you know, "it is ok to discriminate against abortionists"[13] and another mentioned in a follow up email after the interview that "[t]he injustice is very difficult to sit with. We have taken legal actions that haven't helped and have been exhausting and disheartening."[14] Another owner also stated "I would hate to say we have an adversarial relationship with the state but because the state is politically driven, there is the hint of an adversarial relationship here … [The city] just did away with the parade law. We don't have any ordinance that says [the protestors] can't picket in great numbers out front … [We] are responsible for catching them, documenting it and then calling the police out." She ventured that if protestors where behaving this way outside a local hospital, the police would quickly have them move to the opposite side of the street "in a minute."[15]

## Spatial Experiences

Speaking with Charlotte Taft, director of the Abortion Care Network, she posed the question "how do buildings function culturally?" In other words, what role can buildings contribute to the abortion experience? Her question struck a nerve and was one of the original motivating factors as to why I decided to begin this research years ago. You do not find many architects designing abortion clinics and in fact, many clinics can't even afford to consult an architect because of the extremely tight budgets most operate within. Although this research does not pursue this question directly, I found that each clinic I visited has had to negotiate their specific cultural terrain and the influences this has had on the literal site and space of the clinic is apparent in small and thoughtful ways. Although this project's primary focus is not about medical building typologies, healthcare aesthetics or how clinics spatially work, I have found these concerns are important in understanding the larger issues around reproductive healthcare access. In fact it is at this scale that I have found clinics operating in thoughtful ways. As an architect I am continually aware of design's impact on spatial relationships and the user's experience and how this reflects the larger questions I am interested in pursuing.

All of the clinics visited in the south are located in free-standing buildings not initially designed to be an abortion clinic. Some are located in vibrant areas of cities in mixed-use neighborhoods; others are located adjacent to residential communities near interstate access, while others are located in industrial parks. Often when trying to find the clinics, I mistakenly passed them as I was driving by. As buildings, none of the clinics aggressively pronounce what they do and blend in well with their surrounding contexts. When asked about how the clinic found their particular building location, one clinic owner mentioned that she thinks most abortion providers end up where they are due to either political reasons or other constraints.[16] Often people would not rent or sell to an abortion provider. So once providers find a location that can be made to work and is as accessibly located as possible, they typically jump at the property.

I found many attributes distinguishing these clinics from one another and all are invested beyond mandatory state requirements. The additional investments greatly contribute to the overall experience each clinic creates for their patients. Several included quiet or sanctuary rooms for those patients wanting a space for reflection or prayer. Several used color and plants to help create more vibrant spaces one would not typically associate with a medical facility. Only one of the clinics visited seemed to have little concern for spatial aesthetic quality and the clinic's overall environment.

One clinic particularly stands out. Having recently acquired the practice in the past year, the owner felt that in addition to the much needed roof repairs, the interior desperately needed a major improvement. Prior to the renovations, the interior was painted what the owner referred to like a "nasty hospital." This clinic has the best interiors of any I have seen. Immediately upon entering the clinic, you feel that you are in some other world. There are red leather-like chairs and sofas in the waiting room, lavender-purple countertops at the reception area and as one moves farther back into the private realm of the clinic, the walls vary between a soft yellow to a lavender-purple. The exam and procedure rooms have red vinyl floor tiles. The feeling is contrary to any medical facility or hospital I have ever visited and it works because you do not feel like you have entered into a healthcare space. Through the most minimal of efforts of colors and material finishes, the clinic was dramatically transformed and improved.

### Technology

The advent of telemedicine where doctors are not physically present but in the room via teleconference has opened up a new way to practice medicine and deliver healthcare. In areas of the country with few healthcare providers, telemedicine is proving an effective way to bring care to more people. Medical fields such as cardiology, psychiatry, emergency medicine and adult and neonatal intensive care have all benefited from this technology. Recently abortion has also begun to use this technology.[17]

In a recent study published in *Obstetrics and Gynecology* August 2011, researchers at a Planned Parenthood affiliate in Iowa found that medical abortion administered telemedically is both effective and acceptable among those who selected to use this method.[18] Once the woman has had an ultrasound by a technician and proceeded through the various requirements before being seen by the doctor, she then has her consultation with the doctor via video teleconference on a secured connection. Although not physically in the room, the consultation proceeds normally. Once it is time for the doctor to provide the abortion medication, the doctor remotely enters a password to dispense the medication. Offering a much more convenient way for women to access abortion services, telemedicine greatly reduces both time and distance a woman must travel to seek reproductive healthcare.[19]

Telemedicine offers a way to challenge the restrictive legislative systems in place across specific regions of the country. Providing a way for a safe medically induced abortion is an alternative to the common surgical procedure often used in the United States. One of the southern clinic owners mentioned her reticence in telemedicine and why her clinic does not use it. Unlike in Iowa where medical abortions can be given without a doctor physically present, many of the highly restrictive southern states do not allow telemedicine because the doctor is required to be physically present for both the consultation and surgical procedure. Her larger concern, however is with liability and due diligence. People are only human and mistakes can be made. She is quite concerned about whether a doctor is able to see the ultrasound and double-check the technician's ultrasound results. Sometimes a pelvic examination would also need to be done in order to double-check what the ultrasound is showing. When extremely obese women are pregnant, it requires a more experienced doctor and medical staff to read these results, and grave mistakes have been made. Ultimately the patient must be protected and for her, the concern about the possible mistakes that could be made through the use of telemedicine overrides her desire to use the technology. She supports it in theory but not yet in practice.[20]

### Protestors, Demonstrations and the Police

Due to the sheer volume and tenacity of protests in the south that some of the clinic providers I interviewed receive, countless experiences were described to me that seem unbelievable and outright incredible the extremes some of these protestors would go to trying to prevent women from entering abortion clinics. In two particularly highly protested clinics, providers mentioned the vitriolic language, name calling, screaming, use of megaphones and speakers all directed toward the patients. In addition protestors have been known to use hover-arounds, the motorized scooters that enable them to move more quickly around clinic sidewalks and driveways, use ladders to perch above clinic fences in order for noise to carry farther back into the clinic spaces, position fake clinic escorts and nurses out in front to reroute incoming patients, and bombard cars approaching entrances in hopes of preventing the cars from continuing onto the clinic property. One clinic manager mentioned she had "no problem with them protesting but what they are doing is crazy ... even when we prepare the patients, we let them know what is going on, until you see it, until you're in it, you can't understand it." Even representatives from the Feminist Majority could not believe the police allowed this type of protesting to happen.

One heart-wrenching example described by another clinic owner involved an older African American couple that brought in their daughter who was probably 16 or 17 years old. The protestors had really started barraging them with comments on their way into the clinic and by the time they entered the daughter was just sobbing. But when she left it became even worse with protestors yelling things such as "you killed your baby," "you're leaving without your baby," "you left your baby there!" The daughter broke down again and the protestors took her picture placing it on a wanted poster with a caption to the effect of what kind of father allows his child ... This poster was later found online. Remembering the event, the clinic owner said: "It brings tears to your eyes to watch what they do to a human being ... I want to cry when I see what they do to people. It's horrible ... there's nothing Christian about it."[21]

Clinic owners have responded in a variety of ways, many of which are quite creative and with a sense of humor. Probably the most inventive was turning the negative television coverage of protests outside a clinic into a clinic's advertising advantage by hanging a large "1–800 for an abortion" sign out in front so that every time the news was reporting out in front of the clinic building, the sign was in full view. Other tactics mentioned include the installation of remote activated sprinkler systems conveniently located near areas where protestors stand, doing landscape work such as weed eating during the middle of protests requiring protestors to move or get sprayed with grass, playing music with speakers aimed out toward the street during protests drowning out the protestors' noise, the use of car alarms to help overpower protestors' voices and the more typical responses include the use of noise meters measuring protest noise levels and surveillance video of clinic property.

Repeatedly providers told me that they could not rely on the police for protection from protestors. Although police would be present during their most tumultuous and heaviest protest days, the police were not doing their job of upholding the laws protecting abortion patients and providers. One clinic manager was adamant that they only want the police to "not take sides [but] just do their job." Another provider stated "[w]e know the police aren't there." One particular example clearly demonstrates how difficult it is for providers to receive the police protection they desperately need. In a recent incident last year, protestors were standing closer to the clinic than the injunction allowed therefore breaking the injunction. The clinic owner was informed the day before that the police would be there allowing the protestors to "do whatever they want to do" but will write warrants when the protestors break the law. However, during this day of protesting the protestors would not provide their names and therefore the police were unable to do anything. During this particular event, the provider also called the law department in hopes of getting a warrant. But because there were no names and no real identities, no warrant could be issued. Police were present across the street video-taping the entire ordeal but taking no action whatsoever to protect the patients and employees coming in and out of the clinic. The provider said "[y]ou finally reach a point where you know there is nobody here but you." "When you watch one hundred people standing outside breaking the law and the cops are over there, the chief of police was there. I went over there and said chief, please, you've got to help me. I was crying and said you have to help me. We're doing everything we can mama, we're doing everything we can." Pausing, the provider then said "there is nothing else you can do. They've made it clear. It's mind blowing. No one would believe it if you didn't see it."[22]

When discussing their relationship to the local law enforcement, another clinic owner point blankly stated that the noise ordinance is not being enforced in her city. Police will show up when noise levels increase, even be accosted by protestors blowing horns right into their faces but do not issue any tickets in response. Because it is deemed free speech, it appears that noise levels are not enforceable in this southern city.[23] Another clinic described their weekly application process for the noise permit that they compete for with the protestors. The request must be emailed by midnight Friday for the next week's permit. Whoever's email arrives first is granted the permit. If the protestors receive the permit, they can use the microphone and if the clinic receives it, they do not do anything. In other words, they want the permit so the protestors can't have it.

**Reactions**

All of the people I interviewed stated they believe what they are doing is right and are helping to make women's lives better. One clinic manager emphasized, "we believe in what we do. We really do help women. [Patients] have this whole other idea of what is going to happen and they are just shocked how good they feel, how we help them feel good about themselves. It is a good feeling. They are expected to be treated badly. It's so sad." Another employee said "I feel good knowing that I helped somebody, a teenager that is in school, that knows right now that [she] can't do it right now. I am trying to get better in my life so that I can do it in the future." Or in another case, "[a] young girl that hasn't had the chance to be a young child yet and here you are pregnant and getting ready to be a mom if you don't have this procedure. It just does something to your heart to know that you are helping them."

**Mississippi**

Mississippi is one of the most difficult states for women to practice their legal right to abortion with 99 percent of counties without a provider and 91 percent of women living in these counties according to the Guttmacher Institute. With only one provider in the state, some women must travel great distances to receive reproductive healthcare. As I am finishing this book, there is current concern that Mississippi's republican governor Phil Bryant will sign the most recent restriction requiring any doctor performing abortions to have hospital admitting privileges at a local hospital resulting in the closing of the ONLY clinic remaining in the state. Similar to other states, many of their doctors are flown in from out of state to provide care and admitting privileges are only given to local physicians.[24] With so few providers, women must travel greater distances to a clinic. Because there is a mandatory 24-hour delay law, a woman will need to either return the next day or spend the night, either way increasing the cost of the procedure. If someone does not own a car, then how are clinics accessed? In many of the smaller towns, there are no bus or train services available requiring her to seek alternative modes of transportation.

**Distances to/from Several Cities in Mississippi**

    Clarkson—Jackson 154 miles bus: 6 hr 45min $39 RT
    Hattiesburg—Jackson 88 miles bus: 1 hr 40min $48RT
    Tupelo—Memphis 105 miles bus: 2 hr 15min $62RT
    Biloxi—New Orleans 87 miles bus: 2 hr 35min $48RT

As has been noted by the Guttmacher Institute, the abortion rate in the United States can be directly connected to levels of poverty. According to Census data 13 percent of individuals live below the line of poverty nationally. In Mississippi, the average is 9.8 percent. Where statistics reveal greater disparity is in the percentage of female head-of-households with children under 5 years of age (FhdH c<5) living below the line of poverty. For example in Clarksdale where 36.20 percent of the population lives below poverty, 63.5 percent of FhdH c<5 live below poverty; in the state capital of Jackson 23.5 percent of people live below poverty with 53.5 percent of FhdH c<5 live below poverty; in Biloxi 14.6 percent of people live below poverty and 50.7 percent of FhdH c<5 live below poverty; in Pascagoula 20.7 percent of people live below poverty with 77.8 percent of FhdH c<5 live below poverty and in a less populous city of Brookhaven where 26.9 percent of people live below poverty 77.4 percent of FhdH c<5 live below the line of poverty.[25]

Not only are these statistics extremely high but the state of Mississippi also stipulates that no public funding can be used to provide facilities for abortion unless it is necessary to preserve the woman's life, the pregnancy is the result of rape or incest, or there is a fetal anomaly incompatible with live birth.[26] The result of this legislation makes access almost impossible for women of lower economic means. Connecting this data, the direct correlation between poverty, state restrictions and spatial access becomes apparent.

**List of Mississippi State Restrictions**

- Unconstitutional and criminal abortion bans.
- State prohibits certain state employees or organization from receiving state funds from counseling or referring women for abortion services.

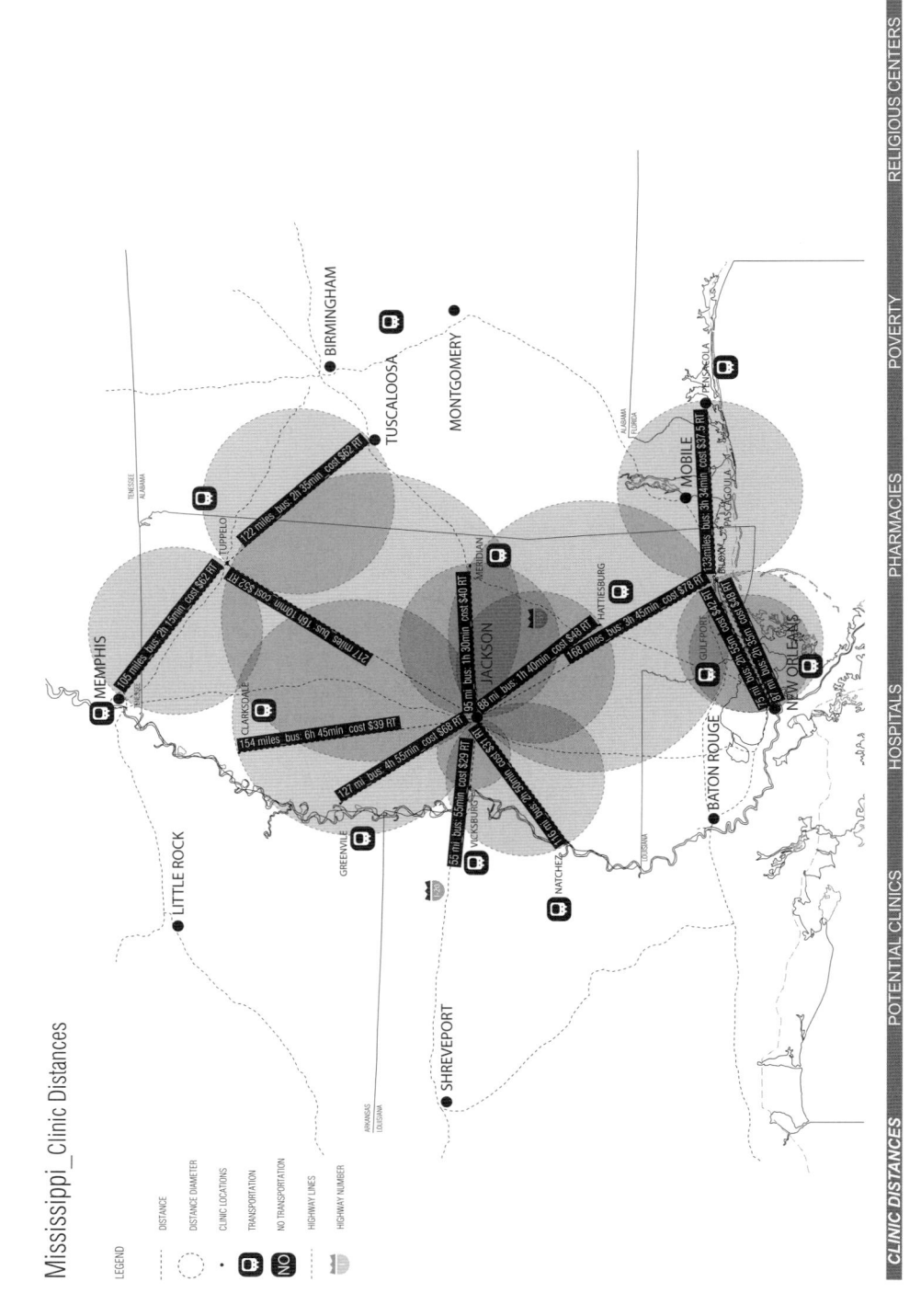

Mississippi_Clinic Distances

LEGEND
- - - - DISTANCE
◯ DISTANCE DIAMETER
• CLINIC LOCATIONS
▣ TRANSPORTATION
NO NO TRANSPORTATION
- - - - HIGHWAY LINES
▥ HIGHWAY NUMBER

Fig. 5.5a  Mississippi clinic distances

CLINIC DISTANCES | POTENTIAL CLINICS | HOSPITALS | PHARMACIES | POVERTY | RELIGIOUS CENTERS

The above diagram contextualizes the location of the only clinic in Jackson within the state. Distances and transportation cost where available are provided. The diagram opposite locates several potential clinics with dashed circles when considering the intersections of poverty levels, locations of hospitals and pharmacies in order to serve the greatest number of women possible.

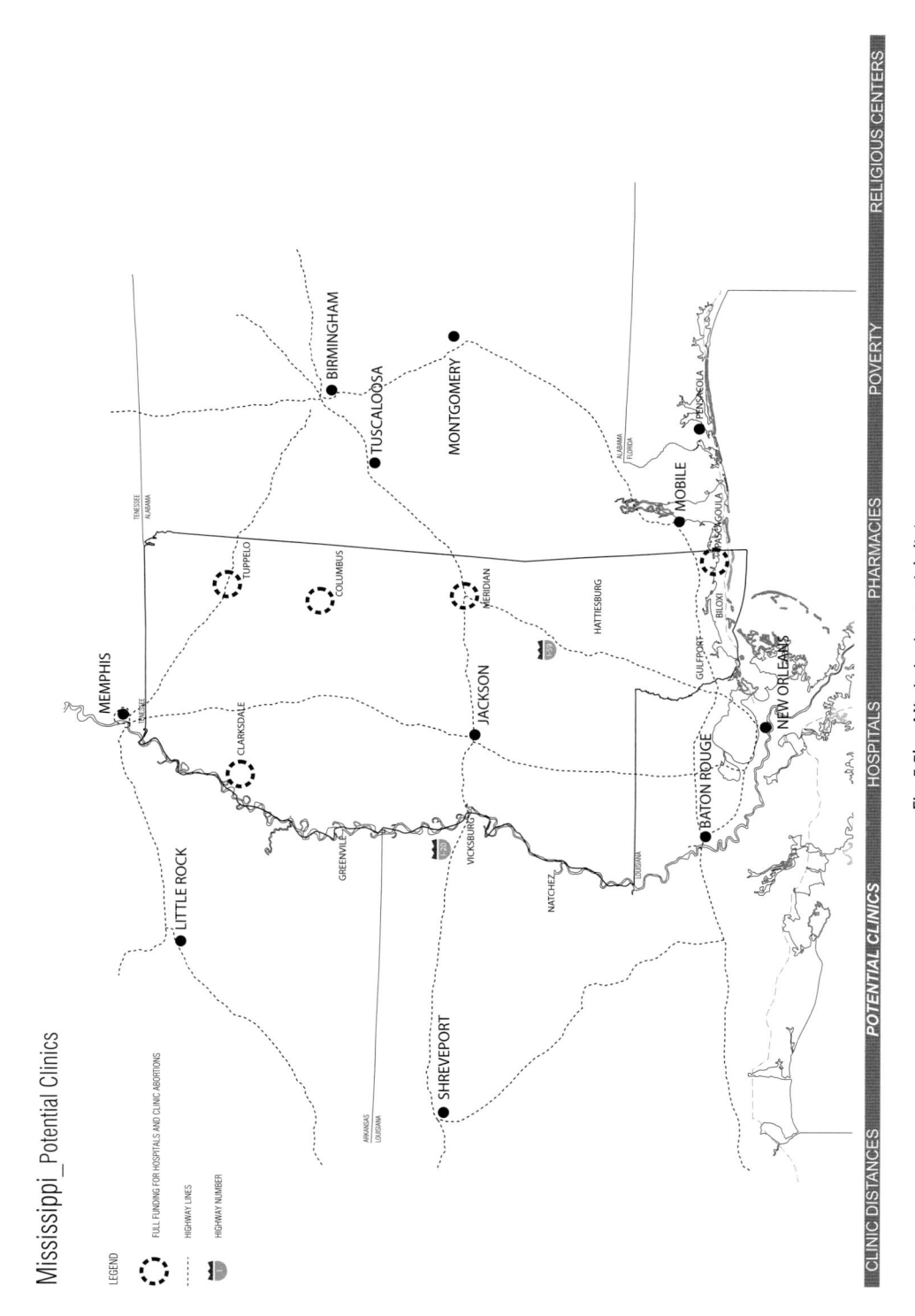

Fig. 5.5b  Mississippi potential clinics

Fig. 5.6a  Mississippi poverty statistics

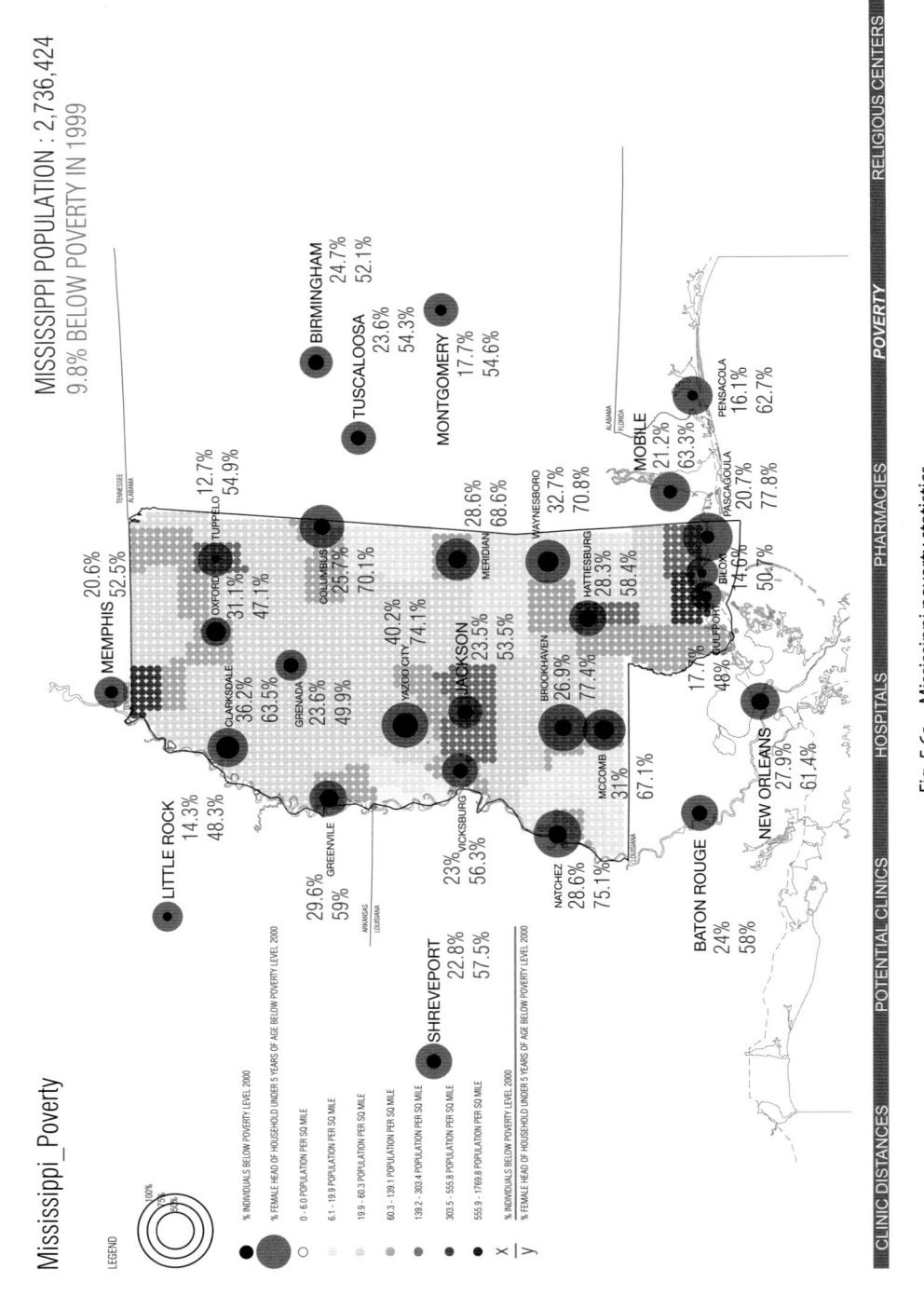

Using 1999 Census data, the diagram above compares poverty statistics for individuals (small dark circles) to single women head of household with children under five (FhdH c<5) against population (smaller background gray dots) throughout the state (large lighter gray circles). You will note how large the percentage of FhdH c<5 are statewide. The diagram opposite illustrates how many religious centers there are throughout all of Mississippi.

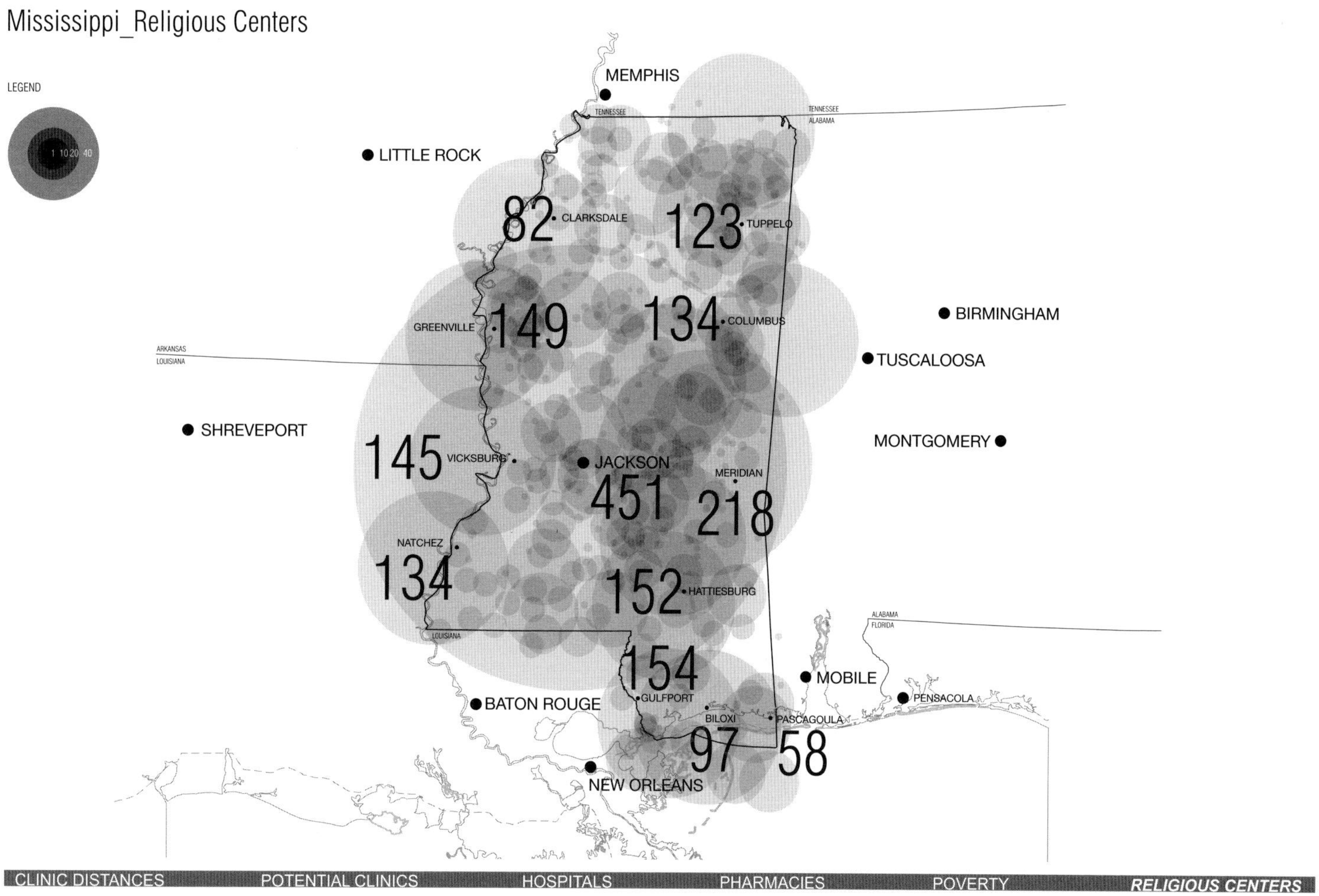

Mississippi_Religious Centers

Fig. 5.6b  Mississippi location of religious centers

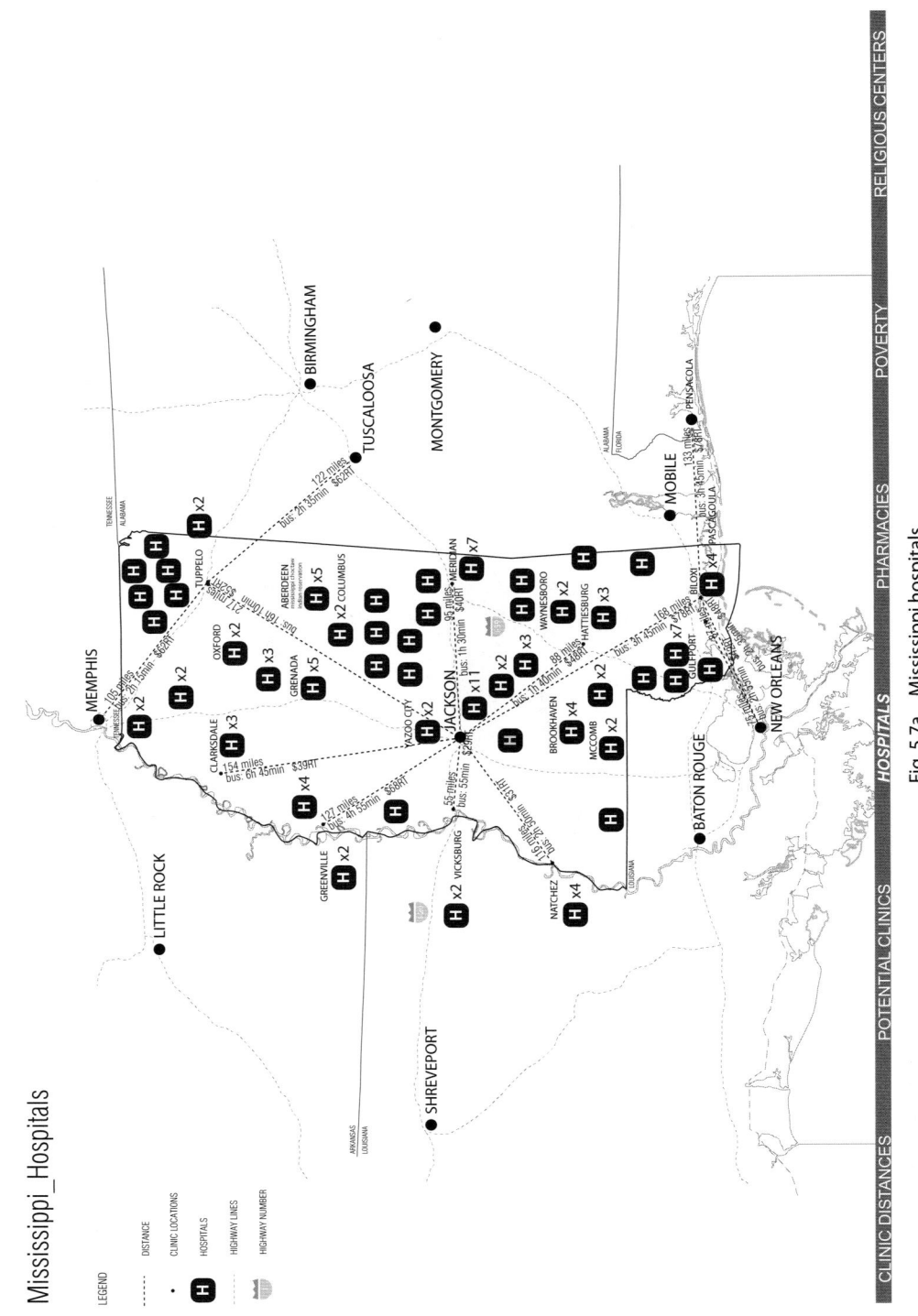

Fig. 5.7a  Mississippi hospitals

The diagram above locates all the hospitals throughout the state and the diagram opposite locates all the pharmacies noting how many stock and sell EC.

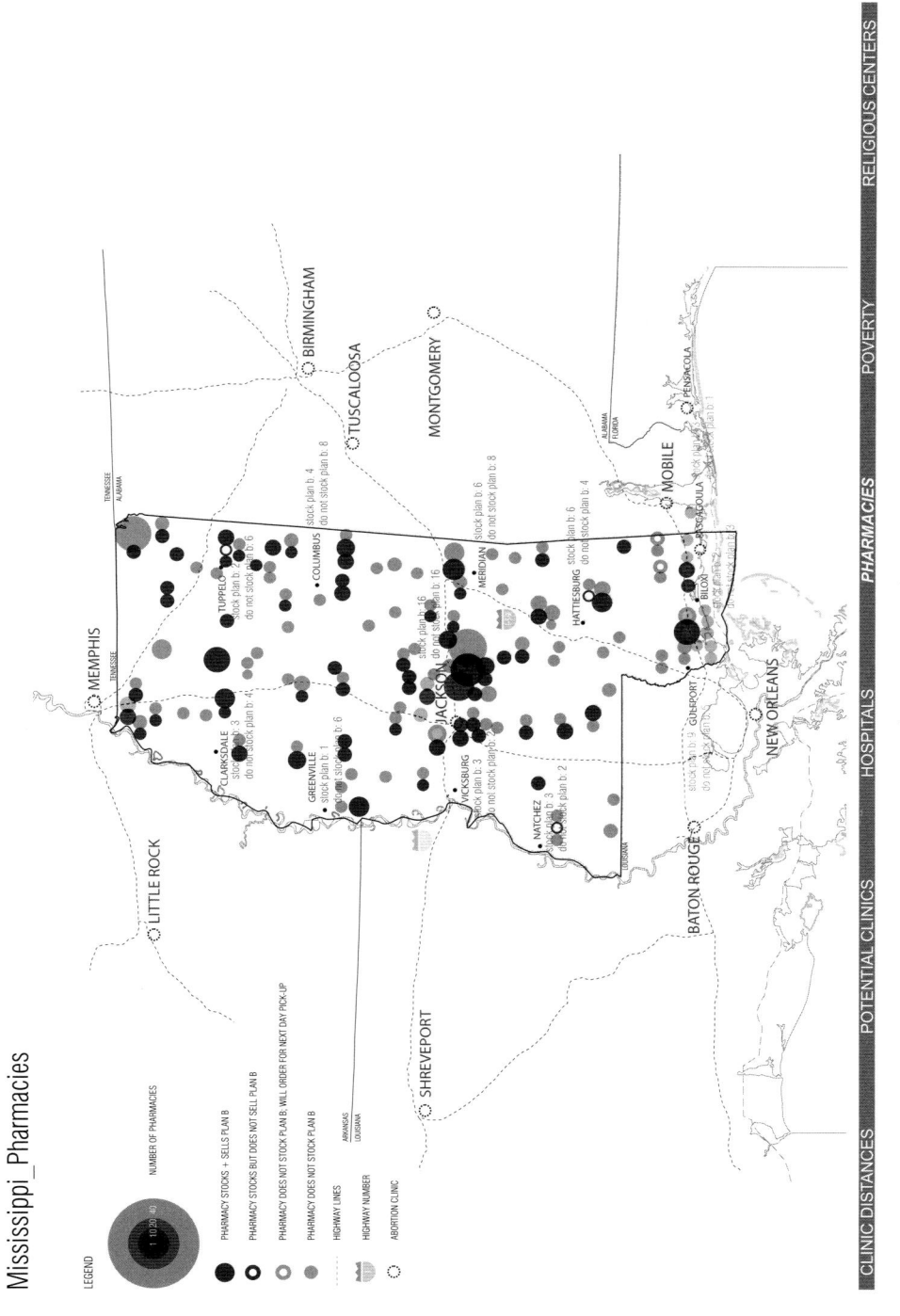

Fig. 5.7b  Mississippi pharmacies

# Mississippi_Pharmacies

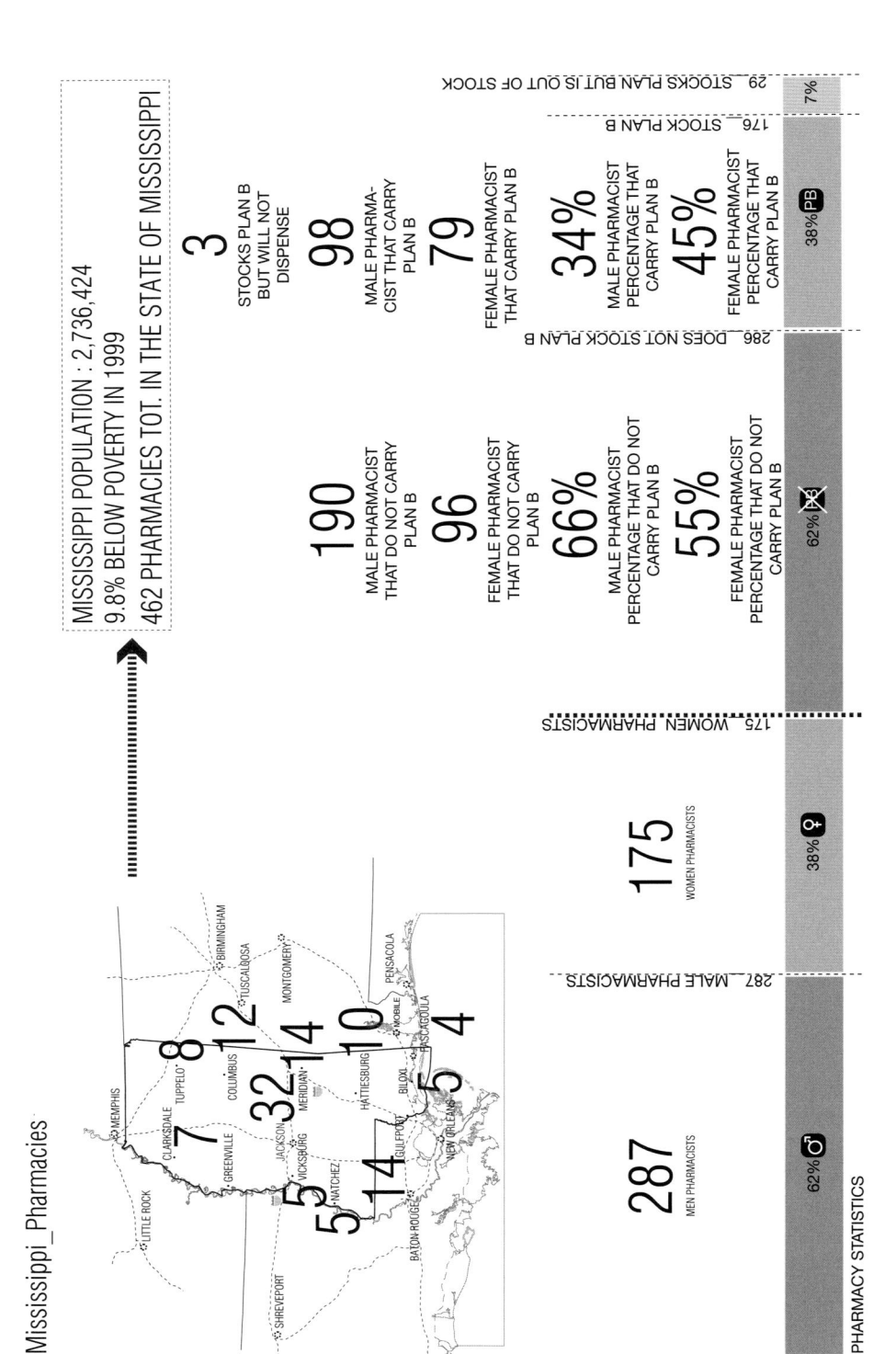

**MISSISSIPPI POPULATION : 2,736,424**
**9.8% BELOW POVERTY IN 1999**
**462 PHARMACIES TOT. IN THE STATE OF MISSISSIPPI**

**3** STOCKS PLAN B BUT WILL NOT DISPENSE

**98** MALE PHARMACIST THAT CARRY PLAN B

**79** FEMALE PHARMACIST THAT CARRY PLAN B

**34%** MALE PHARMACIST PERCENTAGE THAT CARRY PLAN B

**45%** FEMALE PHARMACIST PERCENTAGE THAT CARRY PLAN B

**190** MALE PHARMACIST THAT DO NOT CARRY PLAN B

**96** FEMALE PHARMACIST THAT DO NOT CARRY PLAN B

**66%** MALE PHARMACIST PERCENTAGE THAT DO NOT CARRY PLAN B

**55%** FEMALE PHARMACIST PERCENTAGE THAT DO NOT CARRY PLAN B

29 STOCKS PLAN BUT IS OUT OF STOCK — 7%
176 STOCK PLAN B — 38% PB
286 DOES NOT STOCK PLAN B — 62%

175 WOMEN PHARMACISTS
**175** WOMEN PHARMACISTS — 38% ♀
287 MALE PHARMACISTS
**287** MEN PHARMACISTS — 62% ♂

**PHARMACY STATISTICS**

Fig. 5.8a  Mississippi pharmacy data

The statistics are based on the results from calling all the pharmacies in the state in 2007 and documenting their response to our question "Do you sell emergency contraception? Can I fill my prescription?" At the time we were calling in Mississippi, you still needed a prescription to access this medication if younger than 18 years of age.

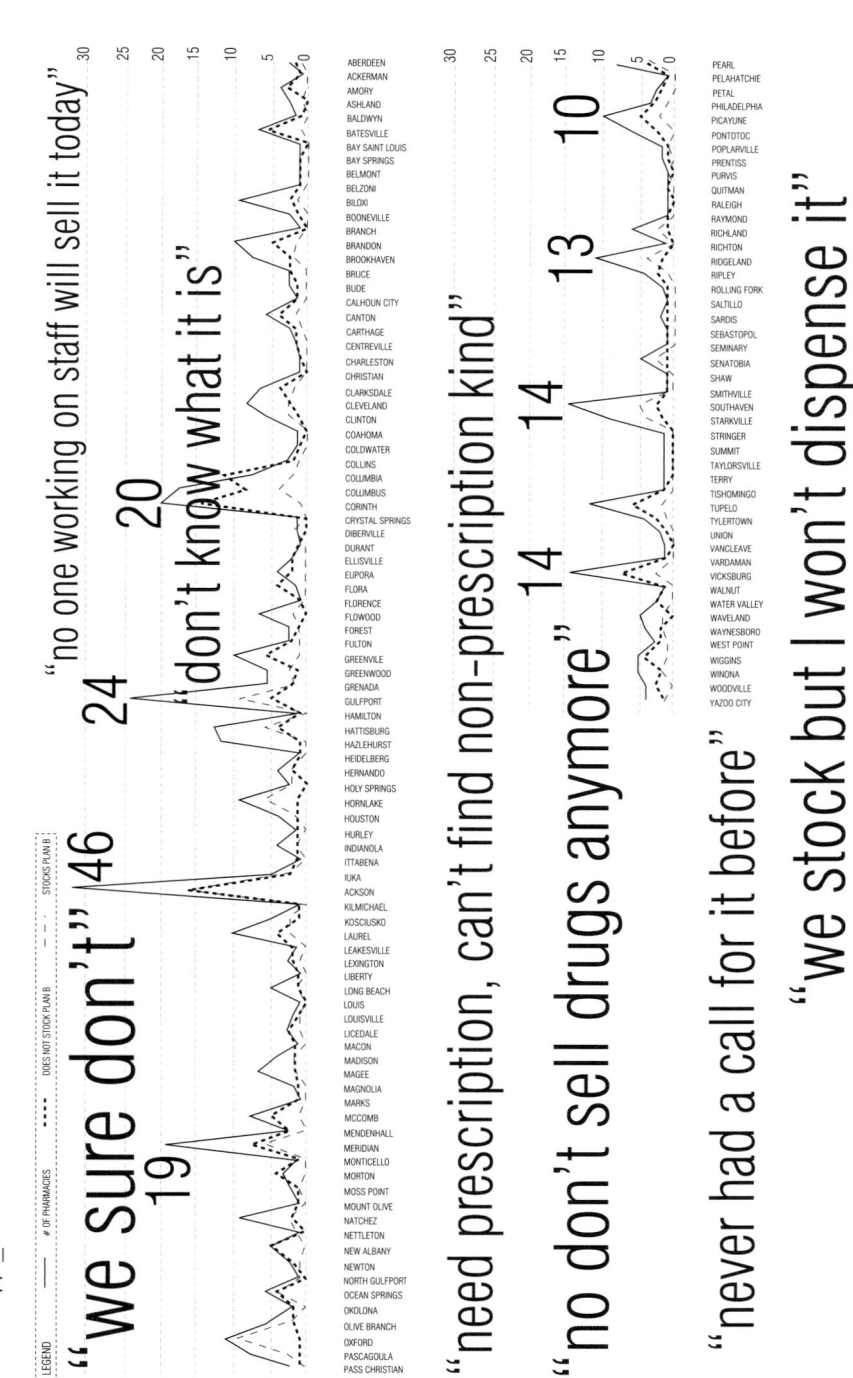

Fig. 5.8b   Mississippi pharmacist replies

- Targeted regulation of abortion providers (TRAP), state subjects providers to burdensome restrictions not applied to other medical professions.
- Physician-only restriction; state prohibits certain qualified health care professionals from performing abortions.
- State restricts insurance coverage of abortion; new state exchange health insurance policies cannot include abortion coverage, except to save a woman's life or if pregnancy is result of rape or incest.
- State allows certain entities to refuse specific reproductive health services, information or referrals.
- State prohibits use of public facilities for performance of abortions.
- Women are subjected to state-directed and biased counseling requirements; must occur in person prior to delay period.
- State requires mandatory 24-hour delay before receiving an abortion.
- State requires mandatory parental consent of a minor.
- State prohibits public funding for women eligible for state medical assistance for general health care unless procedure is necessary to preserve the woman's life, or the pregnancy is the result of rape or incest or fetal abnormality incompatible with live birth.
- Mississippi State Code makes being the parent of an illegitimate child a misdemeanor, and requires that the State Health Department report out-of-wedlock births each month.
- State provides increased access to reproductive health care services. The waiver allows the state to cover family planning services for women of childbearing age with incomes at or below 185 percent of the federal poverty level.[27]

In considering ways to possibly increase and expand contraception access to help reduce the need for abortion, all of the hospitals in the state of Mississippi have been located. In addition, thinking about EC or Plan B® as another possible opportunity to broaden reproductive healthcare, all the pharmacies have been called and asked whether they stock and sell Plan B®.

### Kentucky

With only three abortion providers throughout the state, Kentucky is one of the more difficult states for women to exercise their legal right to abortion with 98 percent of counties without a provider and according to the Guttmacher Institute, 77 percent of women live in these counties. With so few providers, women must travel greater distances to a clinic. Similar to Mississippi, if someone does not own a car, then how are clinics accessed? Because there is a mandatory 24-hour delay law in Kentucky, a woman will need to pay for another round-trip ticket or spend the night in the clinic city, either way increasing the cost of the procedure. Once again, in many of the smaller towns, there are no bus or train services available requiring her to seek alternative modes of transportation.

## Distances to/from Several Cities in Kentucky

    Madisonville—Louisville 207 miles bus: 6 hr 30min $81 RT
    Bowling Green—Louisville 125 miles bus: 2 hr 5min $71RT
    Hazard—Lexington 122 miles bus: no transportation
    Paducah—Nashville 175 miles bus: 2 hr 45min $88RT

In Kentucky, the average level of poverty is 15.8 percent compared to the national average of 13 percent. Female head-of-households with children under 5 years of age living below the line of poverty once again reveal greater disparities. In Louisville, the most populous city in the state, 21.6 percent of individuals live below the line of poverty but 50.7 percent of FhdH c<5 live below the line of poverty. In Bowling Green, 21.8 percent of individuals and 70.1 percent of FhdH c<5 live below the line of poverty; in Paducah 22.4 percent of individuals and 64.7 percent of FhdH c<5 live below the line of poverty. In a far less populated and remote city like London, 20.7 percent of individuals and 84.9 percent of FhdH c<5 live below the line of poverty.[28] Not only are these statistics extremely high but the state of Kentucky also restricts public funding for abortion and prohibits publicly owned hospitals or other publicly owned health care facilities from performing abortions unless it is necessary to preserve a woman's life.[29] The result of this legislation makes access almost impossible for women of lower economic means.

## List of Kentucky State Restrictions

- Unconstitutional and criminal abortion bans.
- State prohibits certain state employees or organization from receiving state funds from counseling or referring women for abortion services.
- TRAP, state subjects providers to burdensome restrictions not applied to other medical professions.
- Physician-only restriction; state prohibits certain qualified health care professionals from performing abortions.
- State restricts insurance coverage of abortion.
- State allows certain entities to refuse specific reproductive health services, information or referrals.
- State prohibits use of public facilities for performance of abortions.
- State allows certain entities to refuse specific reproductive health services, information or referrals.
- State restricts post-viability abortions.
- Women are subjected to biased counseling requirements that can be done via telephone.
- State requires mandatory 24-hour delays before receiving an abortion.
- State requires mandatory parental consent.
- State prohibits public funding for women eligible for state medical assistance for general health care unless procedure is necessary to preserve the woman's life, or the pregnancy is the result of rape or incest or fetal abnormality incompatible with live birth.[30]

# Kentucky_Clinic Distances

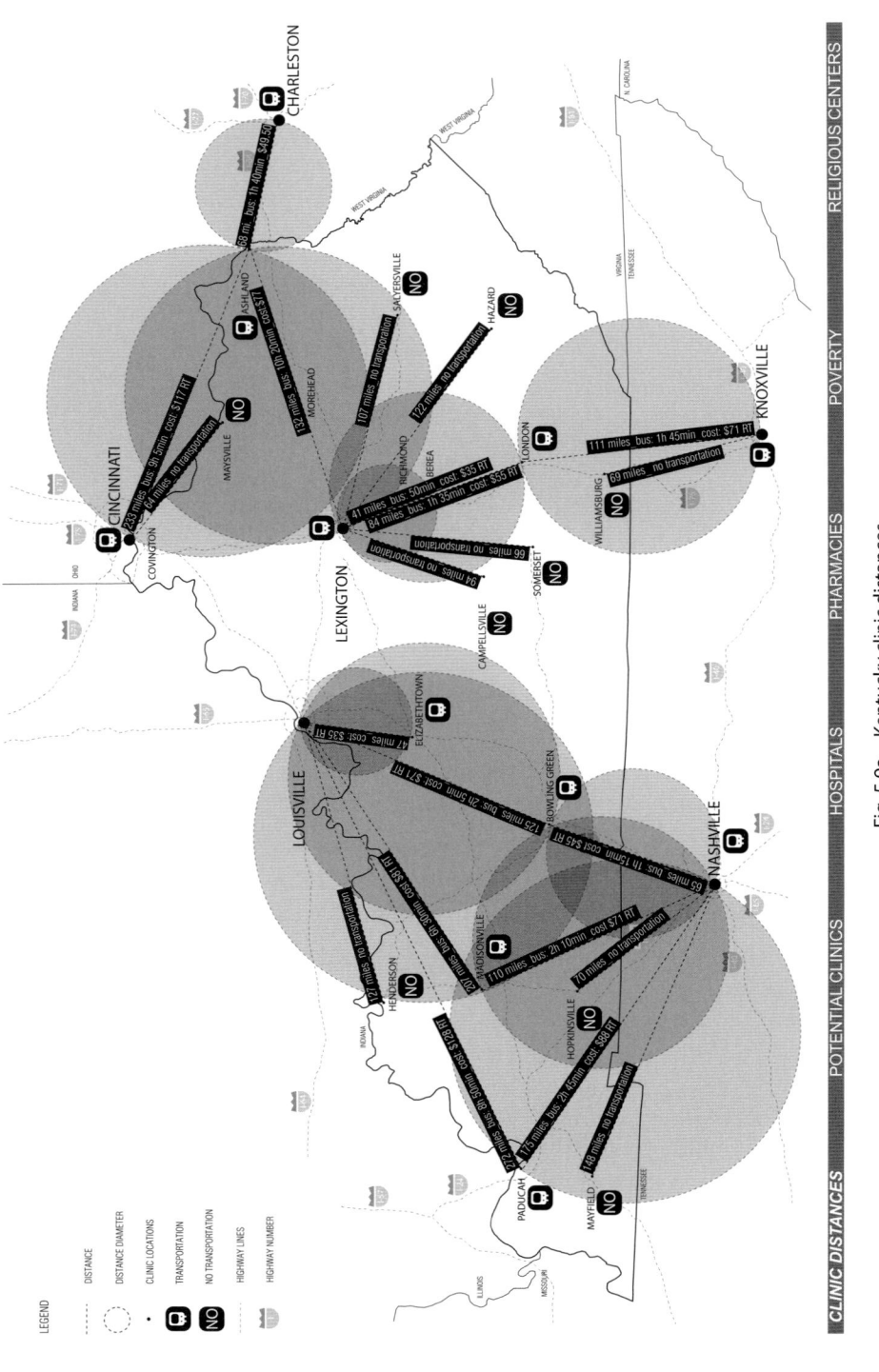

LEGEND
- ---- DISTANCE
- ◯ DISTANCE DIAMETER
- • CLINIC LOCATIONS
- ▣ TRANSPORTATION
- NO NO TRANSPORTATION
- ---- HIGHWAY LINES
- 🛡 HIGHWAY NUMBER

Fig. 5.9a  Kentucky clinic distances

The diagram above contextualizes the location of the clinics within the state. Distances and transportation cost where available are provided. The diagram opposite locates several potential clinics with dashed circles when considering the intersections of poverty levels, locations of hospitals and pharmacies in order to serve the greatest number of women possible.

**CLINIC DISTANCES** | POTENTIAL CLINICS | HOSPITALS | PHARMACIES | POVERTY | RELIGIOUS CENTERS

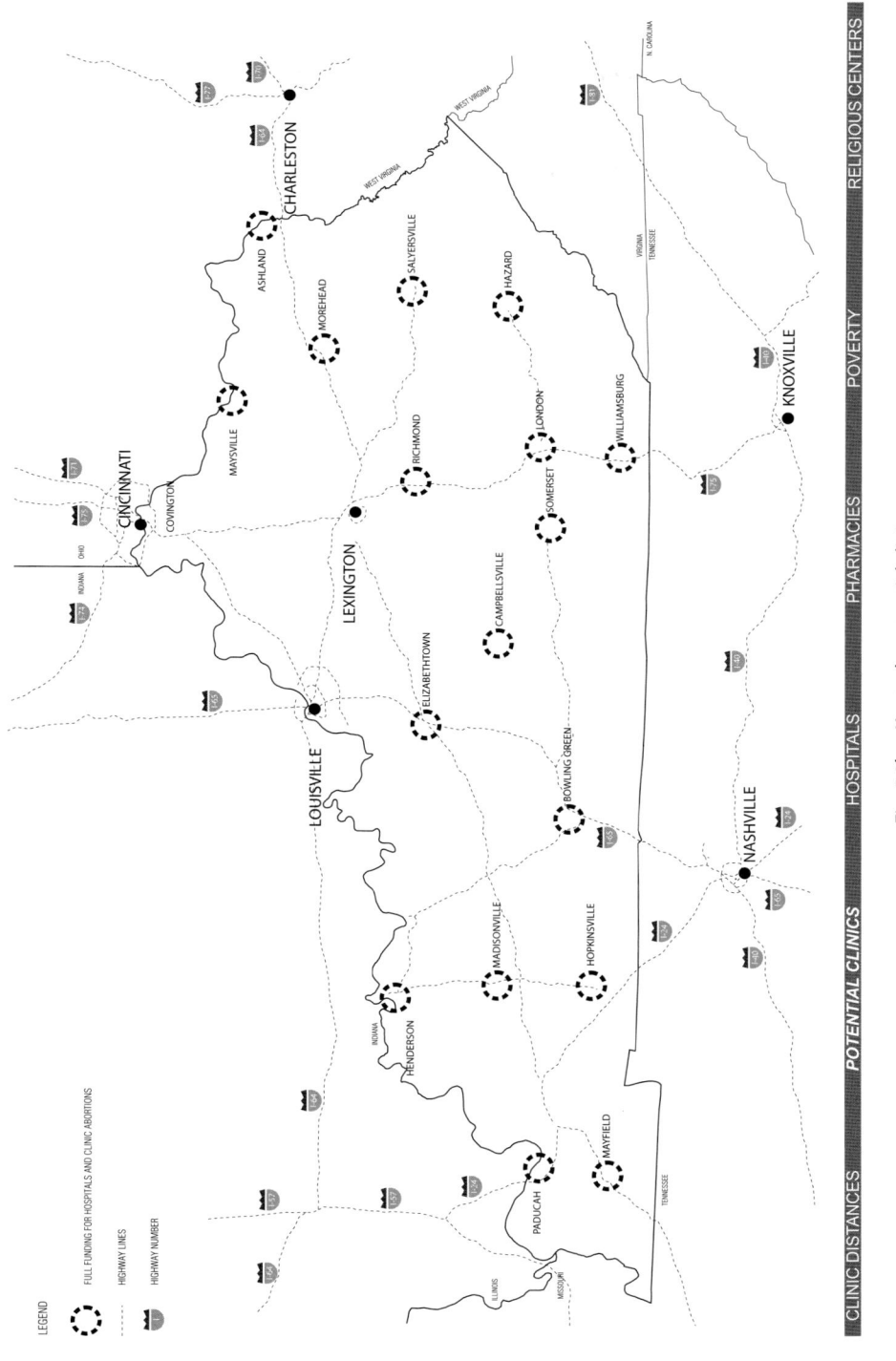

Fig. 5.9b  Kentucky potential clinics

## Kentucky_Poverty

### KENTUCKY POPULATION : 4,206,074
### 15.8% BELOW POVERTY IN 1999

**LEGEND**

- MEASUREMENT OF PERCENTAGES (100%, 50%, 5%)
- % INDIVIDUALS BELOW POVERTY LEVEL 2000
- % FEMALE HEAD OF HOUSEHOLD UNDER 5 YEARS OF AGE BELOW POVERTY LEVEL 2000
- 19.9-60.3 POPULATION PER SQ MILE
- 60.3-139.1 POPULATION PER SQ MILE
- 139.2-303.4 POPULATION PER SQ MILE
- 303.5-555.8 POPULATION PER SQ MILE
- 55.9-1769.8 POPULATION PER SQ MILE
- % INDIVIDUALS BELOW POVERTY LEVEL 2000
- % FEMALE HEAD OF HOUSEHOLD UNDER 5 YEARS OF AGE BELOW POVERTY LEVEL 2000
- x / y

**City statistics:**

- CINCINNATI
- COVINGTON 18.4% / 59.5%
- MAYSVILLE 18.9% / 85%
- ASHLAND 18.4% / 76.9%
- CHARLESTON 16.7% / 64%
- MOREHEAD 26% / 68%
- PIKEVILLE 25.4% / 70.5%
- LEXINGTON 12.9% / 48.1%
- FRANKFORT 13.9% / 54%
- JEFFERSONTOWN 4.3% / 27.2%
- LOUISVILLE 21.6% / 50.7%
- SALYERSVILLE 40.7% / 63.6%
- RICHMOND 25% / 60.4%
- HAZARD 30.5% / 60.9%
- ELIZABETHTOWN 12.1% / 51.6%
- CAMPBELLSVILLE 21.6% / 64.2%
- SOMERSET 22.1% / 58.9%
- LONDON 20.7% / 84.9%
- WILLIAMSBURG 35.4% / 62.5%
- KNOXVILLE 20.8% / 61%
- OWENSBORO 15.9% / 63.9%
- BOWLING GREEN 21.8% / 71.1%
- NASHVILLE 13.3% / 48.1%
- HENDERSON 16.5% / 55.1%
- MADISONVILLE 16.4% / 66.5%
- HOPKINSVILLE 16.8% / 48.9%
- PADUCAH 22.4% / 64.7%
- MAYFIELD 27.5% / 85%

CLINIC DISTANCES | POTENTIAL CLINICS | HOSPITALS | PHARMACIES | POVERTY | RELIGIOUS CENTERS

**Fig. 5.10a   Kentucky poverty statistics**

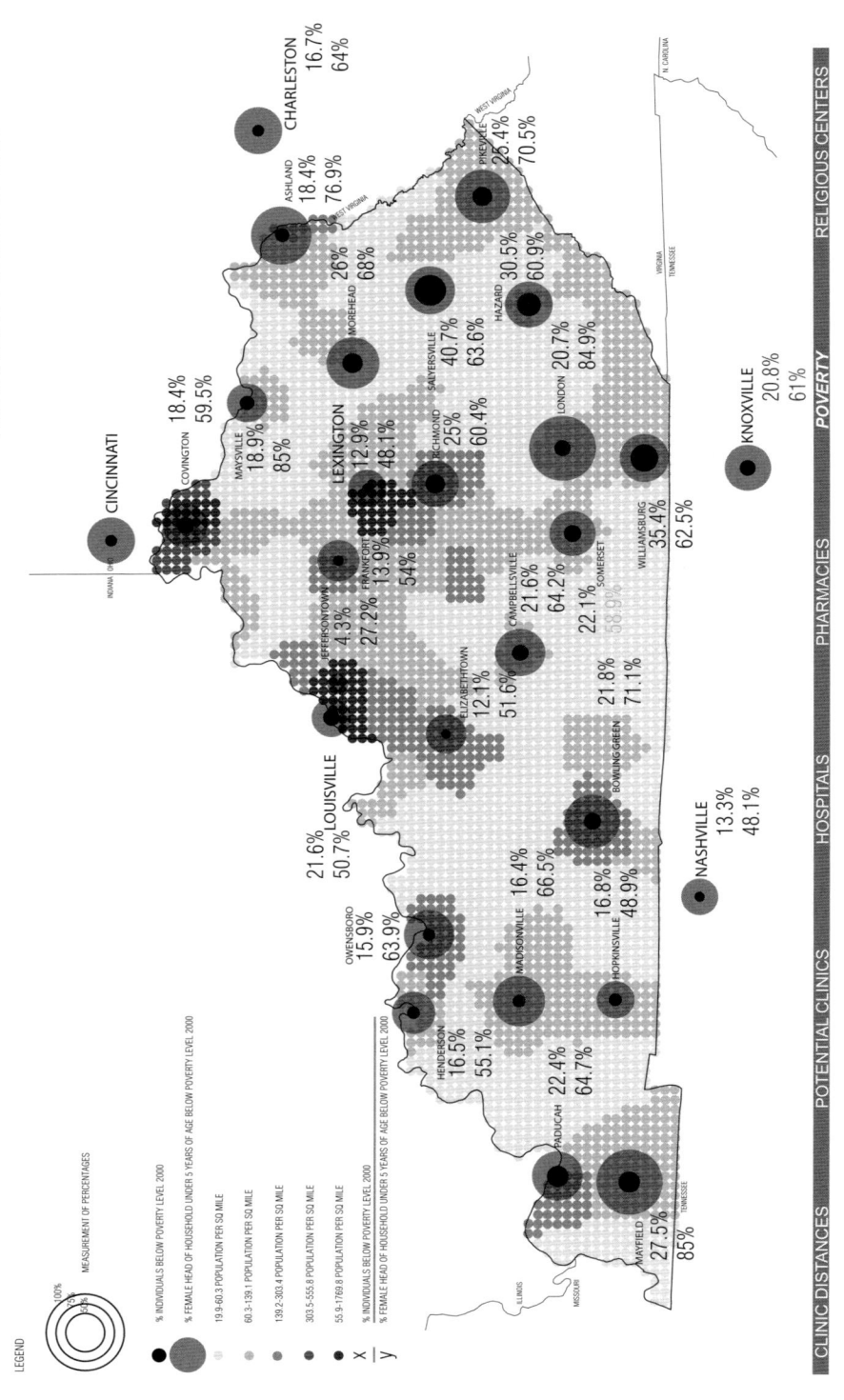

Using 1999 Census data, the above diagram compares poverty statistics for individuals (small dark circles) to single women head of household with children under five (FhdH c<5) against population (smaller background gray dots) throughout the state (large lighter gray circles). You will note how large the percentage of FhdH c<5 are statewide. The diagram opposite illustrates how many religious centers there are throughout all of Kentucky.

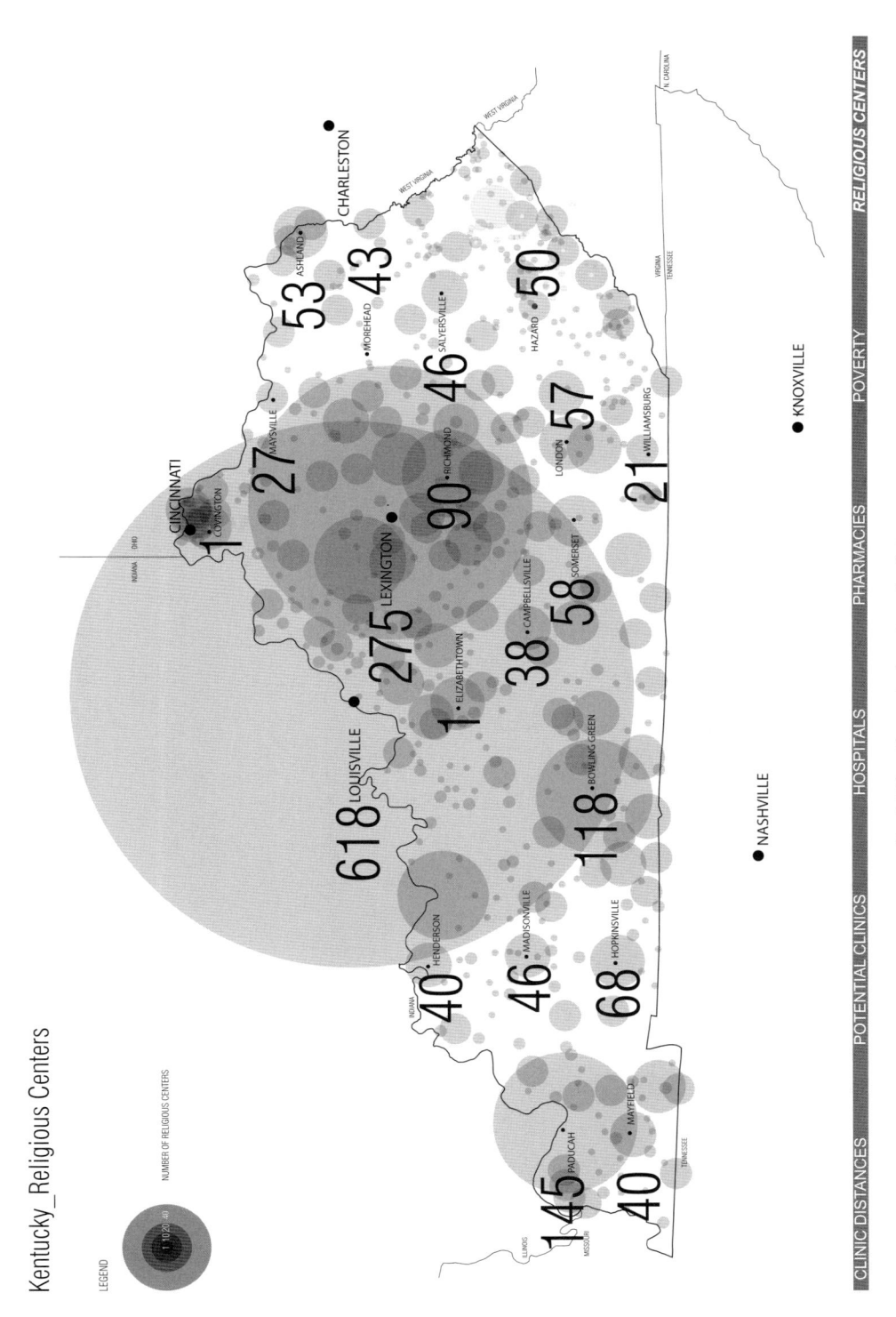

Fig. 5.10b  Kentucky location of religious centers

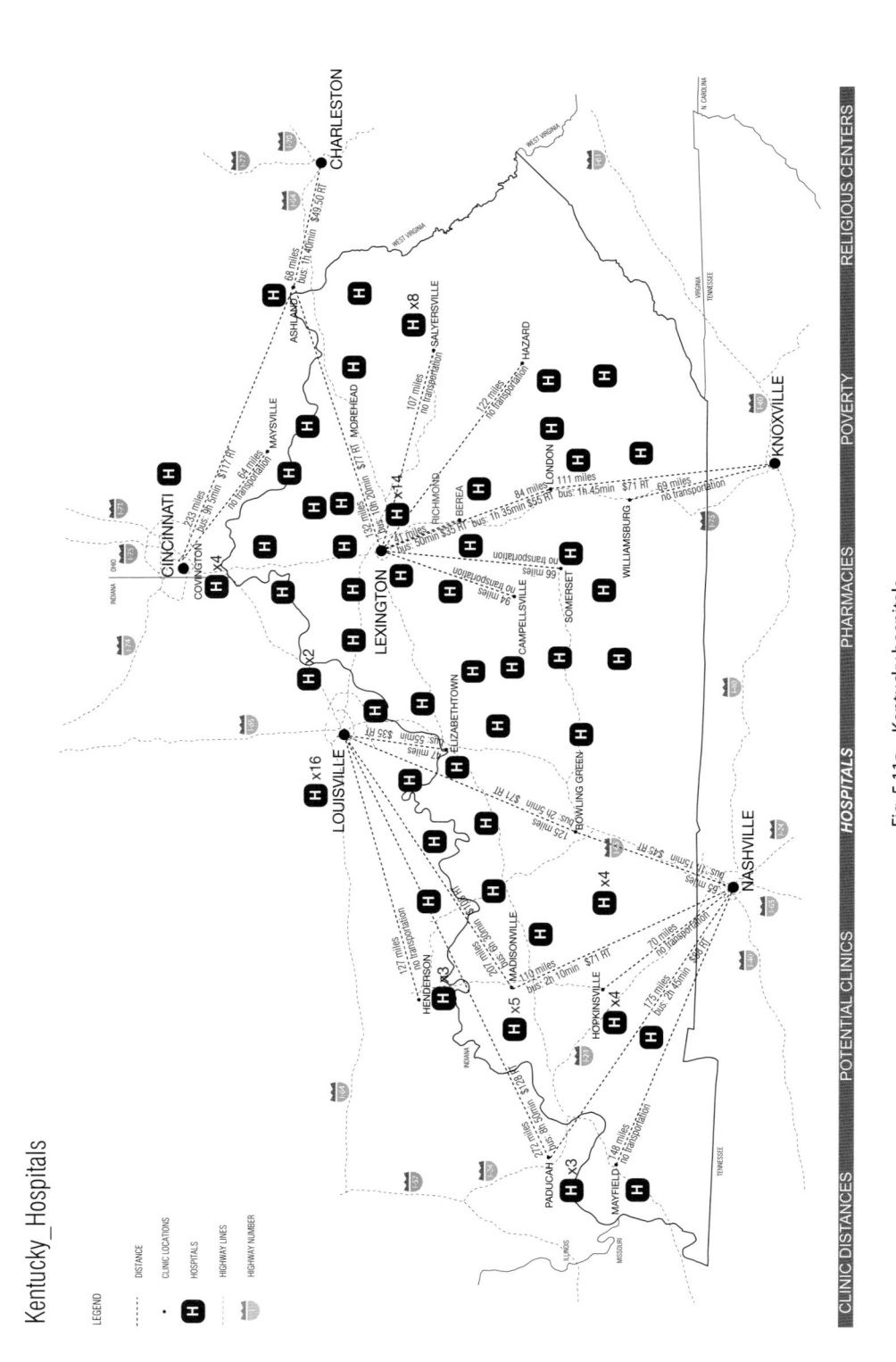

Fig. 5.11a  Kentucky hospitals

The diagram above locates all the hospitals throughout the state and the diagram below locates all the pharmacies noting how many stock and sell EC.

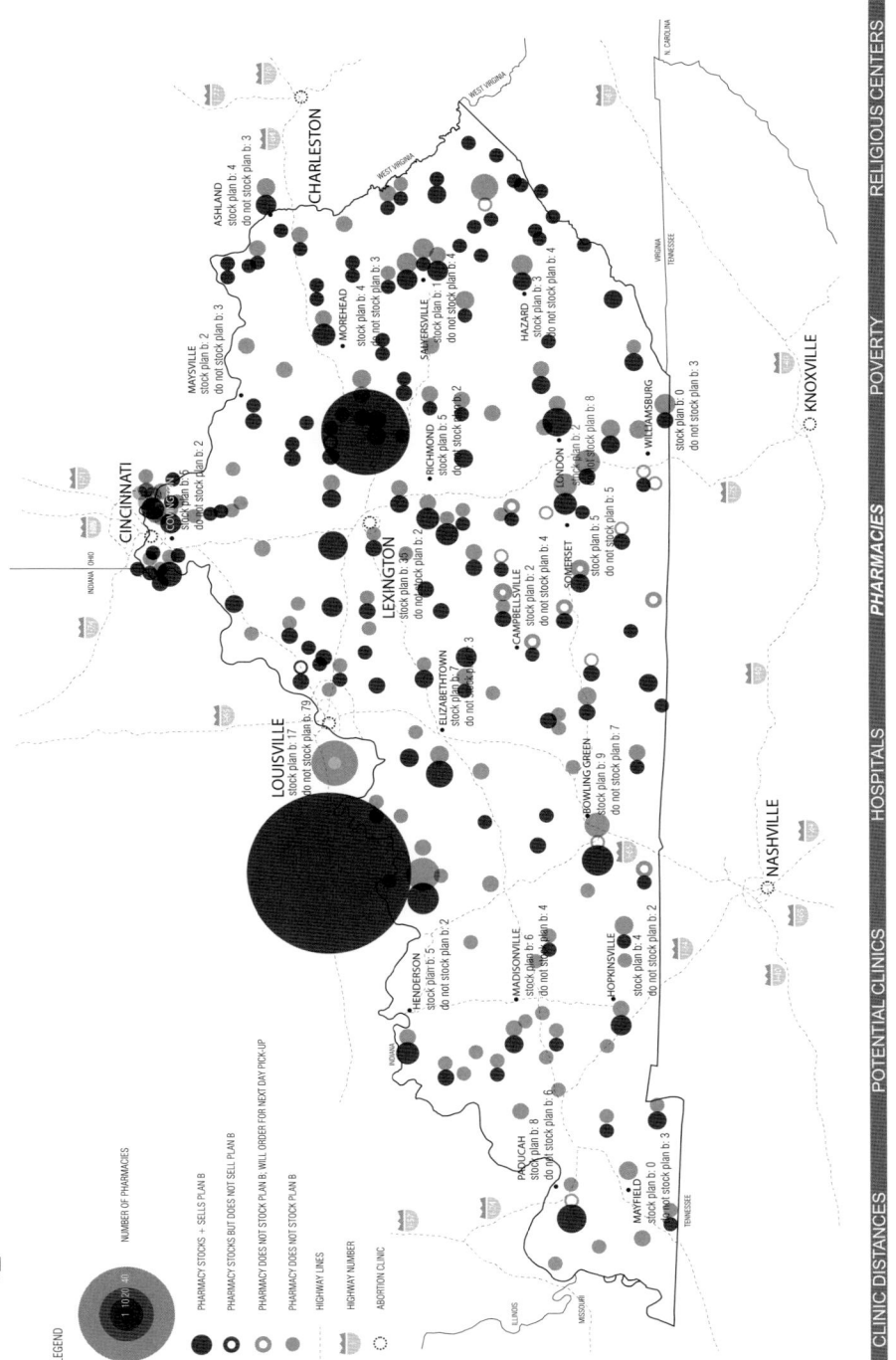

Fig. 5.11b  Kentucky pharmacies

# Kentucky_Pharmacies

**KENTUCKY POPULATION : 4,206,074**
**15.8% BELOW POVERTY IN 1999**
**680 PHARMACIES TOTAL IN THE STATE OF KENTUCKY**

*NUMBER OF PHARMACIES IN LARGER CITIES

Map values:
- PADUCAH 14
- MAYFIELD 3
- HENDERSON 7
- MADISONVILLE 6
- HOPKINSVILLE 6
- BOWLING GREEN 16
- LOUISVILLE 96
- ELIZABETHTOWN 10
- CAMPBELLSVILLE 6
- LEXINGTON 37
- COVINGTON 7
- MAYSVILLE 5
- MOREHEAD 7
- ASHLAND 7
- ST. CHARLESTON 5
- RICHMOND 7
- SOMERSET 10
- LONDON 10
- SALYERSVILLE 7
- HAZARD 10
- WILLIAMSBURG 3

**3** STOCKS PLAN B BUT WILL NOT DISPENSE

**185** MALE PHARMACIST THAT CARRY PLAN B

**205** FEMALE PHARMACIST THAT CARRY PLAN B

**55%** MALE PHARMACIST PERCENTAGE THAT CARRY PLAN B

**60%** FEMALE PHARMACIST PERCENTAGE THAT CARRY PLAN B

**151** MALE PHARMACIST THAT DO NOT CARRY PLAN B

**137** FEMALE PHARMACIST THAT DO NOT CARRY PLAN B

**45%** MALE PHARMACIST PERCENTAGE THAT DO NOT CARRY PLAN B

**40%** FEMALE PHARMACIST PERCENTAGE THAT DO NOT CARRY PLAN B

343 WOMEN PHARMACISTS
335 MALE PHARMACISTS

**335** MEN PHARMACISTS
**343** WOMEN PHARMACISTS

290 DOES NOT STOCK PLAN B
387 STOCKS PLAN B
45 STOCKS PLAN BUT IS OUT OF STOCK

49% ♂ | 51% ♀ | 43% ✗ | 57% PB | 7%

PHARMACY STATISTICS

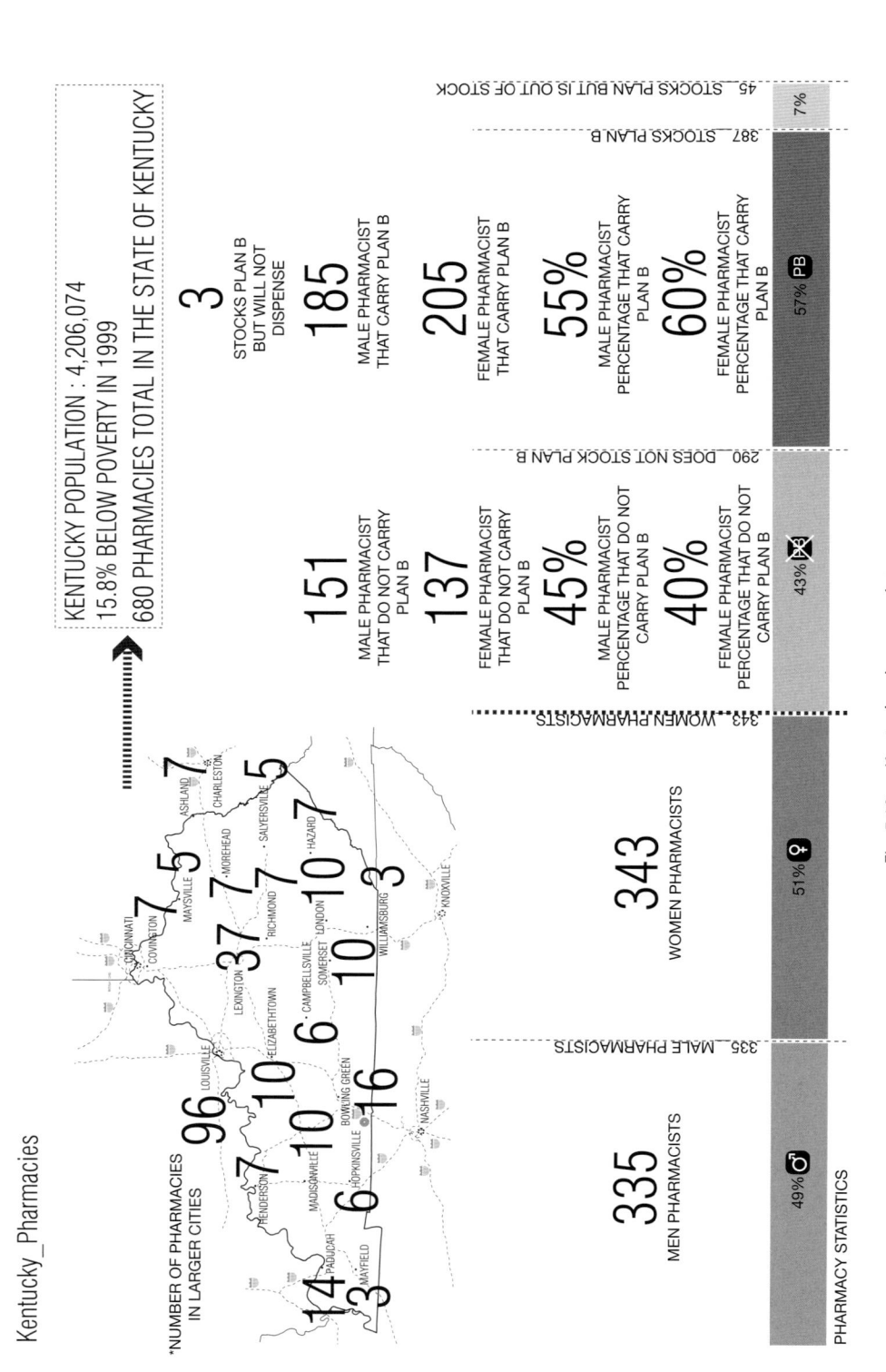

Fig. 5.12a Kentucky pharmacy data

The statistics are based on the results from calling all the pharmacies in the state in 2007 and documenting their response to our question "Do you sell emergency contraception? Can I fill my prescription?" At the time we were calling in Kentucky, you still needed a prescription to access this medication if younger than 18 years of age.

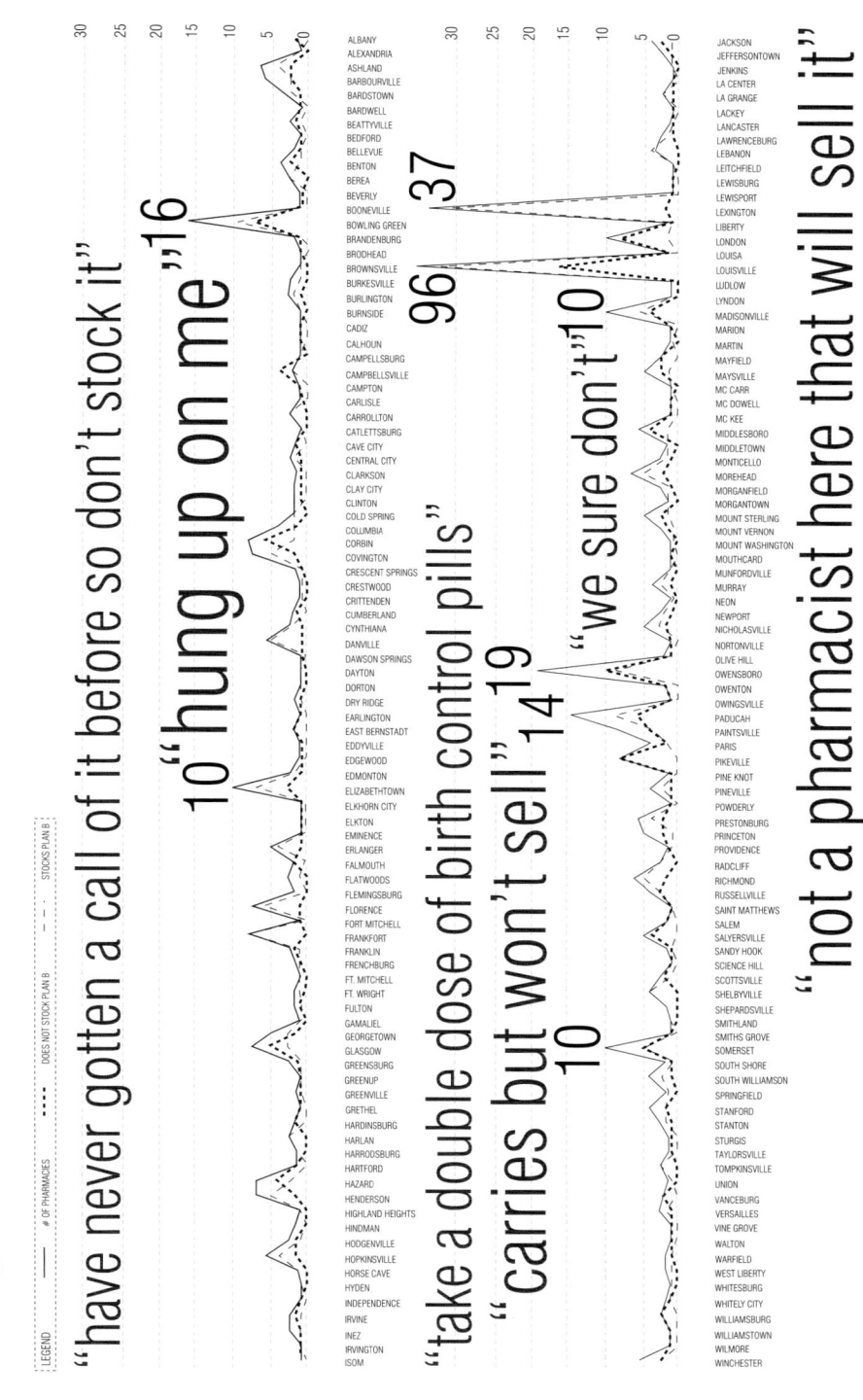

Fig. 5.12b  Kentucky pharmacist replies

**Midwest**

The way a clinic is internally structured has a real impact on the type and scope of services provided. One Midwest clinic director discussed with me why they decided to incorporate as a non-profit when they began back in 1974. It was clear to them that women who have money will always be able to access a safe abortion. Back before *Roe v. Wade*, women would travel to New York, Canada, and Mexico among other places to access abortion care. However, it was poor women showing up in emergency rooms who were the ones unable to access and pay for a safe abortion and needing emergency care after a botched abortion. So when the group decided to become an abortion facility, they determined the clinic would be non-profit to ensure that every woman would be able to afford a safe abortion. The clinic strongly believed that one should not make money on health care, especially for a service like abortion. The vision was strongly connected to the 1970s feminist ideals of being able to serve other women. As a result of their non-profit status, they pay no taxes and can keep their fees low. They have an endowment and through additional fund raising the clinic can subsidize care for about 90 percent of their patients. This type of business model allows a clinic to have far greater control over how they spend their money and what sorts of services they can provide their patients. One advantage mentioned is the thorough counseling and additional support services this clinic is able to provide unlike the other local clinics. Another interesting aspect of being able to keep their fees low is this clinic sets the local market's fee structure. Other clinics are unable to charge much more because the market will not bear it and if the other clinics cannot compete at this fee rate, they will go out of business.[31]

**Expanding Reproductive Justice**

An exciting strategy by one of the Midwest clinics I interviewed is how they use their own building as a test bed for expanding the role and scope of reproductive justice. Incorporating other important social and environmental justice issues, this clinic is expanding their focus to become part of a larger collection of health and human right concerns. I believe this clinic is on to something through positioning abortion within a broader social justice movement gaining more collective leverage and power. In this way, abortion no longer remains an isolated issue but part of a growing body of social justice work.

At the time the clinic was attempting to lease a space in the mid nineties and having difficulty doing so, they came across an abandoned and boarded-up building. After buying the property and undergoing a capital campaign, the building was renovated and paid off in two years. Later because there was so much additional work the building needed and once the clinic began to consider the long-term cost analysis, they decided to make the renovation as innovative environmentally as possible. What really got them thinking about the LEED process was when it was time to replace a 1957-era boiler. They wanted the most efficient boiler as possible, which eventually led to a LEED feasibility study. Working with a LEED AP architect (Leadership in Energy and Environmental Design, Accredited Professional), she helped guide the clinic through the entire process and the clinic hired a design build firm to implement the work. They became the first LEED certified Silver

USA Regions_Midwest

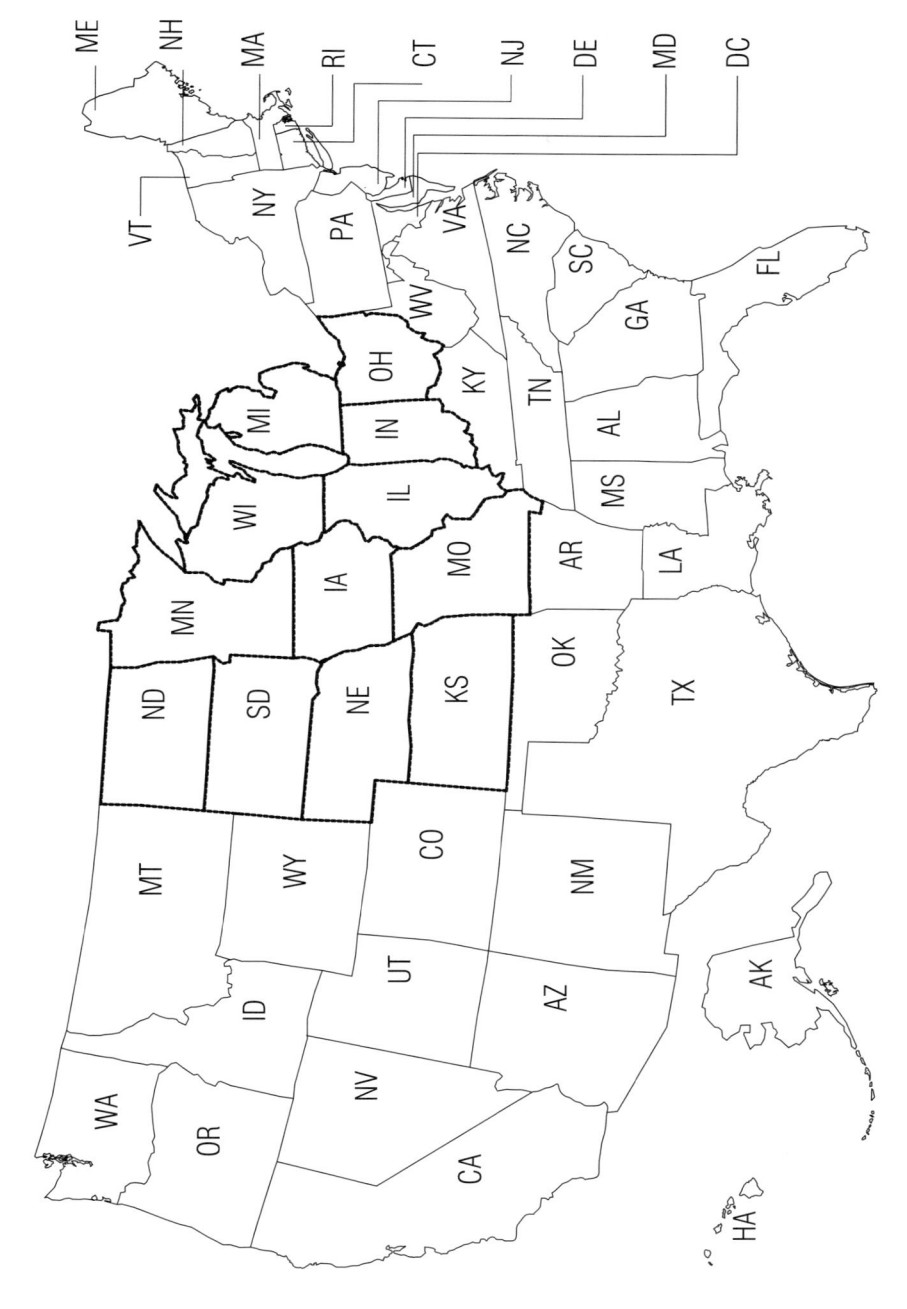

Fig. 5.13  Midwestern region synopsis

USA Regions_Midwest

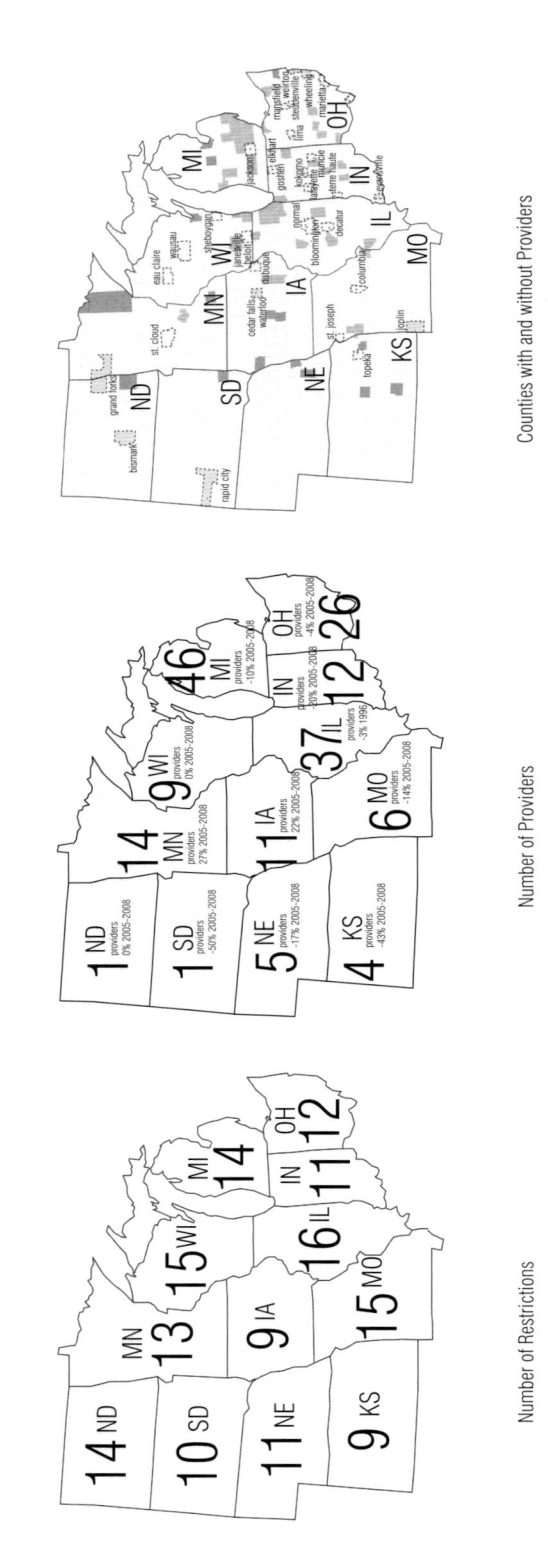

Number of Restrictions

14 ND
10 SD
11 NE
9 KS
13 MN
15 WI
9 IA
15 MO
14 MI
16 IL
11 IN
12 OH

Number of Providers

1 ND providers 0% 2005-2008
1 SD providers -50% 2005-2008
5 NE providers -17% 2005-2008
4 KS providers -43% 2005-2008
14 MN providers 27% 2005-2008
9 WI providers 0% 2005-2008
11 IA providers 22% 2005-2008
6 MO providers -14% 2005-2008
46 MI providers -10% 2005-2008
37 IL providers -3% 1998
12 IN providers -20% 2005-2008
26 OH providers -4% 2005-2008

Counties with and without Providers

Fig. 5.13  Midwestern region synopsis *concluded*

clinic for an existing building renovation receiving a design award for the project. However, this success was not without many obstacles. They encountered numerous sub-contractors refusing to work with them because they are an abortion facility. I have heard similar stories from other Midwestern clinic providers regarding the construction and service trades. Even now, with a LEED Silver building, they have not been fully embraced by the environmental community.

How does this impact their patients and adjacent community? As part of this clinic's investment in the local, they have worked to use their building as a space for larger community engagement. Through an on-site recycle center, both patients and community members can bring in their old belongings and exchange them for other items. Future projects being considered include the installation of solar awnings on the southern and eastern faces of the building, storm water management and the creation of a vegetated roof with staff seating space.

**Spatial Experiences**

One of the biggest attractors for one clinic when deciding to buy their property was that so much of the building was filled with light throughout the day. It completely rebuked the idea of the dark and gloomy abortion clinic. Another clinic director told me "your waiting room reflects how you feel about your patients. It should be tidy and well organized." She clearly connects a patient's experience to the quality of space their experience occurs in. The waiting area is filled with natural light with modern and locally crafted chairs. The space exudes a peaceful aura and is one of the most well considered waiting areas I have been in. She also mentioned the decision to replace the 1990s art hanging throughout the clinic. After visiting many clinics, she realized their art made the clinic appear out of date. Now the walls are filled with large striking photographs of plants and flowers. Their abstract quality and range of muted yet vibrant colors add a level of sophistication. These images also influenced the staff's choice of wall colors moving beyond the typical medical facility color palette of ocean greens, grays and mauves.[32]

Another interesting and successful touch I had never seen before was the use of light diffusers in patient exam rooms. Awarded a grant to improve patient care, this clinic purchased translucent acrylic fluorescent light panel-diffusers printed with pale floral motifs of pale pinks and lavenders. Altering the light quality of the small patient exam rooms, the panels create a more relaxing environment and give the patient something to look at while she lies prostate and stares at the ceiling. These should be used throughout all types of medical facilities. What a difference a patient would have if they entered into a room that no longer had such harsh fluorescent lighting but instead rooms with clouds, flowers, trees, cartoons or even abstract imagery floating above them![33]

During the past 10 years one Midwestern clinic realized more patients were presenting spiritual and religious concerns through their patient feedback forms. In response to this information they were receiving, the clinic renovated an existing space into the Reflection Room. Representing the clinic's investment in sustainability, this new space is made primarily from environmentally friendly materials. Patients seek this space for quiet reflection and solitude.

## Security, Protestors and Demonstrations

Although the providers I interviewed throughout the Midwest did not experience a comparable volume of protestors as those in the south, this is not to say other Midwestern clinics have not experienced such intense scales of protestors. In fact, it is common knowledge that Dr. George Tiller's Wichita, Kansas clinic was a continual focus of anti-abortion sieges and attempted shut downs for years. Clearly Midwestern clinics do receive high levels of protests but the people I interviewed did not mention it being such a great concern. Some have protestors every day there are procedures, others not as often.

Security is handled in a variety of different ways. One clinic has a staff person scan everyone who enters with a metal detector wand and searches all bags and purses. No pocketknives are allowed since Dr. Tiller's 2009 death. Another clinic has a security guard on duty during business hours monitoring everyone and everything entering and exiting the building. None of the people I interviewed have had any real problems with lack of police enforcement or protection as compared to clinics in the south. In fact, one clinic director mentioned that her clinic is considering hiring off-duty policemen for their security in the near future. In her experience, they are more responsive when paying them for off-duty security work. I responded that this seems unfortunate that you would have to pay for a service that should be provided by regular law enforcement but it appears that the expense is not so great and the clinic is willing to spend the extra money to ensure safety.

One clinic mentioned they are the unfortunate recipients of the Image Clear Ultrasound (ICU, pronounced "I see you") RV. Attempting to park as close to a clinic as possible, this form of protest includes a 40-foot-long RV providing free ultrasounds. According to their website, "ICU Mobile is a non-profit ministry of love and grace deploying and supporting a fleet of mobile pregnancy centers so that every woman experiencing an unplanned pregnancy may have a free opportunity to see her unborn child and hear the Gospel in a non-judgmental, non-political and non-coercive environment." ICU states that although they do locate their buses in front of or near abortion clinics and Planned Parenthoods, they try and seek out those in communities who need their services most and go to such places as shopping plazas, community areas, college campuses, beaches or anywhere else there may be a high concentration of women with unplanned pregnancies.[34] Curious about the service they provided, one clinic located near to where an ICU RV was parked had one of their staff seek consultation, saying she recently had a positive pregnancy test but wasn't sure what she wanted to do (she was not actually pregnant). ICU performed an ultrasound and told her "they could hear the baby's heartbeat," yet she was not even pregnant.[35] This is another example of how inaccurate information about women's bodies continues to be propagated.

Another clinic located along a busy street of a Midwestern city feels they are more protected than others I have spoken with. Due to the high visibility and activity around her clinic and the public*ness* of her immediate location, protestors are kept much more in check. The protestors are quite visible due to the relationship between the property line and the sidewalk where they are forced to stand directly in front of the clinic. The downside to the nearness of the property line is that the protestors are so close to the building's entrance and exit because there is no additional space around the building. Although there is complete anonymity for the patients as they park across or down the street, once an observer understands what building the person is going into the patient becomes completely exposed. This has resulted in protestors approaching any woman of reproductive age who passes by in hopes of getting anyone to speak with them.[36] This clinic director made an interesting observation that in this small Midwestern city protestors are more respective than in other parts of the country. She attributes this to the social conventions at play there; people do not typically make eye contact nor do they normally acknowledge passers-by on the street. Protestors are breaking social etiquette by speaking to someone entering a clinic. Unlike in the south, the clinic director feels another advantage is the police station is only about three blocks away.

One comment I have heard from many providers is in regard to the relationship between city governments and abortion protestors. As a result of lawsuits eventually awarded to anti-abortion protestors in one Midwestern city, city government agencies and departments have become far less eager and responsive to requests made by abortion providers. This can include anything from previously discussed police inactivity to the permitting of building renovation work. As one clinic director mentioned, because her local city government is "absolutely terrified of [the protestors]" and "will bend over backwards" for them, she knows that her clinic is being watched and if she wanted to remodel or do any sort of construction work for the clinic, she believes the city would scrutinize so closely and carefully to the point that it could be called a form of harassment.[37]

## South Dakota

With only one provider in the state, the people of South Dakota rejected a ban on almost all abortions in both the 2006 and 2008 elections. Ninety-eight percent of South Dakota counties are without a provider and 76 percent of women live in these counties according to the Guttmacher Institute.

### Distances to/from Several Cities in South Dakota

> Rapid City—Sioux Falls 348 miles bus: 7 hr 15min $175.35 RT
> Pierre—Sioux Falls 225 miles bus: 3 hr 59min $00.88 RT
> Aberdeen—Sioux Falls 204 miles bus: 4 hr 25 min $110.56 RT
> Mobridge—Sioux Falls 304 miles bus: no service

In South Dakota, the average level of poverty is 13.2 percent compared to the national average of 13 percent. Female head-of-households with children under 5 years of age living below the line of poverty once again reveal greater differences. In Sioux Falls, the most populous city in the state, 8.4 percent of individuals live below the line of poverty but 40.4 percent of FhdH c<5 live below the line of poverty; on the Pine Ridge Indian Reservation 53.5 percent of individuals and 68.3 percent of FhdH c<5 live below the line of poverty; in Belle Fourche, 12.6 percent of individuals and 76 percent of FhdH c<5 live below the line of poverty;

South Dakota_Clinic Distances

Fig. 5.14a   South Dakota clinic distances

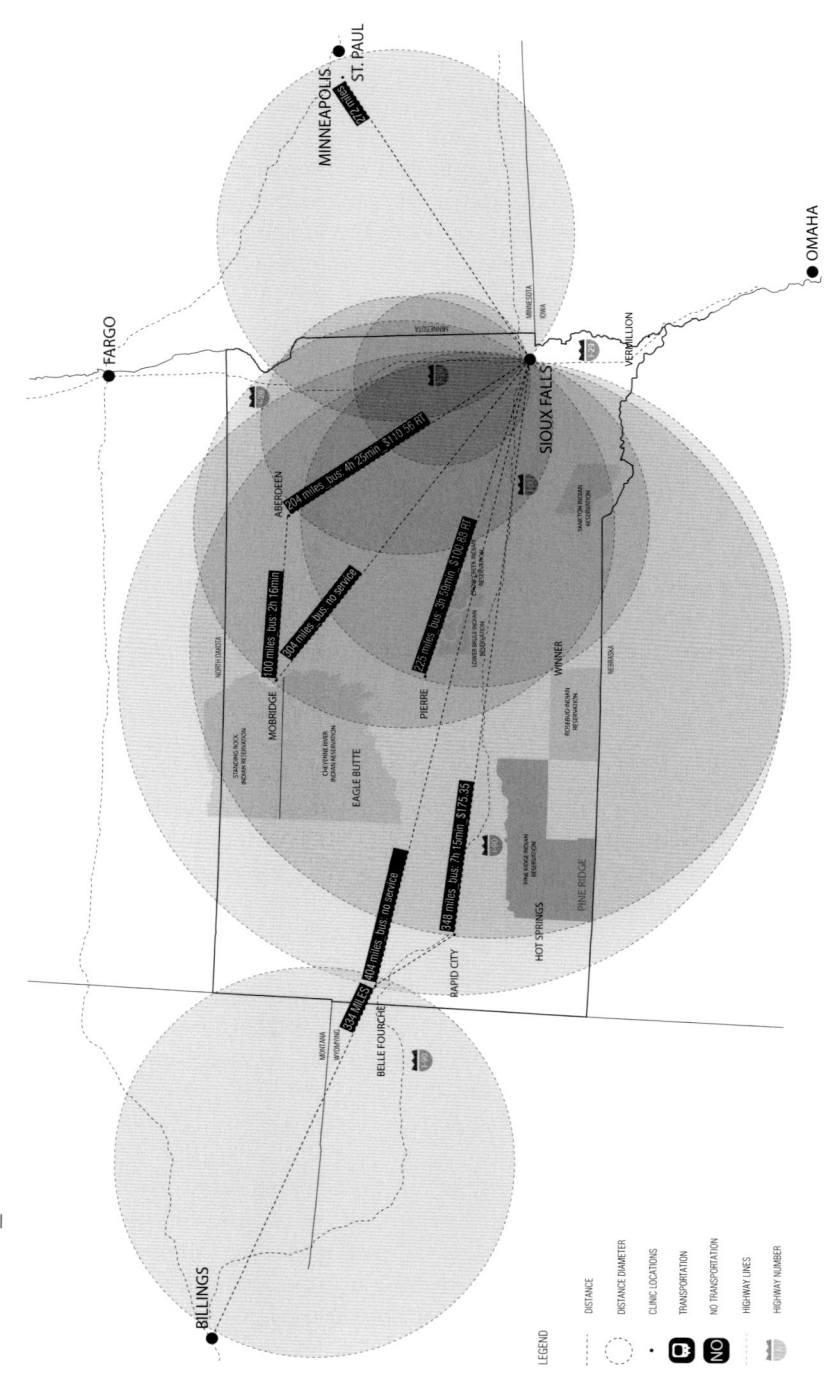

The diagram above contextualizes the location of the only clinic in Sioux Falls. Distances and transportation cost where available are provided. The diagram below locates several potential clinics with dashed circles when considering the intersections of poverty levels, locations of hospitals and pharmacies in order to serve the greatest number of women possible.

*CLINIC DISTANCES*  *POTENTIAL CLINICS*  *HOSPITALS*  *PHARMACIES*  *POVERTY*  *RELIGIOUS CENTERS*

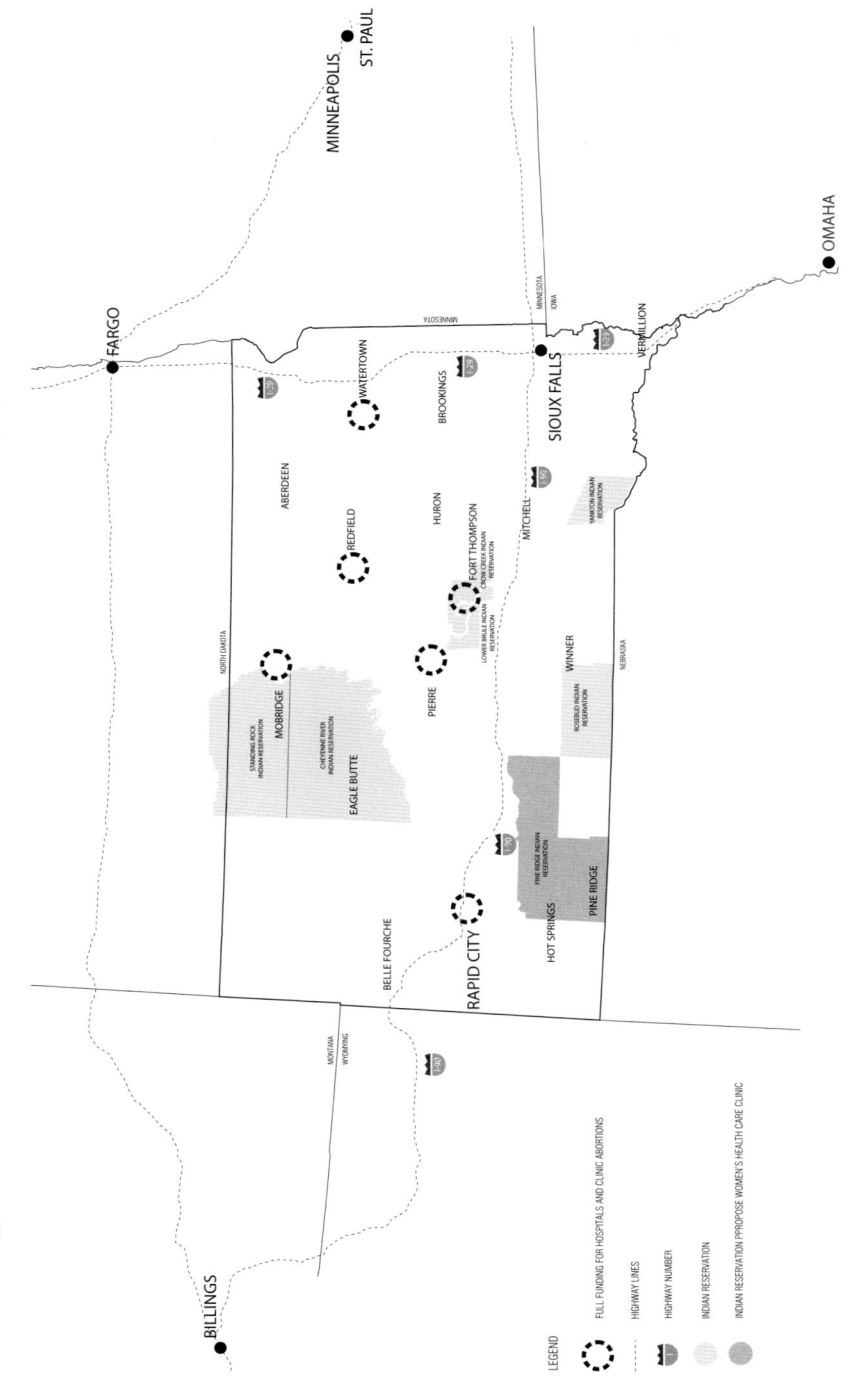

Fig. 5.14b  South Dakota potential clinics

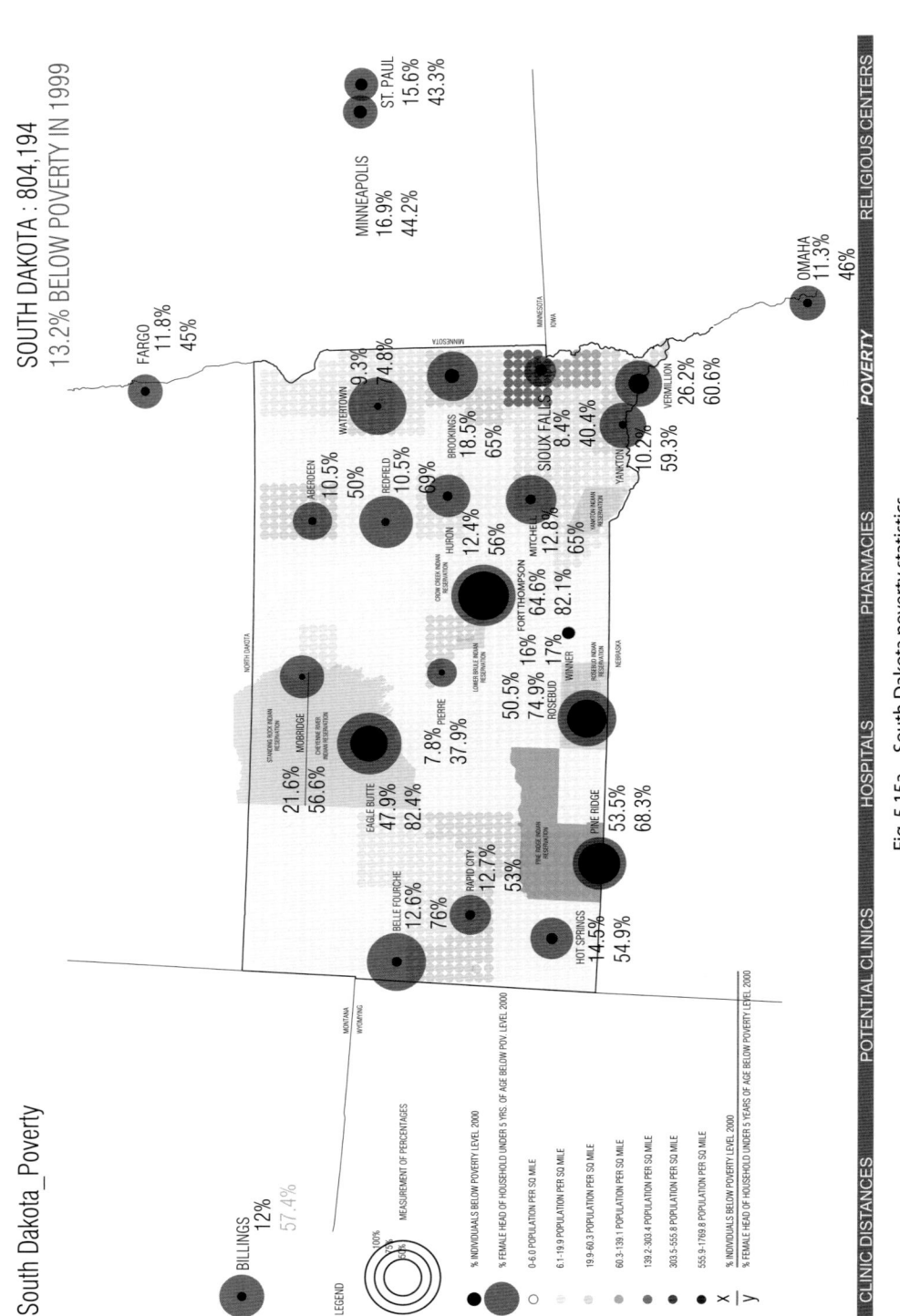

Fig. 5.15a  South Dakota poverty statistics

Using 1999 Census data, the diagram above compares poverty statistics for individuals (small dark circles) to single women head of household with children under five (FhdH c<5) against population (smaller background gray dots) throughout the state (large lighter gray circles). You will note how large the percentage of FhdH c<5 are statewide. The diagram below illustrates how many religious centers there are throughout all of South Dakota.

South Dakota_Religious Centers

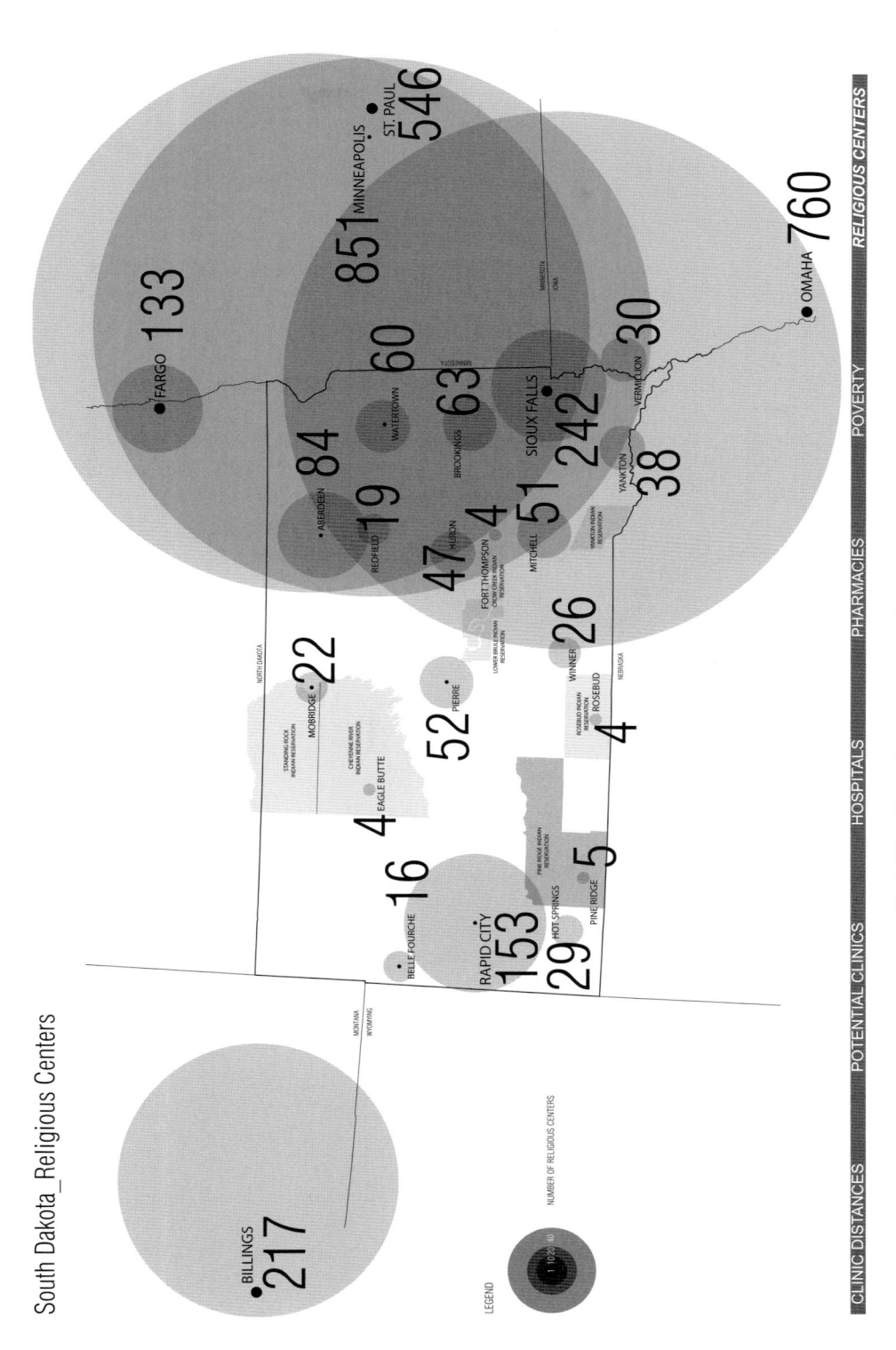

Fig. 5.15b  South Dakota location of religious centers

in a far less populated and remote city like Eagle Butte, 47.9 percent of individuals and 82.4 percent of FhdH c<5 live below the line of poverty.[38] Not only are these statistics extremely high but the state of South Dakota also restricts public funding for abortion. As Supreme Court Justice Ruth Bader Ginsburg observed "There will never be a woman of means without choice anymore … we have a policy that affects only poor women, and it can never be otherwise … the government has no business making that choice for a woman."[39]

**List of South Dakota State Restrictions**

- Unconstitutional and criminal abortion bans.
- TRAP, state subjects providers to burdensome restrictions not applied to other medical professions.
- Physician-only restriction; state prohibits certain qualified health care professionals from performing abortions.
- State allows certain entities to refuse specific reproductive health services, information or referrals.
- State prohibits use of telemedicine for performance of medication abortion.
- State restricts post-viability abortions.
- Women are subjected to biased counseling requirements.
- State requires mandatory 24-hour delay before receiving an abortion; can be provided by phone.
- State requires mandatory parental notice.
- State prohibits public funding for women eligible for state medical assistance for general health care unless procedure is necessary to preserve the woman's life.[40]

Another aspect that differentiates South Dakota from other states is the number and size of Native American reservations located throughout the state. Reservations are beyond federal jurisdiction, subject primarily to internal governance. Given that South Dakota tried to overturn *Roe v. Wade* and thus make abortion illegal in 2006 and 2008, the clinic and additional spaces of access in this state offered an interesting area for investigation because of their political and spatial potential. The proposed illegalization coincided with the announcement in 2006 by Cecilia Fire Thunder, Oglala Sioux tribal president on the Pine Ridge Indian Reservation, of her intention to create a health clinic for women on the reservation.[41] In the event Governor Mike Rounds signed the South Dakota abortion ban into law, the reservation clinic would begin to provide abortions. Because Native American reservations are beyond federal jurisdiction, Cecilia Fire Thunder was dramatically expanding the idea of access beyond federal government intervention. Although this did not happen, the idea of establishing women's reproductive health care services on over 300[42] reservations across the United States completely alters the landscape of access creating a realm beyond government control. This is similar in the way Women on Waves operate beyond international sovereign boundaries.

South Dakota_Hospitals

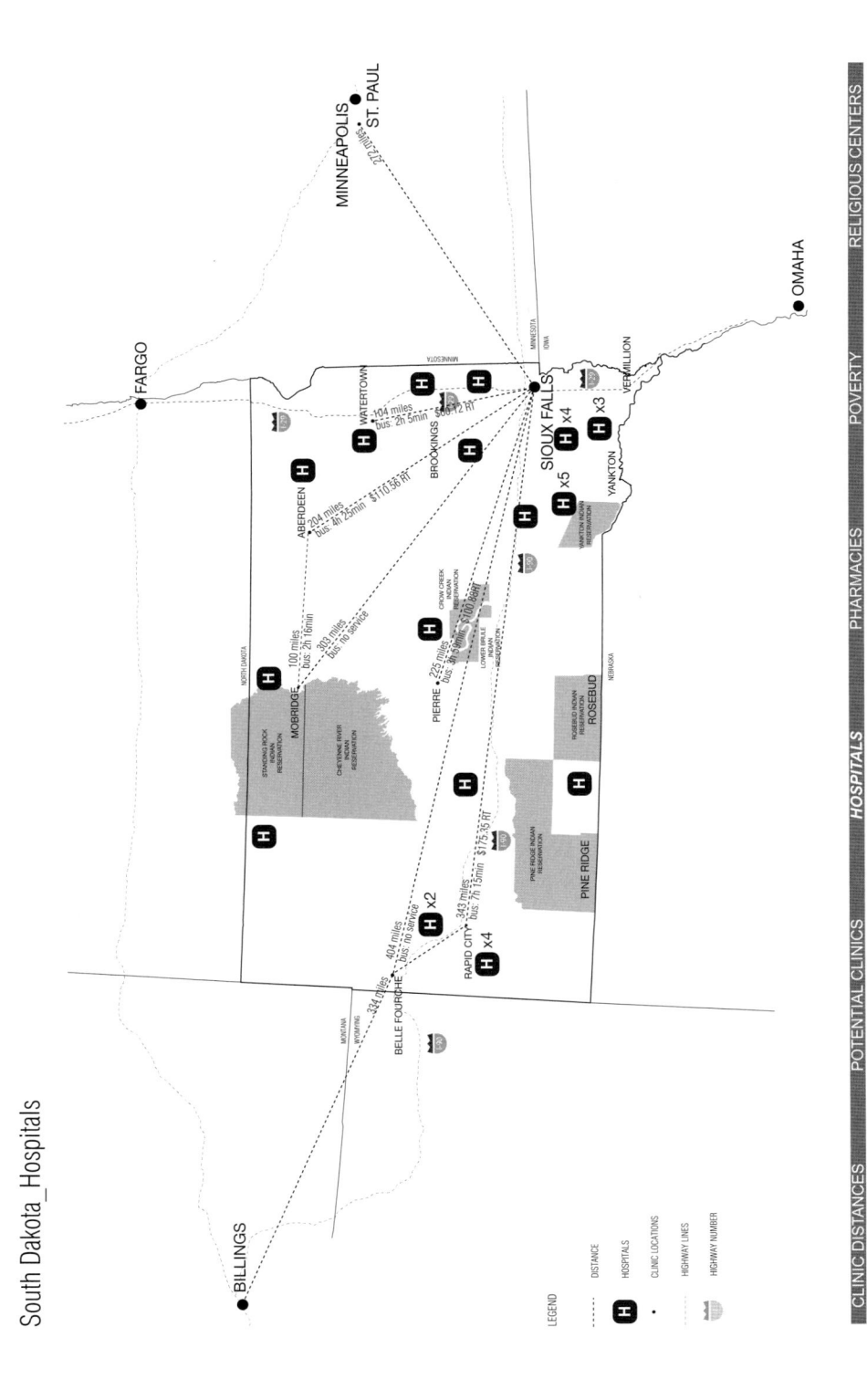

Fig. 5.16a  South Dakota hospitals
This diagram locates all the hospitals throughout the state

CLINIC DISTANCES | POTENTIAL CLINICS | HOSPITALS | PHARMACIES | POVERTY | RELIGIOUS CENTERS

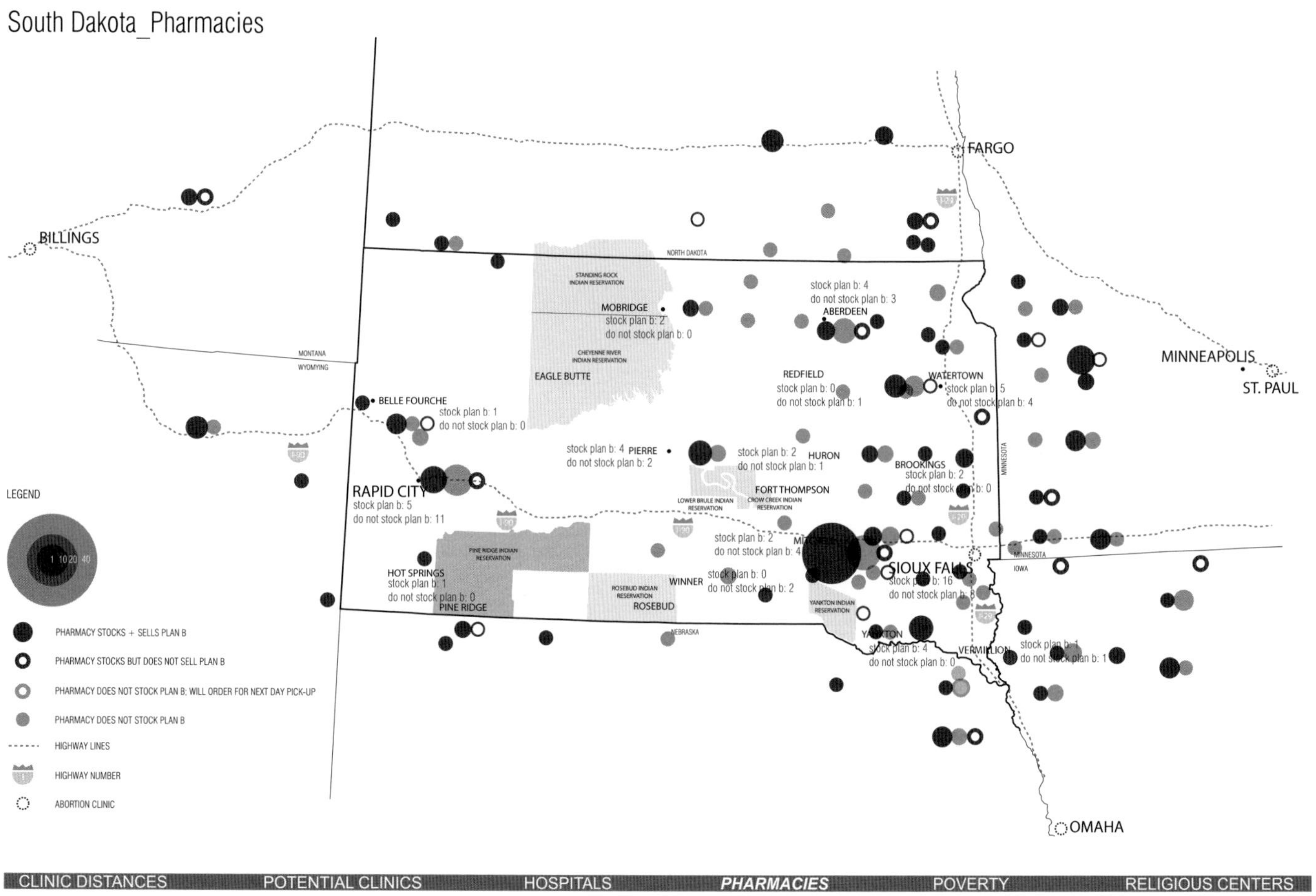

Fig. 5.16b  South Dakota pharmacies
This diagram locates all the pharmacies noting how many stock and sell EC.

South Dakota_Pharmacies

SOUTH DAKOTA POPULATION : 804,194
13.2% BELOW POVERTY IN 1999
145 PHARMACIES TOTAL IN THE STATE OF S. DAKOTA

PHARMACY STATISTICS

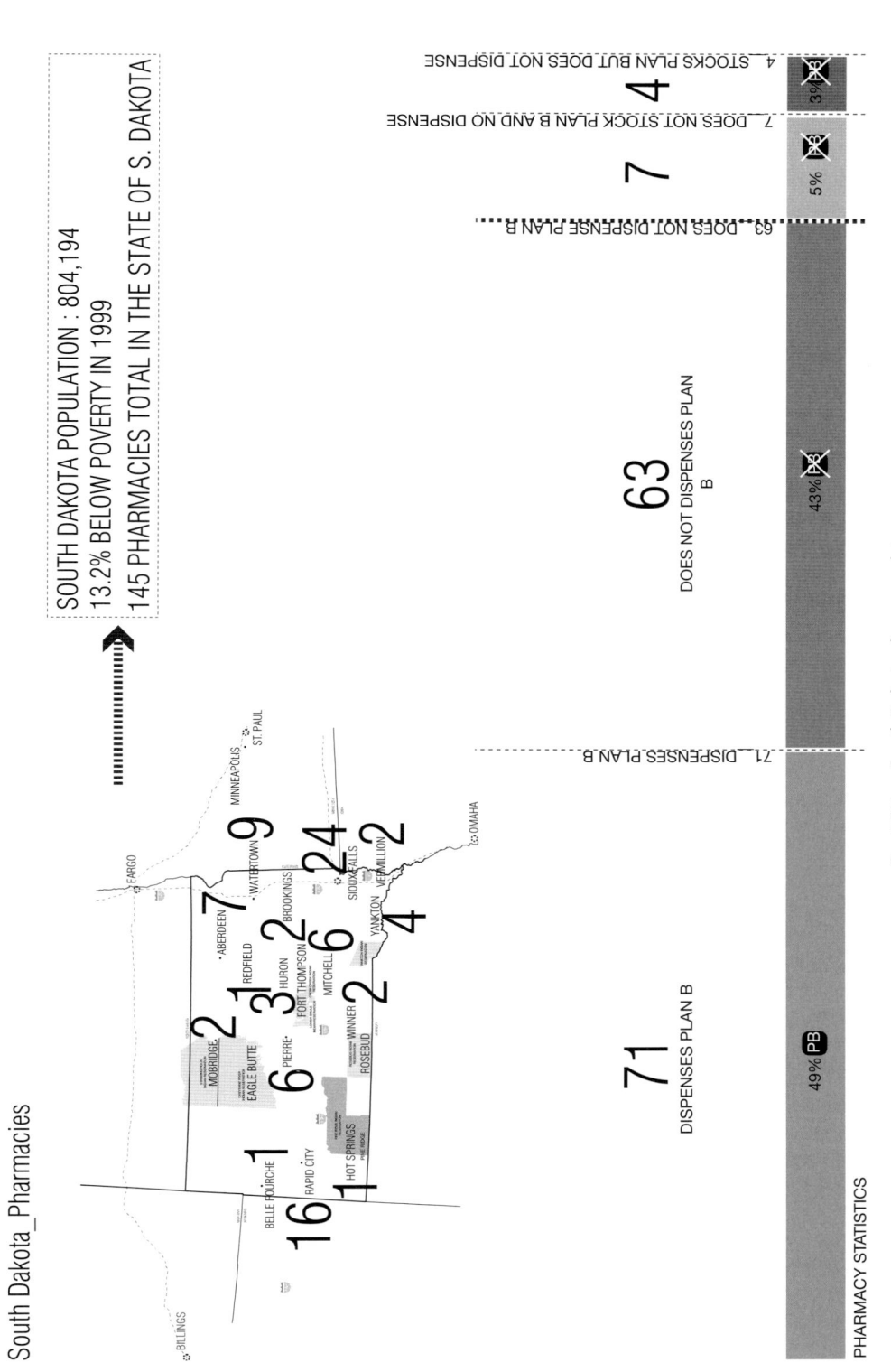

71 DISPENSES PLAN B
63 DOES NOT DISPENSES PLAN B
21 DISPENSES PLAN B
7 DOES NOT STOCK PLAN B AND NO DISPENSE
4 STOCKS PLAN BUT DOES NOT DISPENSE

49% PB
43%
5%
3%

Fig. 5.17a    South Dakota pharmacy data

South Dakota _ Religious Centers

LEGEND
——— # OF PHARMACIES
·········· DOES NOT STOCK PLAN B
– – – STOCKS PLAN B

"don't carry it" 33
"we don't have any but we'll get it tomorrow" 16
"we don't carry it and even if we did we don't dispense it" 9
"will get it tomorrow"
"we don't"
"we carry it but don't dispense it"

ABERDEEN
ARMOUR
BELLE FOURCHE
BERESFORD
BOWDLE
BRANDON
BROOKINGS
CANTON
CHAMBERLAIN
CLARK
CLEAR LAKE
CORSICA
DAKOTA DUNES
DEADWOOD
DELL RAPIDS
ELK POINT
EUREKA
FAULKTON
FLANDREAU
FREEMAN
GETTYSBURG
GREGORY
GROTON
HOT SPRINGS
HURON
IPSWICH
LAKE PRESTON
LEMMON
LENNOX
MADISON
MILBANK
MILLER
MITCHELL
MOBRIDGE
PARKER
PARKSTON
PIERRE
PLATTE
RAPID CITY
REDFIELD
SALEM
SIOUX FALLS
SISSETON
SPEARFISH
STURGIS
TYNDALL
VERMILLION
VIBORG
WAGNER
WATERTOWN
WEBSTER
WESSINGTON SPRINGS
WHITE RIVER
WINNER
YANKTON

Fig. 5.17b  South Dakota pharmacist replies

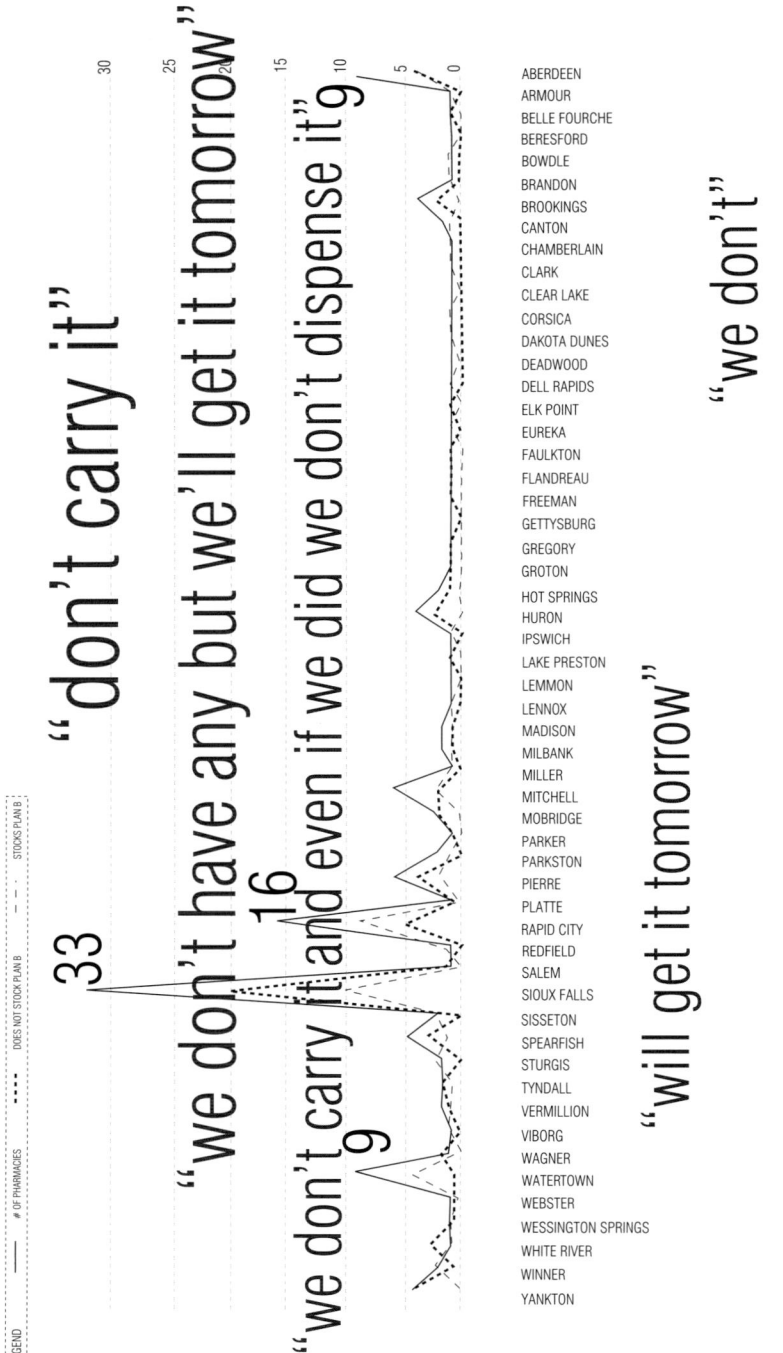

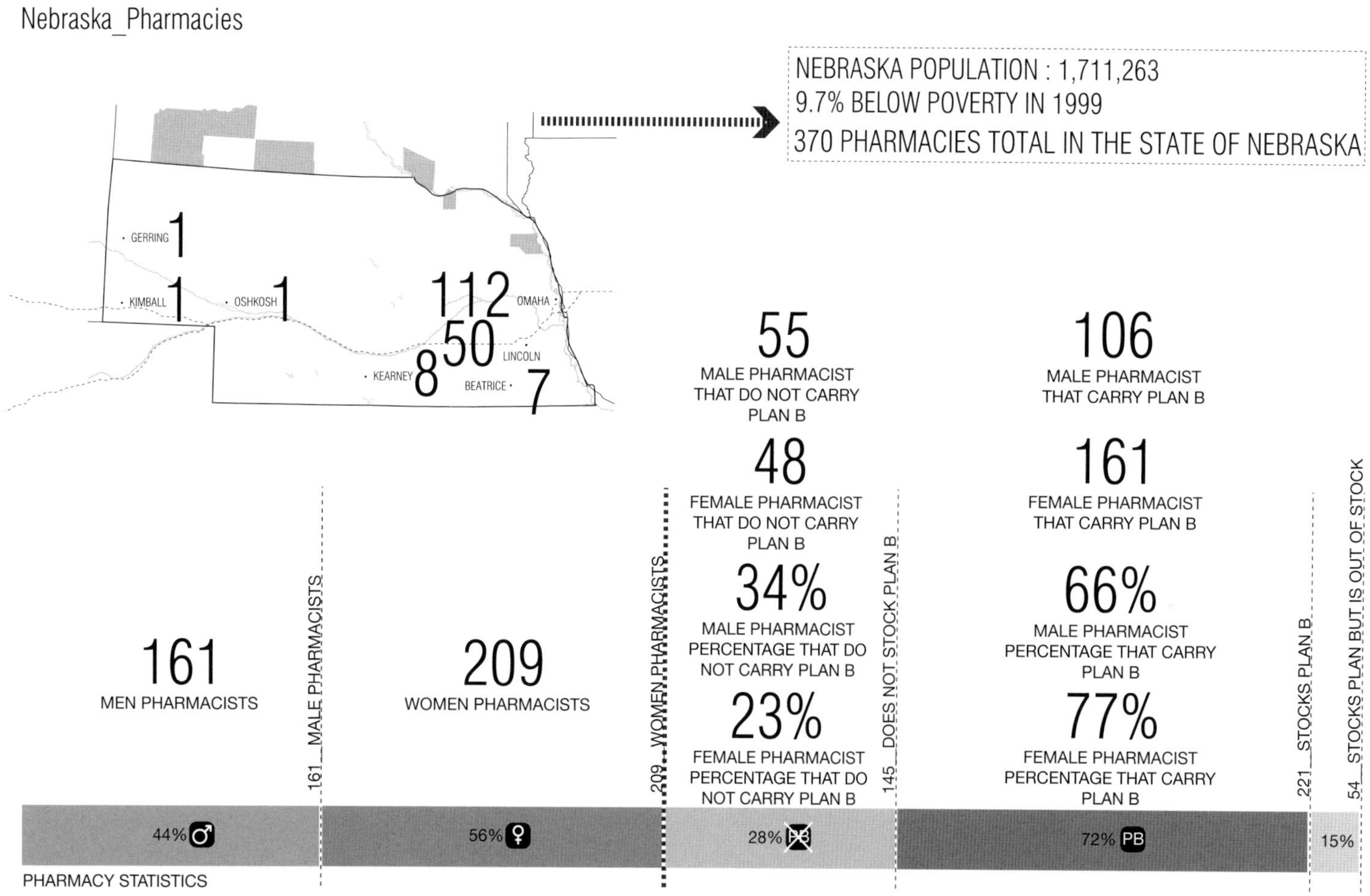

Nebraska_Pharmacies

NEBRASKA POPULATION : 1,711,263
9.7% BELOW POVERTY IN 1999
370 PHARMACIES TOTAL IN THE STATE OF NEBRASKA

- GERRING  1
- KIMBALL  1
- OSHKOSH  1
- OMAHA  112
- LINCOLN  50
- KEARNEY  8
- BEATRICE  7

**106** MALE PHARMACIST THAT CARRY PLAN B

**161** FEMALE PHARMACIST THAT CARRY PLAN B

**66%** MALE PHARMACIST PERCENTAGE THAT CARRY PLAN B

**77%** FEMALE PHARMACIST PERCENTAGE THAT CARRY PLAN B

**55** MALE PHARMACIST THAT DO NOT CARRY PLAN B

**48** FEMALE PHARMACIST THAT DO NOT CARRY PLAN B

**34%** MALE PHARMACIST PERCENTAGE THAT DO NOT CARRY PLAN B

**23%** FEMALE PHARMACIST PERCENTAGE THAT DO NOT CARRY PLAN B

**209** WOMEN PHARMACISTS

**161** MEN PHARMACISTS

161 MALE PHARMACISTS
209 WOMEN PHARMACISTS
145 DOES NOT STOCK PLAN B
221 STOCKS PLAN B
54 STOCKS PLAN BUT IS OUT OF STOCK

PHARMACY STATISTICS

44% ♂  |  56% ♀  |  28% ⌧  |  72% PB  |  15%

Fig. 5.18a    Nebraska pharmacy data

Fig. 5.18b  Nebraska pharmacist replies

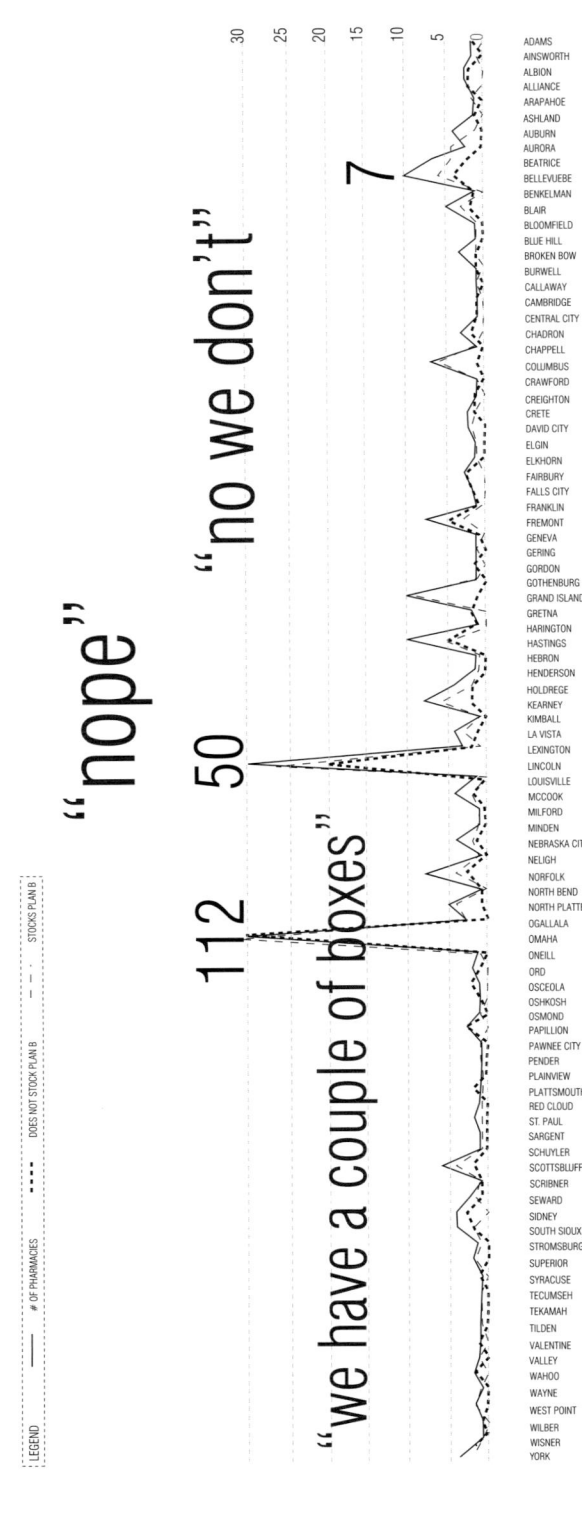

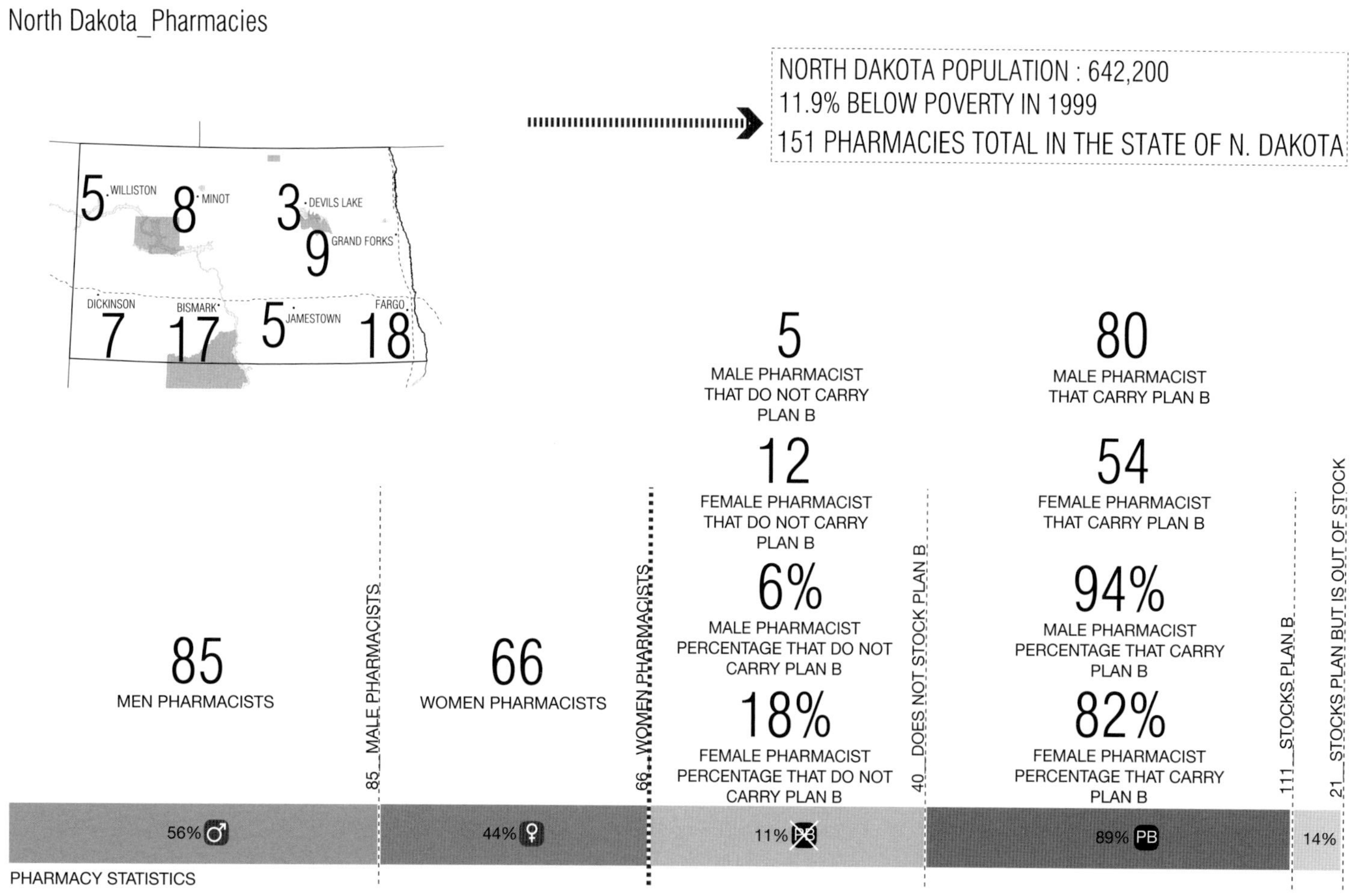

North Dakota_Pharmacies

NORTH DAKOTA POPULATION : 642,200
11.9% BELOW POVERTY IN 1999
151 PHARMACIES TOTAL IN THE STATE OF N. DAKOTA

5 WILLISTON
8 MINOT
3 DEVILS LAKE
9 GRAND FORKS
5 JAMESTOWN
18 FARGO
7 DICKINSON
17 BISMARCK

**85** MEN PHARMACISTS

**66** WOMEN PHARMACISTS

**5** MALE PHARMACIST THAT DO NOT CARRY PLAN B

**12** FEMALE PHARMACIST THAT DO NOT CARRY PLAN B

**6%** MALE PHARMACIST PERCENTAGE THAT DO NOT CARRY PLAN B

**18%** FEMALE PHARMACIST PERCENTAGE THAT DO NOT CARRY PLAN B

**80** MALE PHARMACIST THAT CARRY PLAN B

**54** FEMALE PHARMACIST THAT CARRY PLAN B

**94%** MALE PHARMACIST PERCENTAGE THAT CARRY PLAN B

**82%** FEMALE PHARMACIST PERCENTAGE THAT CARRY PLAN B

85 MALE PHARMACISTS
66 WOMEN PHARMACISTS
40 DOES NOT STOCK PLAN B
111 STOCKS PLAN B
21 STOCKS PLAN BUT IS OUT OF STOCK

PHARMACY STATISTICS
56% ♂ | 44% ♀ | 11% ✗ | 89% PB | 14%

Fig. 5.19a  North Dakota pharmacy data

North Dakota Pharmacies

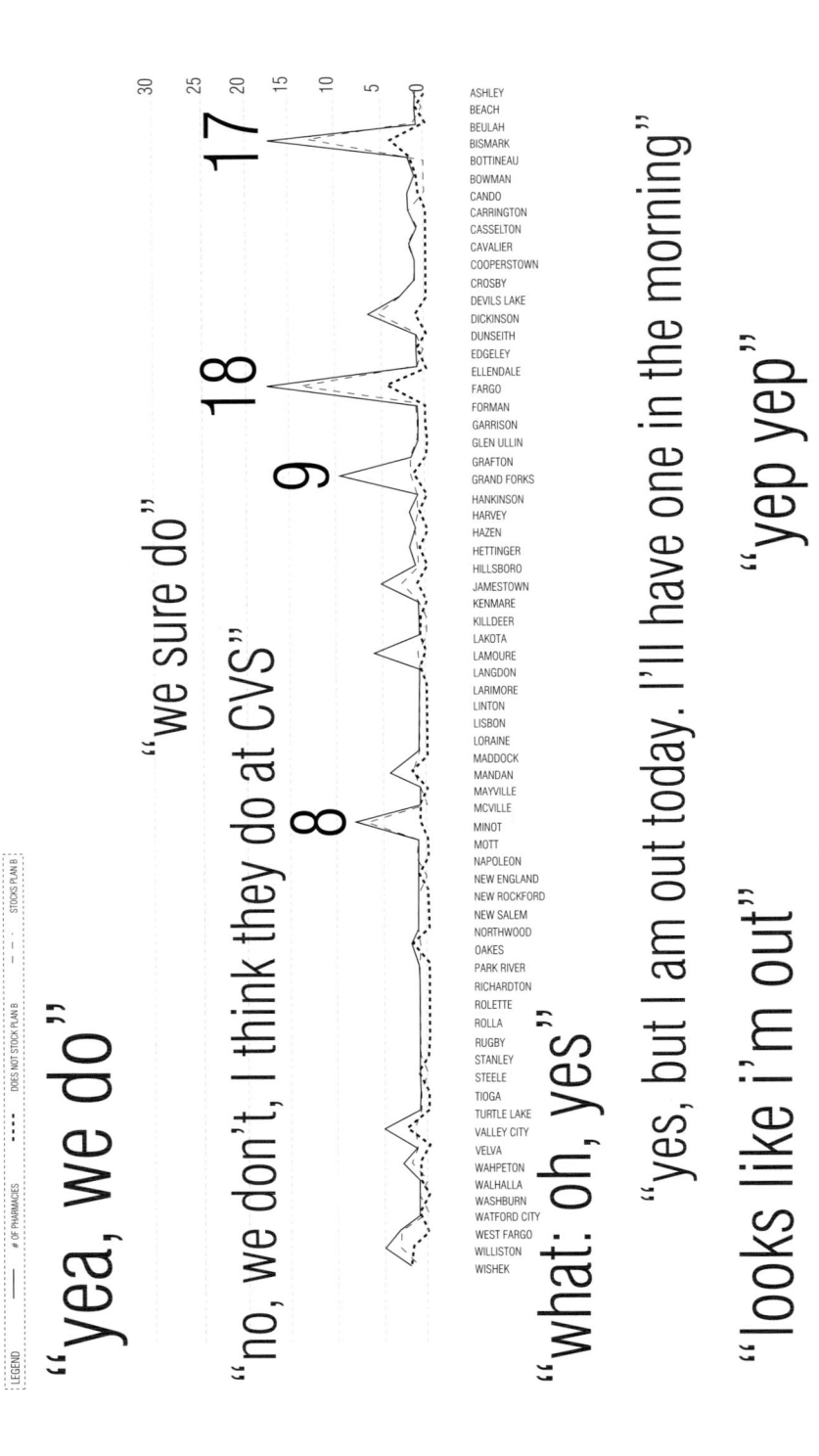

LEGEND
——— # OF PHARMACIES
••••••• DOES NOT STOCK PLAN B
— — — STOCKS PLAN B

"yea, we do"

"we sure do"

"no, we don't, I think they do at CVS"

"what: oh, yes"

"yes, but I am out today. I'll have one in the morning"

"yep yep"

"looks like i'm out"

ASHLEY
BEACH
BEULAH
BISMARK
BOTTINEAU
BOWMAN
CANDO
CARRINGTON
CASSELTON
CAVALIER
COOPERSTOWN
CROSBY
DEVILS LAKE
DICKINSON
DUNSEITH
EDGELEY
ELLENDALE
FARGO
FORMAN
GARRISON
GLEN ULLIN
GRAFTON
GRAND FORKS
HANKINSON
HARVEY
HAZEN
HETTINGER
HILLSBORO
JAMESTOWN
KENMARE
KILLDEER
LAKOTA
LAMOURE
LANGDON
LARIMORE
LINTON
LISBON
LORAINE
MADDOCK
MANDAN
MAYVILLE
MCVILLE
MINOT
MOTT
NAPOLEON
NEW ENGLAND
NEW ROCKFORD
NEW SALEM
NORTHWOOD
OAKES
PARK RIVER
RICHARDTON
ROLETTE
ROLLA
RUGBY
STANLEY
STEELE
TIOGA
TURTLE LAKE
VALLEY CITY
VELVA
WAHPETON
WALHALLA
WASHBURN
WATFORD CITY
WEST FARGO
WILLISTON
WISHEK

Fig. 5.19b  North Dakota pharmacist replies

The statistics are based on the results from calling all the pharmacies in the South Dakota in 2006 and documenting their response to the question "Do you sell emergency contraception? Can I fill my prescription?" At the time I was calling in South Dakota you needed a prescription to access the medication regardless of age. By the time we were calling in Nebraska and North Dakota in 2008, you still needed a prescription to access this medication if younger than 18 years of age.

Based on this data, reproductive healthcare dramatically shifts to women and expands availability especially when you take into account all the hospitals throughout the state. Abortion clinics are no longer the sole place of access.

## WEST

**Spatial Experiences**

Almost all the clinics I have visited and providers I have interviewed were deeply concerned with the feeling their clinics exuded. Architects would normally discuss this in terms of aesthetic choices but it was interesting to notice that providers rarely talked about their clinics in those terms. More often, the discussion centered upon colors and materials used to create spaces of healing and peacefulness, how patients would move through clinic spaces and what sorts of functional issues the clinic must address. Although I would deliberately ask questions that would reveal underlying aesthetic choices, I realized that although providers understand these issues on a more intuitive level, this was not the way they wanted to discuss them. A few providers interviewed in this region worked with architects or interior designers helping them create the types of spaces and spatial workflow they desired for their individual practices.

One particular provider I interviewed, who has practices in neighboring states, strongly believes that security remains an issue for abortion clinics. Clinics are still getting bombed and tampered with in regular frequency.[43] In fact, she thinks it is still as bad as it was in the nineties. In response to her concerns, she worked with an architect in one of her clinics to create a circular spatial flow of patient care. Patients would not exit through the same door they entered in through. This was a small yet clear security measure the doctor required so that no one in the waiting room would know who was leaving and under what circumstances they would be leaving.[44] I believe this is an extremely thoughtful gesture towards patient's privacy, security and anonymity. The spatial organization of her clinic is one of the most thoughtful clinic layouts I have seen.

Another clinic director mentioned intentionally picking colors that would help produce an atmosphere of healing. This clinic also worked with an interior designer on a pro bono basis guiding their choices toward ones helping further create a healing and relaxing environment. Although invested in the positive affect the clinic can have on her patients, this director was quite candid about how her spatial decisions have been made in anticipation of what the anti-choice movement can or may do. She even went as far as declaring that the "anti's dictate a lot of what we do in terms of how we design our building ...."[45]

I would also ask about their considerations of clinic location during interviews. I was interested in understanding how clinic providers understand their location's effect on their practice. More often than not, the clinics I visited were spaces retro-fitted to become an abortion clinic. Many are making the most of the space they have available. Clearly these constraints influence not only the interior workings of the clinic based on their spatial limitations but also affects how a patient is able to access their clinic. Location can hinder and maybe unbeknownst to the providers, facilitate protestors' activities and publicity.

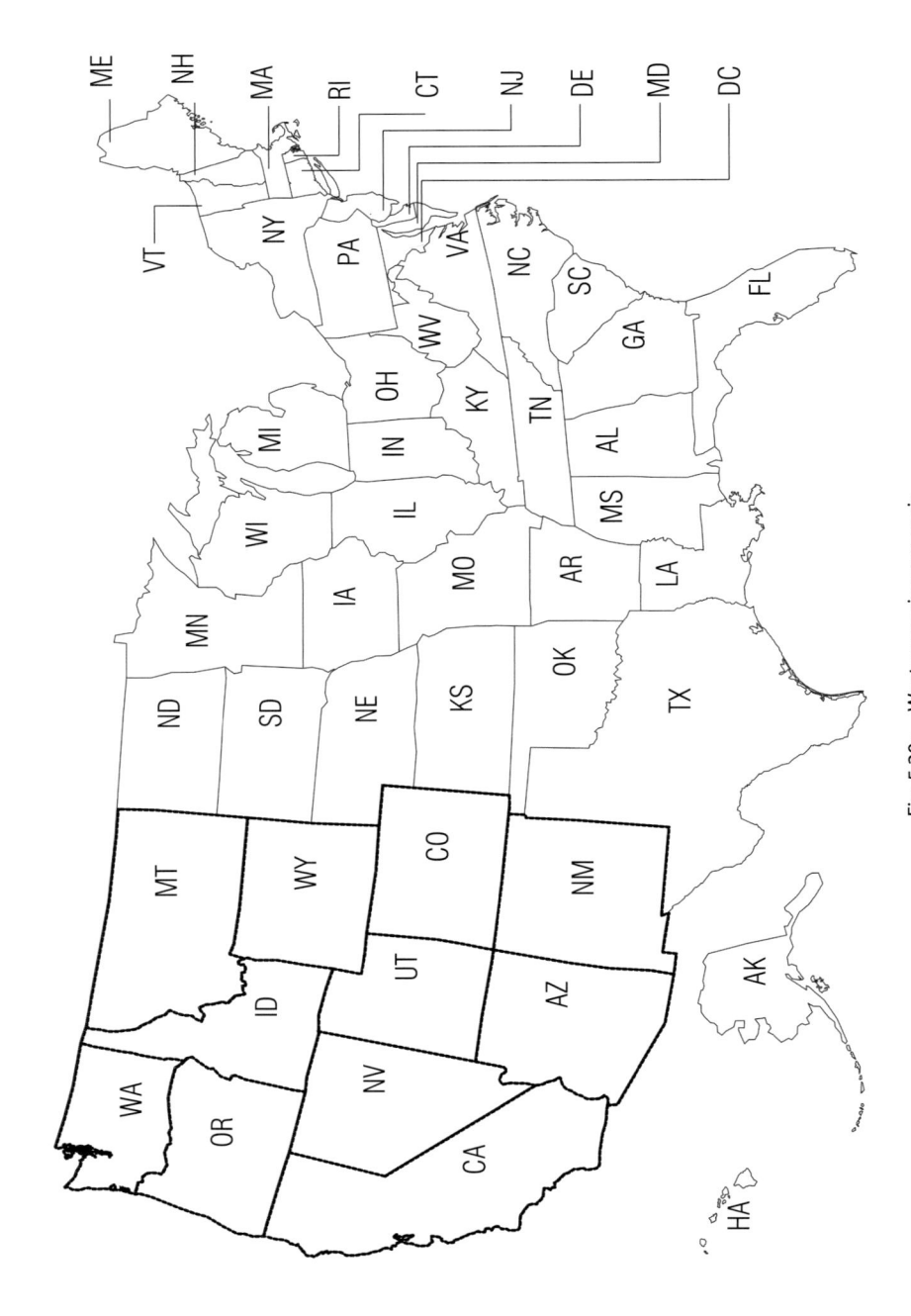

Fig. 5.20a  Western region synopsis

This map excerpt provides an overview of the states officially included as part of the south defined by the US Census Bureau. Included are the number of abortion providers and number of state restrictions.

USA Regions _West

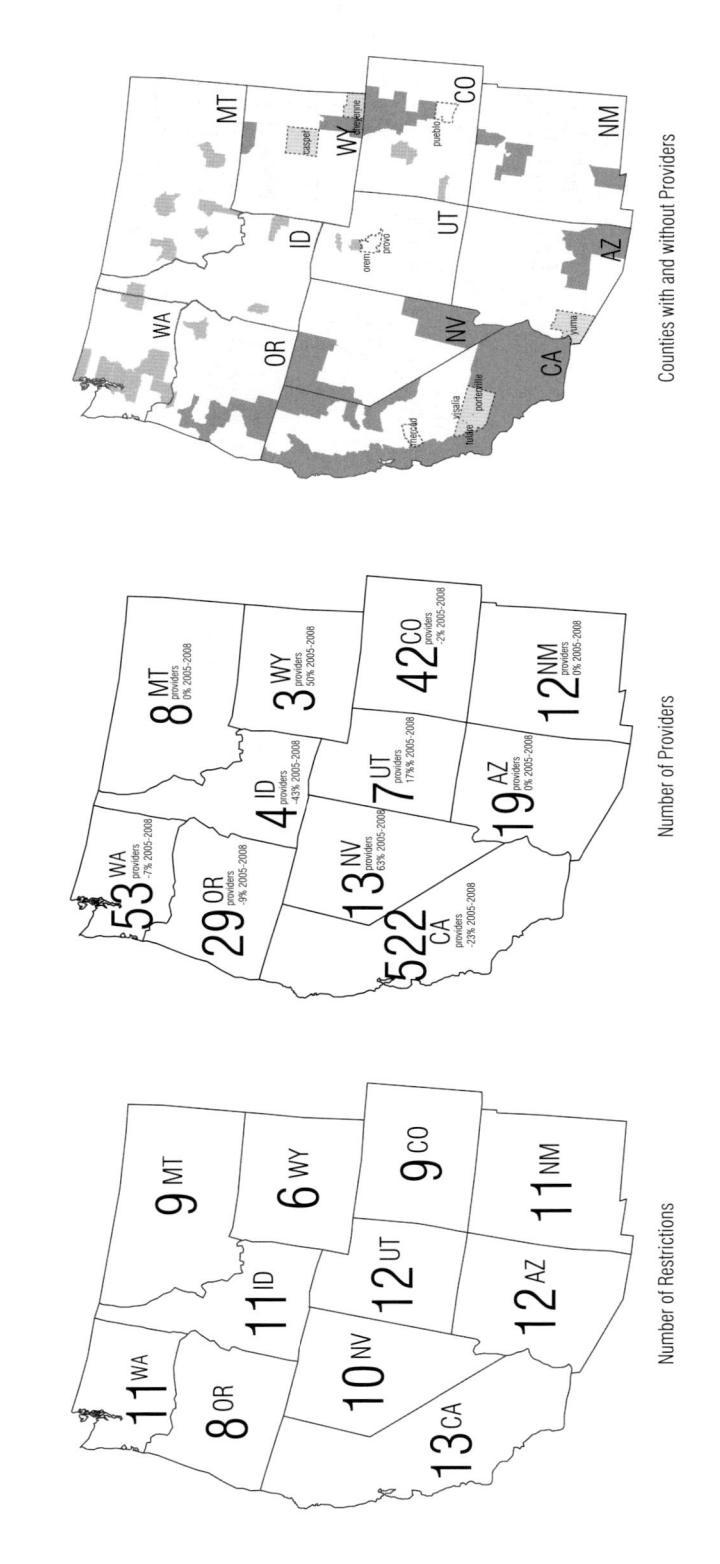

Fig. 5.20b  Western region synopsis

One particular clinic director who began her career in abortion care in the northeast and moved to the west coast had much to say about clinic locations and the differences she experienced between the two coasts. As a non-profit everything is about location and affordability. However, there are cost considerations to everything. As a result of being incredibly vigilant about security, location was always discussed in terms of protection and the ability to create as secure a space as possible. She would prefer to have her clinic not be located on the ground floor because the only point of access is from the front door. If you are located on a higher floor, there is the possibility of being surrounded and trapped in the elevator. As we were discussing the range of location possibilities, it became clear that every space comes with both positive and negative factors. No space is perfect; there will always be challenges to providing the securest space as possible.

She also thought that in their particular case being in a free-standing clinic did not provide as many logistical challenges as being in an office park location. A clinic is less vulnerable as a single entity because there were not as many concerns about how to make their floor or entrance from the hallway more secure.[46] On the other hand, another doctor I interviewed who is part of several abortion practices in neighboring states had a different opinion. Working in both multi-story locations and single story buildings, her varied experiences has led her to believe that being in a multi-practice location with a variety of different types of medical offices is advantageous and provides far more anonymity than other types of locations. One of the issues her practice always considers before seeking new space is where does the property line fall and how far away is this property line from the point of entrance into the clinic. This distance is crucial offering an easy buffer from protestors, patient parking and protest-free patient mobility. Her practice has also considered locating one of their clinics in a shopping mall but does not see this as a long-term expansion strategy. Similar to a free-standing clinic, she believes being located in a mall would be isolating. The primary reason she strongly advocates for the larger medical complex location is this type of site helps keep abortion in the mainstream. You are just another type of doctor practicing medicine among many other types of doctors and medical practices.

Another point this doctor made was regarding hospitals and care. She would gladly perform abortions in her local hospital but they will not allow her to do so. She believes that hospitals are acting as "moral arbiters of care." Hospitals in this particular city will not allow for the services to be paid for through insurance. With a voter referendum saying no to abortion care in this state hospital, the hospital board voted and decided to not allow abortions. Hospitals walk a fine line because they can lose their accreditation when there are no abortion providers to teach interns. It is common practice to have hospitals find independent local providers to provide this teaching component.[47]

**Separation of Church and State**

A sad but clear example of the necessity of maintaining separation between Church and state is demonstrated by the 2009 case in Phoenix, Arizona where a woman needed an abortion to save her life. Eleven weeks pregnant, this woman was admitted to St. Joseph's Hospital and Medical Center, a Catholic hospital, with pulmonary hypertension where her body was unable to deliver enough oxygen. If her pregnancy continued, she would die. The administrator at the time the patient was admitted, Sister Margaret McBride, gave her approval for the abortion and the woman's life was saved. As a result of this nun's decision granting permission for an abortion to be performed at a Catholic hospital, Sister McBride was excommunicated. The rational for the excommunication as Rev. John Ehrich, medical ethics director for the Diocese of Phoenix, stated: "There are some situations where the mother may in fact die along with her child. But — and this is the Catholic perspective — you can't do evil to bring about good. The end does not justify the means."[48] The larger issue this raises addressed by the American Civil Liberties Union is whether religious hospitals are violating the Emergency Medical Treatment and Active Labor Act, 42 U.S.C § 1395dd and the Conditions of Participation of Medicare and Medicaid, 42 C.F.R. § 482.13 by refusing to provide emergency reproductive health care even though these hospitals participate in the Medicare and Medicaid systems. The ACLU argues that "[r]eligiously affiliated hospitals are not exempt from complying with these laws, and cannot invoke their religious status to jeopardize the health and lives of pregnant women seeking medical care." Because Catholic hospitals operate 15 percent of the hospital beds in the United States and often are the only hospital a community has access to, many pregnant women may not receive appropriate or medically necessary care.[49] To try and further legislate this type of action, the House of Representatives passed the Protect Life Act on October 13, 2011 prohibiting women from purchasing health care covering abortion under the Affordable Care Act. Making it legal for hospitals to deny abortion for women with life-threatening conditions, this legislation goes further than any thus far in denying a woman's right to a legal abortion in an emergency.[50]

**Differing Attitudes**

One of the interesting revelations I had as I interviewed people was how doctors and providers in different parts of the country interpret legislation. Clearly support for abortion varies across the United States (and North America for that matter), and there are some who are willing to more liberally interpret legislation. Of all the providers and doctors I interviewed, one older doctor stated point-black that he has no problem broadly interpreting the informed consent law in order to provide care for those who need it most. The state mandated 24-hour informed consent prior to a woman's procedure places an extreme burden on some of his out-of-town patients. He will work with other clinics out of the area to help accommodate women who otherwise cannot afford the 24-hour waiting period. This doctor was adamant that if need be, he would take this all the way to the Supreme Court because as the law states, restrictions cannot create an undue burden on a woman seeking an abortion. Many of his patients travel great distances due to lack of providers nearby as well as in neighboring states and the 24-hour waiting period can create an undue burden. Additionally, he is also willing to wave fees due to hardship.[51]

## UTAH

### Distances to/from Several Cities in Utah

> Brigham City—Salt Lake City 38 miles bus: 45 min $26 RT
> Green River—Salt Lake City 175 miles bus: 3 hr 45 min $74 RT
> Cedar City—Las Vegas 166 miles bus: 3 hr $70 RT
> St. George—Las Vegas 119 miles bus: 2 hr 5 min $38 RT

The Guttmacher Institute reports that in 2008, 97 percent of Utah counties had no abortion provider with 64 percent of Utah women living in these counties. As has been noted by the Guttmacher Institute, the abortion rate in the United States can be directly connected to levels of poverty. In Utah, individuals living below the line of poverty are on average 9.8 percent. In Salt Lake City, the state capital and most populous city in the state, 15.3 percent of individuals live below the line of poverty and 38.4 percent of FhdH c<5 live below the line of poverty. In St. George, 11.6 percent of individuals live below the line of poverty and 64.10 percent of FhdH c<5 live below the line of poverty. In a far less populated and remote city like Roosevelt, 21.1 percent of individuals and 81.8 percent of FhdH c<5 live below the line of poverty.[52]

### List of Utah State Restrictions

- Unconstitutional and criminal abortion bans.
- TRAP, state subjects providers to burdensome restrictions not applied to other medical professions.
- Physician-only restriction; state prohibits certain qualified health care professionals from performing abortions.
- State restricts insurance coverage of abortion.
- State allows certain entities to refuse specific reproductive health services, information or referrals.
- State restricts post-viability abortions.
- Women are subjected to biased counseling requirements in person.
- State requires mandatory 24-hour delay before receiving an abortion.
- State requires mandatory parental notice and consent.
- State prohibits public funding for women eligible for state medical assistance for general health care unless procedure is necessary to preserve the woman's life or the pregnancy is the result of rape or incest or fetal abnormality incompatible with live birth.
- State law ensures women's access to emergency contraception by sexual assault survivors.[53]

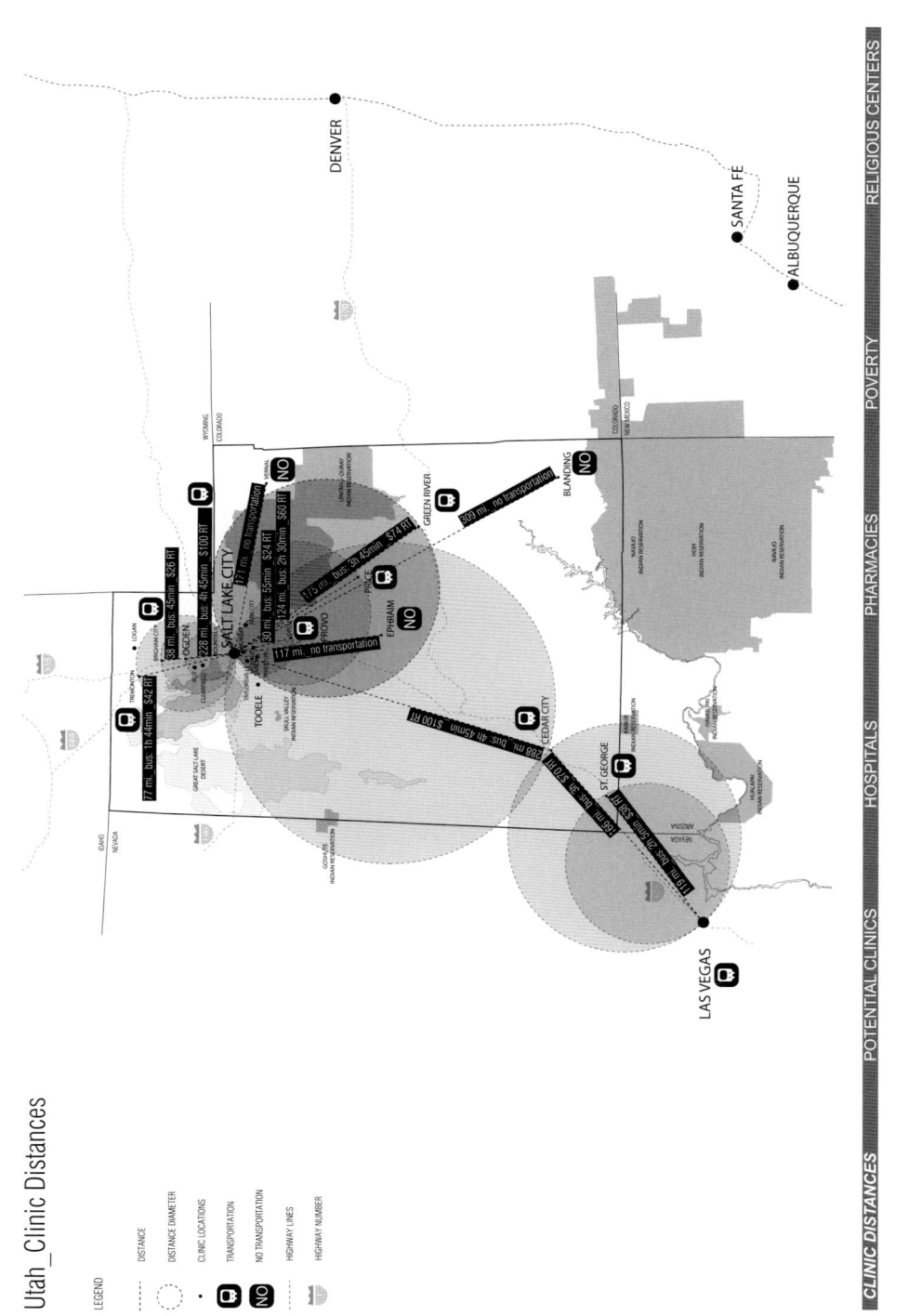

Fig. 5.21a  Utah clinic distances
This diagram contextualizes the location of the clinics within the state. Distances and transportation cost where available are provided

# Utah_Potential Clinics

**LEGEND**

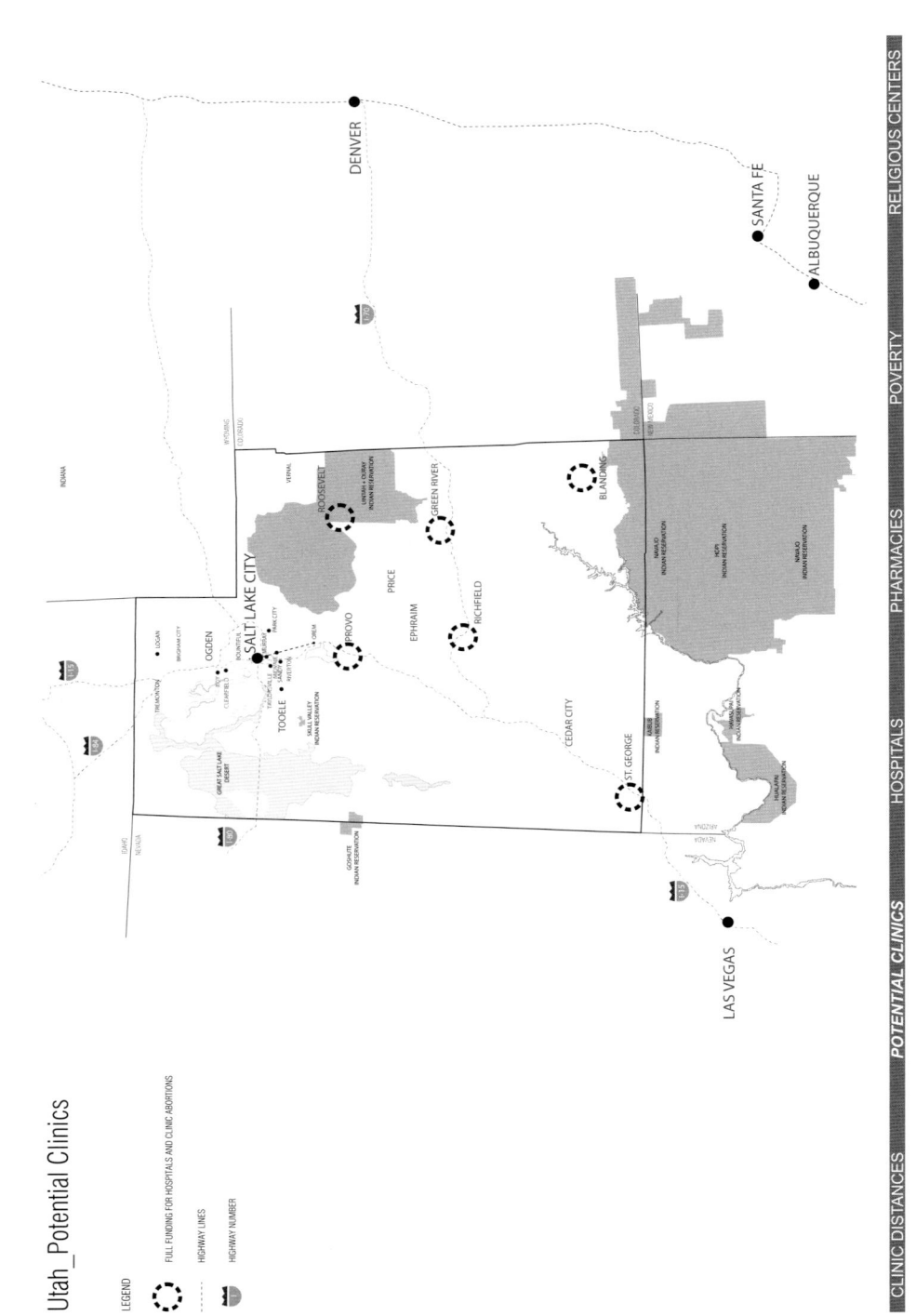

◯ FULL FUNDING FOR HOSPITALS AND CLINIC ABORTIONS
---- HIGHWAY LINES
🏠 HIGHWAY NUMBER

**Fig. 5.21b   Utah potential clinics**

This diagram locates several potential clinics with dashed circles when considering the intersections of poverty levels, locations of hospitals and pharmacies in order to serve the greatest number of women possible.

CLINIC DISTANCES | POTENTIAL CLINICS | HOSPITALS | PHARMACIES | POVERTY | RELIGIOUS CENTERS

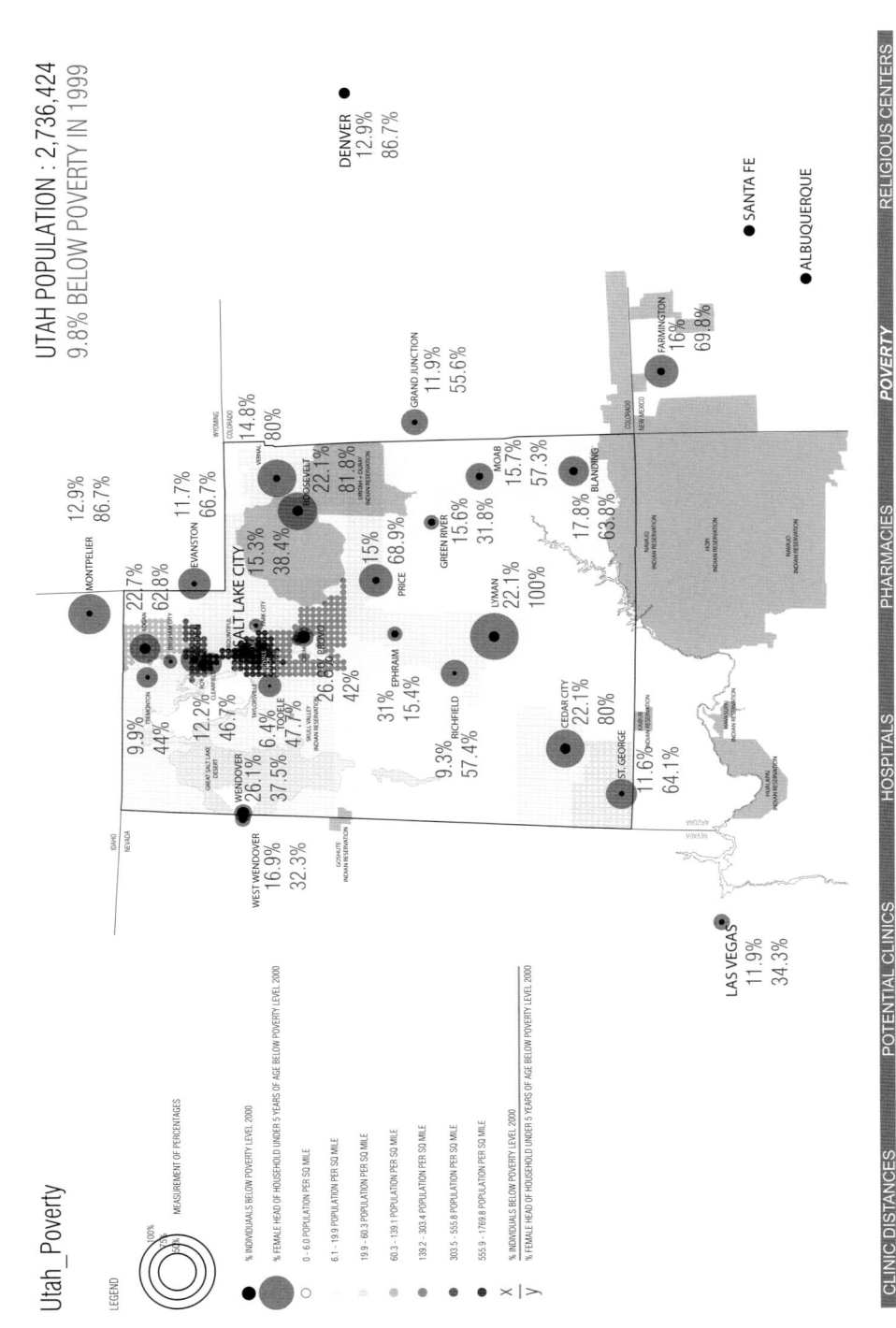

Fig. 5.22a  Utah poverty statistics

Using 1999 Census data, this diagram compares poverty statistics for individuals (small dark circles) to single women head of household with children under five (FhdH c<5) against population (smaller background gray dots) throughout the state (large lighter gray circles). Utah is a sparsely populated state. You will note how large the percentage of FhdH c<5 are statewide.

## Utah_Religious Centers

LEGEND

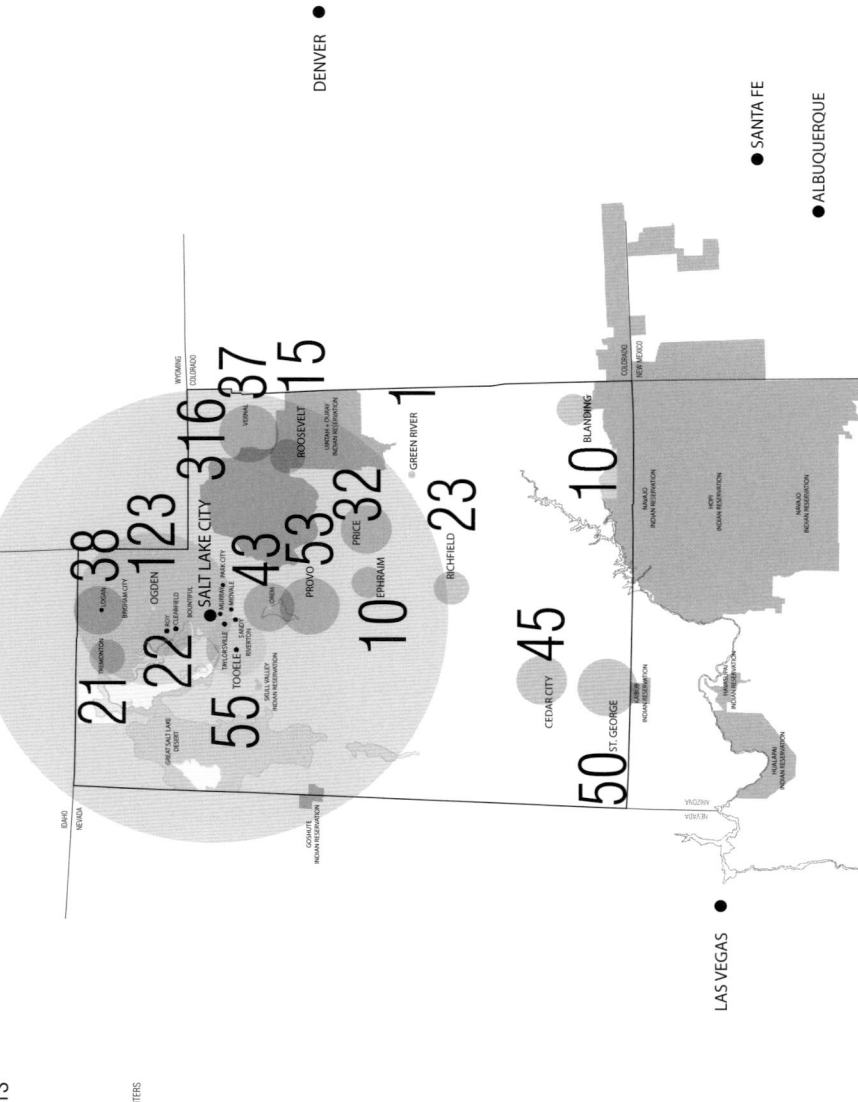

NUMBER OF RELIGIOUS CENTERS

Fig. 5.22b   Utah location of religious centers
This diagram illustrates how many religious centers there are throughout all of Utah.

CLINIC DISTANCES | POTENTIAL CLINICS | HOSPITALS | PHARMACIES | POVERTY | RELIGIOUS CENTERS

## OTHER POSSIBLE LANDSCAPES OF ACCESS

### Pharmacies, Contraception and Emergency Contraception

One way to think more broadly about reducing the need for abortions is through broad-based accurate sex education and access to contraception including Plan B® or what is commonly referred to as the morning-after pill or EC. In 1999, Plan B® was approved for prescription use. In 2003 the drug's manufacturer applied for non-prescription status but in 2004 was denied. In 2006, Plan B® was approved for over-the-counter availability for women 18 years and older and in 2009, this was expanded to include women 17 years and older. Although the FDA has recommended emergency contraception as a non-prescription drug, the Secretary of Health and Human Services Kathleen Sebelius overruled the FDA's decision thus continuing the intrusion of politics into science.[54]

Most people do not want to deal with this facet of sex; it is not glamorous, not particularly easy and therefore most do not do much about it. One doctor mentioned how she believes there is still a real stigma around EC as well as contraception. She hears from patients all the time "it just happened." Neither EC nor contraception is used widely enough. She suggests a marketing push with redesigned packaging to have more aesthetic appeal towards women. If EC were in every woman's medicine cabinet it would become far more effective. As this doctor noted, because people have to ask for it, because there is an additional step to access, it makes the whole encounter uncomfortable and discourages women from purchasing it. Some abortion clinics do sell EC making it easier to access if only women were more aware of this. Now available as an over-the-counter medication for women 17 years and older and as prescription-only for other minors, the local pharmacy is an indispensable tool in lowering the abortion rate and expanding access. Having called all the pharmacies in the state, the data collected includes whether each pharmacy stocks and sells Plan B®, stocks but does not sell Plan B®, does not stock but will order Plan B® for next day pick-up, or flatly refuses to stock and sell Plan B®. An important difference between hospital and pharmacy locations is that pharmacies are located in much smaller towns and are more widely accessible. Pharmacies have the potential of reaching a far greater number of people at a much earlier stage, potentially eliminating the need for an abortion.

One doctor speculated about the ease of purchasing EC or abortion pills as commonly referred to on the black market, especially across the border in Mexico. Selling them by the pill, they are less expensive than Plan B and work just as well. If these pills do not work then a woman can seek medical care and just say she is bleeding.[55] Recalling the pre-*Roe* days when women would seek emergency care for botched abortions, is this what women are forced to do again, even though abortion is legal in the United States?

### Hospitals

There are several ways to rethink the issues around access. The first is to reconsider the use of hospitals as places where abortions could be performed. As per Figure

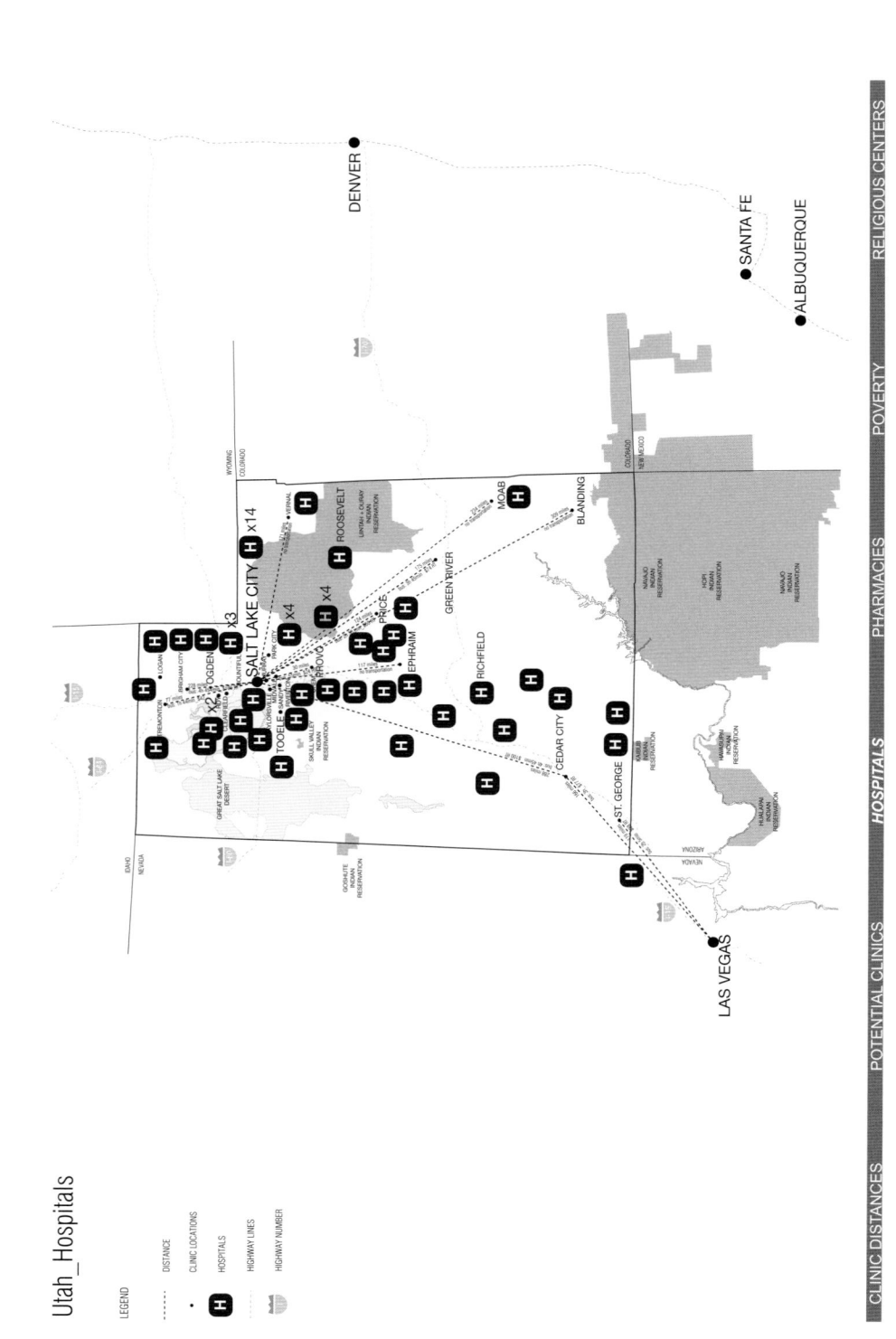

Fig. 5.23a  Utah hospitals

The diagram above locates all the hospitals throughout the state and the diagram below locates all the pharmacies noting how many stock and sell EC.

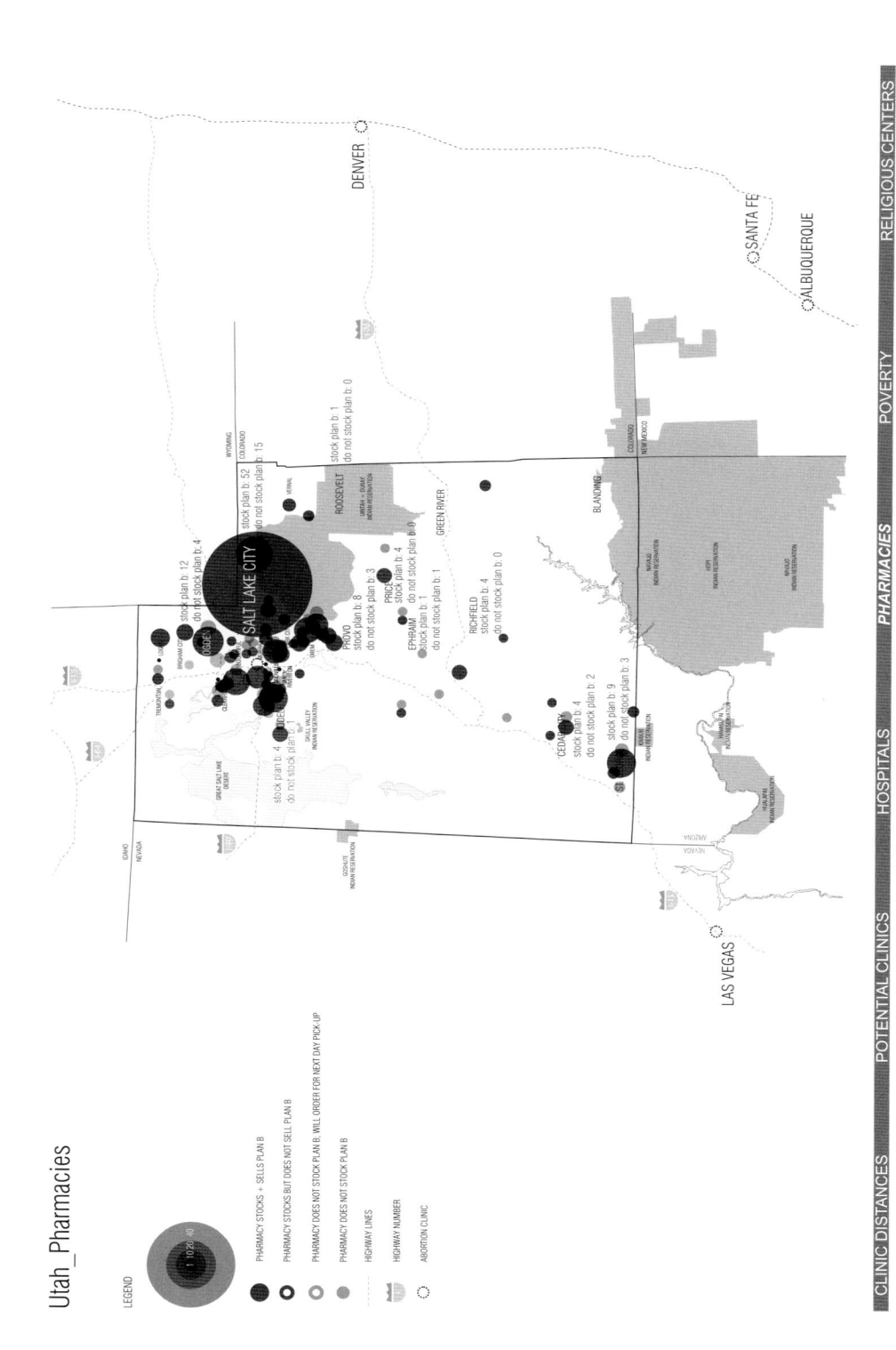

Fig. 5.23b  Utah pharmacies

Utah_Pharmacies

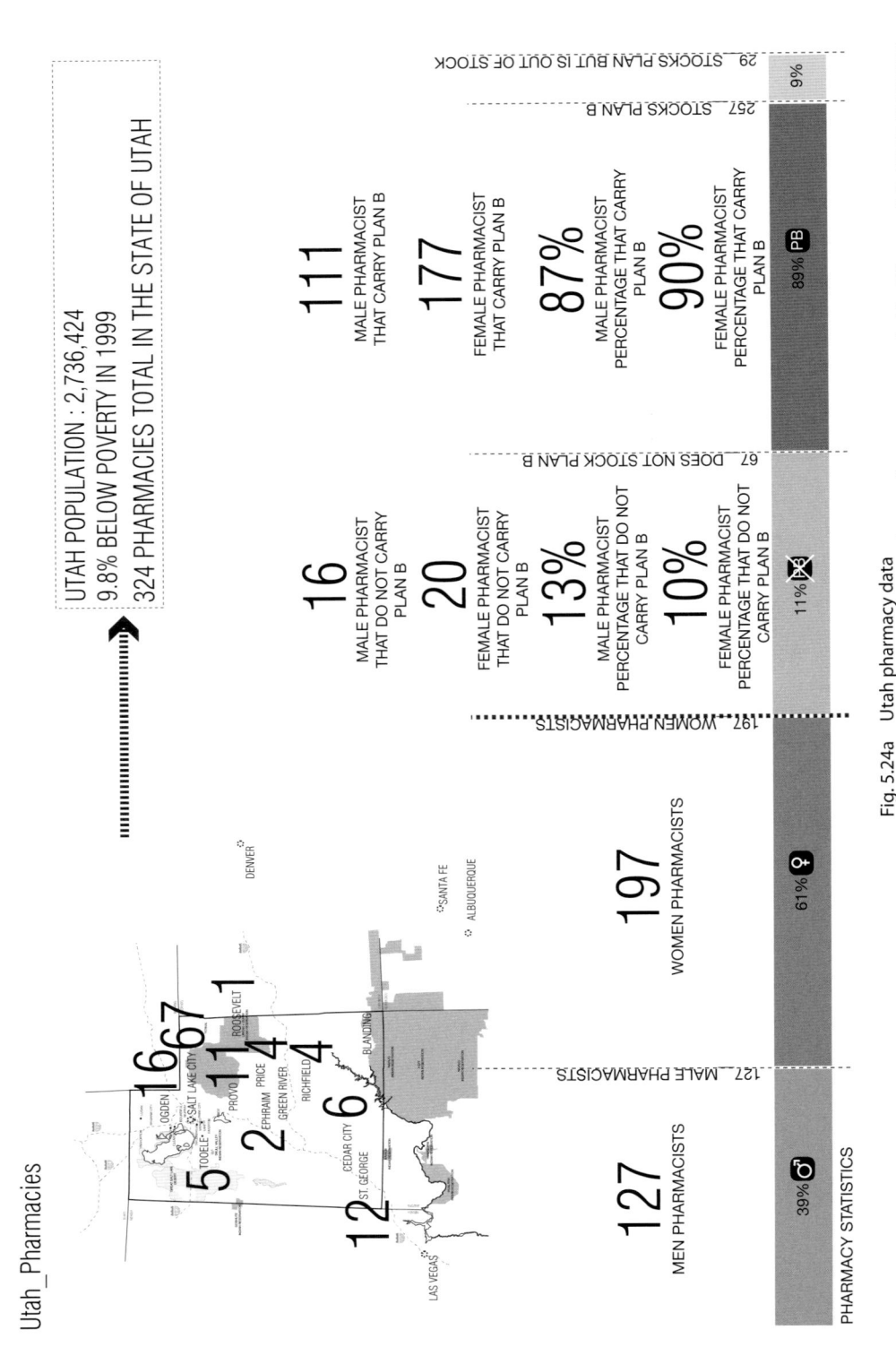

UTAH POPULATION : 2,736,424
9.8% BELOW POVERTY IN 1999
324 PHARMACIES TOTAL IN THE STATE OF UTAH

16 OGDEN
5 TOOELE
67 SALT LAKE CITY
11 PROVO
1 ROOSEVELT
2 EPHRAIM
4 PRICE
4 GREEN RIVER
4 RICHFIELD
6 BLANDING
12 ST. GEORGE
CEDAR CITY

DENVER
SANTA FE
ALBUQUERQUE
LAS VEGAS

127 MALE PHARMACISTS
197 WOMEN PHARMACISTS

127 MEN PHARMACISTS
197 WOMEN PHARMACISTS

16 MALE PHARMACIST THAT DO NOT CARRY PLAN B
20 FEMALE PHARMACIST THAT DO NOT CARRY PLAN B
13% MALE PHARMACIST PERCENTAGE THAT DO NOT CARRY PLAN B
10% FEMALE PHARMACIST PERCENTAGE THAT DO NOT CARRY PLAN B

111 MALE PHARMACIST THAT CARRY PLAN B
177 FEMALE PHARMACIST THAT CARRY PLAN B
87% MALE PHARMACIST PERCENTAGE THAT CARRY PLAN B
90% FEMALE PHARMACIST PERCENTAGE THAT CARRY PLAN B

62 DOES NOT STOCK PLAN B
257 STOCKS PLAN B
29 STOCKS PLAN BUT IS OUT OF STOCK

PHARMACY STATISTICS

39% ♂    61% ♀    11% ⊠    89% PB    9%

Fig. 5.24a  Utah pharmacy data

The statistics are based on the results from calling all the pharmacies in the state in 2008 and documenting their response to the question "Do you sell emergency contraception? Can I fill my prescription?" At the time we were calling in Utah you still needed a prescription to access this medication if younger than 18 years of age.

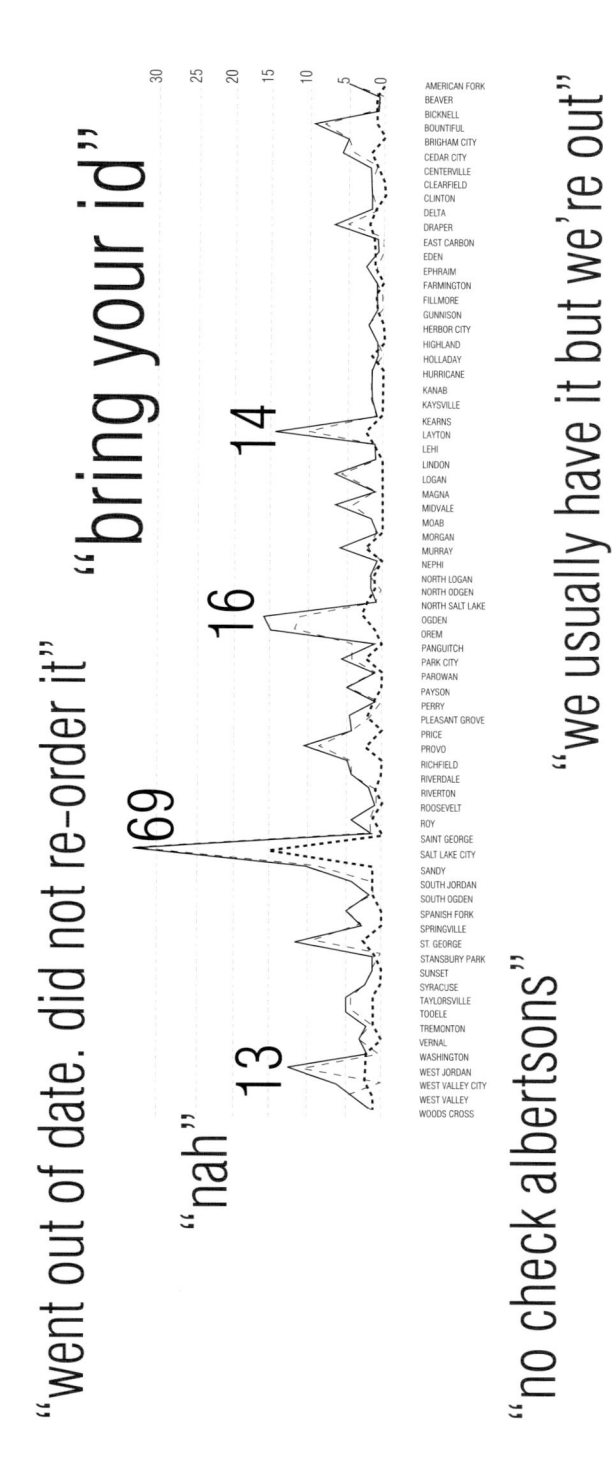

Fig. 5.24b  Utah pharmacist replies

5.21, Utah goes from a state with four abortion providers to one with over almost 50 providers! Not only does the provider number increase but also the locations of hospitals cover the majority of the state's geography, decreasing the distance a woman must travel to a find a provider.

**Planned Parenthood**

One of the surprising discoveries revealed through interviewing concerns independent providers relationship with Planned Parenthood. Synonymous with reproductive healthcare and a woman's right to choose in the media, Planned Parenthood has become a household name and probably the most recognized in relation to abortion. In the last two to three years Planned Parenthood has become a lightning rod for the conservative right's attack on women's healthcare. Just this past year, Congress attempted to entirely defund Planned Parenthood during the budget debates with the House of Representatives passing an amendment to eliminate funding to Planned Parenthood 240 to 185 in February 2011.[56]

According to Planned Parenthood's most recent Annual 2009–2010 report, only 3 percent of their services involve providing abortions. The remaining 97 percent are allocated in the following distribution: 33.5 percent include contraception, 38 percent include STI/STD testing and treatment, 14.5 percent include cancer screening and prevention, almost 10.5 percent are other women's health services including pregnancy tests and prenatal services and the last .5 percent are for other services including family practice services for both women and men, adoption referrals to other agencies and other procedures for both women and men. Overall Planned Parenthood cared for 3 million people in 2010.[57] Hailed as an assault on women and women's healthcare, the defunding of Planned Parenthood would eliminate numerous services including contraception, cancer and STD screenings and newborn nutritional support among others.[58] Although this did not pass at the federal level during 2011, several states including Kansas, Indiana, North Carolina, New Hampshire and Texas have taken it upon themselves to defund Planned Parenthood at the state level during 2011.[59] However states trying to restrict a Medicaid beneficiary's freedom of choice for family planning services "risk losing federal support."[60]

Although several providers interviewed said they have a working relationship with their local Planned Parenthood clinic borrowing supplies and informing one another if any unusual things are going on and are overall on amicable terms, I found the general consensus to be that independent providers are quite skeptical of Planned Parenthood. Many voiced concern regarding Planned Parenthood's business practice of going into areas where there are already established independent providers, ones deeply connected with their communities, and often eventually putting these smaller clinics out of business. This sort of conduct has produced a real distaste for Planned Parenthood's "national plan."[61] This was a side of Planned Parenthood I had not been familiar with prior to interviewing. These comments come from across the US reflecting not an individual bias but a collective experience.

Another director echoed these remarks stating Planned Parenthoods "aren't going to places where the needs are." They have the financial resources to do this yet seem to lack an understanding of the bigger picture around access. When this happens, it places a strain on the other existing providers in an area. This director also mentioned the concern that one day the only provider left may be Planned Parenthood because they are such a large organization. Private clinics do not have the same financial and resource security.[62]

It was also mentioned that Planned Parenthoods are probably the only providers who can meet all of the new stricter regulations being passed by state legislatures. I was informed Planned Parenthoods are building surgery centers in a variety of states.[63] Whether this is a preemptive attempt to circumvent potential future restrictions it is yet to be seen. However, these types of facilities are expensive to build and I doubt many of the people I interviewed would be able to afford the sort of upgrades being required by the recent onslaught of ever stricter legislation. There are many restrictions being passed that are not improving medical care, only making operating an abortion facility more difficult and increasingly burdensome. An example of this was seen in the state of Kansas in June 2011. The state passed stricter legislation dictating room size, emergency equipment required on site, stocking of medication and blood supplies as well as connections to local hospitals. Formally issued in June and approved later the same month, this left almost no time for clinics to respond and alter their facilities. Only one of the three clinics in the state actually received a license and this clinic was the local Planned Parenthood.[64] Although on paper these new restrictions sound completely reasonable, in practice when one begins to consider what it really means to stipulate such things as closet size or hallway widths that would already accommodate storage and free and clear wheelchairs movement. They are anything but reasonable. One clinic owner mentioned when she was first retrofitting her building she was required to move a 22-foot-long wall just one inch in order to have the hallway to code. One begins to wonder, what is really the point? Restrictions are becoming far too onerous. They are not improving abortion care only making obtaining a clinic license more costly and difficult if not sometimes impossible as demonstrated in Kansas this past year. These political gymnastics camouflaged as medical necessities continue to proliferate across this country. As Center for Reproductive Rights lawyer Bonnie Scott Jones has stated, these extensive regulations and spatial requirements abortion clinics are forced to adhere to and accordingly alter clinic spaces by in order to maintain their licenses are often largely unrelated to the actual procedure itself. These TRAP bills single out abortion clinics, creating extreme burdens.[65]

Interestingly, one provider mentioned that soon after abortion became legal in 1973 and the clinic where she worked had opened, Planned Parenthood would not touch the abortion issue "with a ten-foot pole." Planned Parenthood turned down a request to open a clinic in their city. Even when medication abortion became practiced, Planned Parenthood still refused. However, this provider surmised that once realizing they could make money on medication abortion, then the local Planned Parenthood started to offer this service.[66]

The many complaints I heard about Planned Parenthood made me reflect upon my own experience when I first began this research and was hoping to work with them. I had sought permission to conduct interviews with employees and patients to better understand the impact space was having on the services being provided both outside and within the clinic. After regularly checking in with my contact at Planned Parenthood for over a year and half, I was eventually informed that my request would not be granted. There was never an opportunity provided to understand what Planned Parenthood's concerns were and whether I could work with them to redefine the scope of my study. Their response was just no. As a result, I was forced to reframe what and how this research would progress. I feel confident that the no from Planned Parenthood actually helped to strengthen and expand the focus of the research. On the one hand, I completely understand Planned Parenthood's denial. Abortion is such a contested issue and people's lives are at stake. I in no way want to compromise someone's safety. However, on the other hand, I believe the pro-abortion movement needs to reclaim and take back the ground the anti-abortion movement has usurped. This requires more discussion, more outreach, and far more visibility of those supporting and working in the abortion rights movement. I only wish Planned Parenthood had been more willing and more responsive to my request. I believe my research would have benefited from their feedback and engagement. It is a widely known fact that Planned Parenthood is a highly bureaucratic organization and their reluctance and eventual denial seems only to reconfirm this. Their insularity, although understood, is not always beneficial to the image being projected publicly.

When I began to consider with whom and where I would like to conduct interviews across the country, I again attempted to contact local Planned Parenthoods in hopes of being able to interview some of their clinic directors. Once again I was unable to penetrate through the tight control of their regional affiliates. I was disconnected a number of times from the general 1–800 number, left many voicemails that were either never returned or returned weeks later. This behavior made me wonder what someone must feel like, especially a teenager who is calling to schedule an abortion. How difficult, frustrating and time consuming the process must be trying to just get through to a Planned Parenthood. Maybe my experience is an anomaly but I am not so sure it is. Many of the providers I interviewed said they often receive former patients from Planned Parenthood who decided not to continue their care there because they were dissatisfied.

## Security

*Abortion clinics*
Since the 1980s, security has become a far greater concern and unfortunate reality for abortion providers. All but one of the people interviewed discussed their concerns and requirements in creating a secured space for both their patients and employees. Many of the providers interviewed believe the employees, doctors and owners are now the primary targets of more aggressive, dangerous and extremist protestors. Although patients still receive an inordinate amount of attack making their way into and out of clinics, these tend to be more verbal assault

and obstruction of cars attempting to block the entrance onto the properties of abortion providers.

The requirement for increased security has been born out of the intensified use of violence by anti-abortion protestors. As cited earlier, the Feminist Majority's 2010 National Clinic Violence Survey finds there has been an increase of severe clinic violence against 23.5 percent of all clinics. This is the highest recorded level of violence since 1997 when 25.0 percent of all clinics reported one or more occurrences of severe violence. The survey also revealed an increase by almost a third of clinics reporting three or more incidents of severe violence and harassment. The Violence Survey found that there has been a shift to more "intensive targeting of doctors and clinic personnel and staff." This confirms what the providers I interviewed have noticed. In addition, the survey discovered clinics with "poor" experiences with local law enforcement were two times as likely to experience high levels of violence in 2010 than clinics who had "good" or "excellent" experience with their local law enforcement. Their survey also demonstrates that the FACE law is not being used to its full extent. Clinics have reported an increase in FACE violations in 2010, a rise for the first time since 1999, yet the number of opened investigations resulting from these violations decreased.[67]

Typical security protocols for independent clinics are to both document and report any activity that falls within security concerns including such events as protestors infringing upon clinic property lines, breaching secured spaces and accosting patients and employees, breaking noise variances and noise level limits. These activities are reported to the local police and the Feminist Majority. Begun in 1989 in response to Operation Rescue's hope to turn Los Angeles into the first "abortion-free city," the Feminist Majority's National Clinic Access Project (NCAP) has trained and mobilized over 56,000 community volunteers. The largest of its kind in the United States, these volunteers help keep reproductive health centers open in the midst of sometimes extreme harassment and intimidation. Having served 47 cities in 26 states, NCAP is a vital component creating visual support for providers. In addition NCAP also provides security assessments and training for clinic staff.[68]

Security protocols vary from clinic to clinic. Immediately upon entering some clinics require all people to walk through a metal detector, others hand-scan those who have entered once they arrive at the front desk, while other clinics do not allow any handbags and cell phones inside. At one clinic, the director is insistent that no knives of any kind are allowed on the premises and they must be left in the car. It appears that since 9/11 people are far more receptive to heightened security measures. As one provider acknowledges, it is the reality of our situation now. It should be noted that it is not uncommon for people to be required to pass through metal detectors for other medical services in locations where there are greater risks for safety. With all the negative publicity that both the New Jersey and Virginia Planned Parenthoods received in response to undercover videos of purported pimps and prostitutes seeking abortions for minors by Live Action in 2011,[69] clinic owners have become far more concerned about the ease and ability of filming. Therefore many clinics do not allow cameras or phones with cameras into their spaces. One never knows what will be uploaded to YouTube and how out of context it may be taken.

Another clinic has had ongoing struggles with their local law enforcement about three separate fences installed in the front of their property over a period of time. For years the clinic had a mature hedge creating a zone of privacy all along the clinic's walkway entrance. Law enforcement urged the clinic to remove this hedge so that the clinic would not remain hidden from their view or provide people a place to hide or to place explosives. Eventually the clinic agreed and had the privacy hedge removed. Initially, the clinic used rebar staked in the ground with horizontally running wire marking the line where protestors could not pass. The clinic noticed that the rebar boundary would magically move closer and closer to the building, at least a foot or more forward, positioning protestors closer to the clinic entrance. Every time the clinic realized the rebar boundary had been moved closer to the building, a clinic employee would go out, remeasure and relocate the rebar "fence." After a while the local police "suggested, recommended and urged" the clinic to build a real protective fence assuring the clinic that if the fence was built, the police would be better able to keep the peace and enforce the law. Eventually, against the clinic owner's better judgment, a six-foot tall wooden fence was built. This last fence has resulted in protestors standing on the top of ladders in order to be vertically higher than the top of the fence so their noise can better carry into the clinic. Protestors will also use ladders to climb and perch in trees near the fence so they will be positioned above the fence. Of course these are all illegal activities. Protestors are never arrested, receive only a warning and a second chance, and then the cycle repeats. The laws are not being followed. The clinic feels imprisoned by the fence. The law is not enforced, people continue to use ladders and the clinic owner told me that the fence feels like a joke.[70]

*Security concerns*
Some clinics have undergone FBI security and threat assessments to know more precisely what needs to be added to their security protocols. The FBI told one clinic owner that they want her clinic wide open urging her to not install any fencing. She had been contemplating installing a fence but the FBI convinced her not to. Insisting there should be nothing around her clinic that can be used to place a bomb in, even her dumpsters are padlocked closed in hopes of preventing them from being used to house explosives.[71]

One of the most difficult balances to make is between a clinic's security concerns and the environment, spatial qualities and desired experience created inside. A clinic does not want to come across as creating a lock-down experience. One clinic provider said, "you don't want to make your clinic feel like a fortress." One wants to demonstrate a secure space without being too extreme. This includes communicating with patients about what they should expect prior to arriving, what are the security measures in place, how many doors will a patient go through before being admitted into the clinic, informing a patient about a security guard at the entrance, and so on. But "how do you define too much these days?" This is an extremely difficult question to answer and most people I interviewed agreed this was a moving target. Clearly communication with staff and patients is critical to ensure all involved are aware of why the space is configured and securitized the way it is. Layers of security systems are expensive. Bullet-proof glass, gates, fences, window guards, security guards, elaborate locking systems, surveillance cameras all add up. This is coupled with where in the country the clinic is located and what level of threat they regularly receive.[72] Over the past many years clinics in Florida, Mississippi, Alabama, North Carolina, South Dakota, Virginia and Kansas have received much higher levels of protestor activity. According to the 2010 Feminist Majority clinic violence survey, "[a] strong, positive relationship with law enforcement continues to be crucial for abortion clinics threatened by violence and harassment." However, this is not possible in some of these most contentious states because law enforcement refuse to do their job to uphold and enforce the law.

## CANADA

At first glance, the grass always seems greener on the other side and this was definitely the case with what I perceived about abortion in Canada. Canada remains the only country to have completely decriminalized abortion.[73] The assumption was that because of Canada's more liberal social programs and policies combined with their universal healthcare, all women would have access to abortion in Canada. My research has shown that unfortunately access in Canada, as with the United States, while it may appear on paper to be far more available for all women, there are major gaps and barriers to access in certain provinces in Canada as there are in certain states across the United States.

Compared to the United States, there are far fewer abortion providers overall throughout Canada. There is at least one location to access abortion services, either in a hospital or clinic, in each of the provinces and territories except in Prince Edward Island (PEI) where there are no providers whatsoever. PEI also restricts payment to only one Halifax hospital if the Department of Health and Social Services deems the procedure as "medically necessary" and there is only one hospital in Halifax willing to accept referrals from PEI women. Although all remaining provinces and territories do have at least one place a woman can seek abortion care, due to the time sensitivity of abortion and possible wait times this is not enough access. A woman may have to wait up to four weeks in the eastern provinces of Newfoundland and Labrador and between three to five weeks in Manitoba, Ontario and Saskatchewan. Combine waiting times with the concern whether provincial insurance will offer reciprocal coverage if you are out of province or decide to seek care at a clinic rather than a hospital and a woman begins to have a more difficult time accessing abortion. More to be discussed about provincial insurance coverage shortly. Out of the 13 provinces and territories, there are only 43 private clinics and only 114 hospitals where a woman can seek access in Canada. What is even more revealing is that there are five provinces/territories without a private clinic and of these five, only three have one hospital where the procedure is performed. There is not one province or territory where every hospital will perform the procedure; in fact not even half of all hospitals will do so. A throwback to pre-1988, New Brunswick is the only province requiring a woman to have approval from two physicians prior to her receiving an abortion.[74]

**Barriers to Access**

Although completely legal since 1988, abortion in Canada still remains difficult to access across the country and availability depends upon where in Canada you live. In "Barriers to Access to Abortion Through a Legal Lens," Downie and Nassar list both legal and non-legal barriers to abortion access. For example since the majority of abortions are provided in hospitals, women can encounter difficulties in the doctor referral process. If one's primary care physician is unwilling to make the referral, a woman may not be aware of alternate places to seek another one. When trying to self-refer, a woman may be asked to provide unnecessary and private information before being able to access a provider preventing her own anonymity.[75] It should be noted abortion is the only medical procedure providing a "conscience clause" for Canadian doctors.[76]

Abortion is a time-sensitive procedure. Difficulties in referrals equate to delays in the time a woman has to actually access the procedure. The earlier the better and the longer she has to wait, the greater the increase in possible risk. When women are confronting difficulties accessing medically necessary procedures similarly not faced by men, this is discrimination based on sex as determined by Canada's Supreme Court.[77] As per Canadian Medical Association (CMA) policy a doctor can claim "right of consciousness" and not provide a woman a referral for an abortion. However, as described by Jeff Blackmer, Executive Director of the Office of Ethics, CMA policy also stipulates that a doctor "should not interfere in any way with this patient's right to obtain the abortion." Blackmer's assumption that a woman will have an alternate doctor for a referral is not always possible particularly in regions with fewer doctors. Therefore under these circumstances a "physician has an obligation under CMA policy to provide the referral …."[78] So which is it? A patient requests a referral but due to a doctor's moral, ethical or religious beliefs does not want to provide one and can refuse, and yet the patient is requesting it. As Blackmer concludes, "[t]here should be no delay in the provision of abortion services."[79] As Downie and Nassar point out there is an inherent contradiction in this logic. On paper an alternative is provided for by another doctor but in practice, as illustrated, this is not always the case if another doctor cannot be found.

Another problem being experienced in both the United States and in Canada is the lack of medical students selecting to go into abortion care and the severe lack of training all medical students receive in abortion while in medical school. Considered optional, abortion education is not a standard part of Canadian medical school curriculum where abortion procedures are discussed less than an hour on average.[80] Combine less doctors with fewer hospitals providing abortions, women have even fewer and more limited options. Comparing statistics found in the 1977 Badgley Report where only 20.1 percent of all public hospitals provided abortion care with the 2003 Canada Abortion Rights Action League (CARAL) finding where 17.8 percent of public hospitals and with the 2006 Canadians For Choice (CFC) finding one observes a further drop where only 15.9 percent of all public hospitals are now providing the service.[81] The consequences of fewer doctors with fewer hospitals translate into much longer waiting times with women being confronted with gestational limits as yet another factor that must be considered.[82] Please see Fig. 3.11 Abortion in Canada for further details.

In addition to less availability, distances women are required to travel seeking abortion care have increased and are considered a major obstacle in accessing reproductive healthcare. In a study conducted by Sethna and Doull in 2007 with the Toronto Morgantaler Clinic (TMC), two series of questionnaires were given to patients coming to the clinic in order to document distances, cost and time women spent in seeking abortion care. Their pilot study found 73.5 percent of all respondents traveled an hour or more to the clinic with a little more than 15 percent traveling between 101 km and more than 1,000 km to the clinic. Women making less than $30,000 per year were found to travel greater distances ranging from 200 km to more than 1,000 km than those whose incomes where greater. They also found that about 90 percent of women paid less than $50 on transportation and 93.6 percent did not have to spend any money on accommodations. However, they did find a significant increase in expenditure for those traveling with a companion especially when considering the additional costs of childcare, meals and loss of income from missed work.[83]

Insurance coverage can become a roadblock if you are either living out of province or prefer to seek care outside a hospital with delays and manipulated flows of insurance monies to and from different provinces and territories for funding abortion. Abortion has been deemed a medically necessary procedure and is supposed to be covered by the Canada Health Act, however women are finding it difficult in some particular provinces and territories in Canada to have the procedure covered under their insurance. Only 5 of the 13 provinces provide full funding for the procedure if performed in any of the approved hospitals, clinics or community health centers (CLSC in Quebec). Four provinces/territories provide full funding for procedures performed only in hospitals. The remaining provinces all have some sort of restriction in place depending on where the procedure is performed.

In Manitoba coverage only includes full funding in hospitals and one clinic in Winnipeg. In Alberta out of province women must pay a facility fee and in Saskatchewan provincial insurance only covers abortions performed in hospitals. There is full funding in hospitals and clinics but there is a quota on the number of procedures funded at the Calgary clinic. A lawsuit won in Manitoba overruled the government's policy of funding hospital-only abortions due to the fact this went against access to timely services under the Canada Health Act. In Quebec if the procedure was performed in a hospital or community health center it would be fully covered but women have about 50 percent of abortions performed in Montreal clinics where the government partially pays for these procedures requiring a woman to pay approximately $200. New Brunswick will only fully fund the procedure if deemed medically necessary by two doctors and performed in a hospital. Dr. Morgantaler is currently challenging this funding policy.[84] Nova Scotia, similar to Quebec, hospital procedures are fully covered but women must pay the remainder of the service if it is sought in a clinic. There are no clinics or hospitals that will perform abortions in PEI and the province will pay only one Halifax hospital if deemed medically necessary by the Department of Health and Social Services. The Yukon Territory has a reciprocal agreement with funded hospital abortion services in British Columbia; and in both the Northwest and Nunavut Territories they fully fund only hospital abortions.[85]

There are further restrictions on insurance coverage. As Downie and Nassar point out, women on work or student visas are not covered and women in British Columbia have a minimum residence requirement prior to being insured for abortion coverage. Other women living near provincial borders who have medical care performed across a provincial border often have to pay out of pocket and hope they will be reimbursed from their own province afterwards. The authors also mention one particular troubling aspect of inter-provincial insurance. Abortion is not included on the Inter-Provincial Health Insurance Agreement Coordinating Committee (IHIACC), the unit deciding what services will be medically covered for billing across provinces.[86] Whether politically driven or not, the exclusion of abortion on inter-provincial coverage is deeply troubling and creates further hurdles to overcome for women seeking reproductive healthcare.

Similar to concerns requiring doctors to provide referrals for abortion and some declining to do so, there have been reports of hospital staff and switchboard operators withholding or not providing accurate information about abortion to patients. Uninformed about costs and insurance billing for both in and out of province patients, it has been noted that these staff sometimes direct women to anti-abortion counseling centers.[87] There must be more reliable and accurate information required from hospital staff. It is reprehensible that medical institutions would allow personal beliefs to interfere or even prevent medical treatment. Clearly there are many gaps in abortion access across Canada as demonstrated by the varying policies of each province and territory. Depending upon where in the country you live, you may have to pay out of pocket for travel to access an abortion. Although it is federally declared a legal right, many of the provinces and territories have created additional difficulties making it more complicated for women to actually receive care.

**Emergency Contraception**

Emergency contraception (EC) or Plan B® if used effectively could greatly reduce the abortion rate. In theory the easier to access emergency contraception, the more women will use it. Once EC was first approved in Canada in 2000, there became a big push for the drug to be available over-the-counter (OTC) in order for more women to have access. Britain began OTC availability late in 2000 and in 2001 British Columbia offered EC without a prescription.[88] Researchers found the change through this public health policy initiative in British Columbia (the first province providing prescriptive authority to pharmacists), significantly increased the use of emergency contraception during the provincial study period during

1996 to 2002. By the second year the policy had been implemented, the number of women accessing emergency contraception more than doubled.[89] Once Health Canada reclassified emergency contraception as a non-prescription drug in April 2005 any woman could walk into a pharmacy, pay a consultation fee, consult with a pharmacist, and then have access to the drug and purchase it. However, in May 2008, emergency contraception was given full over-the-counter status by the National Association of Pharmacy Regulatory Authorities, no longer requiring a medical consultation with a pharmacist prior to being able to purchase the drug. Providing greater access, Canada became the fifth country behind Norway, the Netherlands, Sweden and India allowing women to purchase emergency contraception without any barriers to access.[90]

## MEXICO

Unlike in the United States and Canada, abortion in Mexico is incomparably far more restrictive while the country has one of the highest rates of unsafe abortions in the world. From 2006 data, abortion is 40 percent higher in Mexico than in the United States.[91] High rates of maternal mortality are traced to illegal and unsafe abortion practices resulting in the fourth highest cause of hospital admissions in public hospitals in Mexico.[92] Statistically it has been reported there is a correlation between higher maternal morbidity and mortality rates in countries with stricter abortion laws than in countries with more liberal policies.[93] The United Nations has determined that "health, reproduction, and sexual self-determination" are basic human rights and has further stated that a significant marker of the level of a country's inequality and poverty can be indicated through maternal mortality rates.[94] The UN Convention on the Elimination of all Forms of Discrimination Against Women (CEDAW) calls for reviewing laws where abortion is illegal. Mexico, as a participant in UN treaties and conventions, is supposed to be bound to these standards yet the country does not ensure abortion access as a gender equality issue.[95]

Like the United States, Mexico is a federal system comprised of 31 states and the Federal District of Mexico City, the country's capital. On a federal level, abortion is legal only as a result of rape. Each state then further legislates access to abortion due to their own penal code with Mexico City having the most liberal policies in the entire country.[96] Since 2007, 30 out of 32 states allow abortion due to an accident, 29 out of 32 states allow if there is a risk to a woman's life, 13 out of 32 states allow for fetal impairment, 11 out of 32 states allow if there is a risk to the woman's health and 12 out of 32 states allow abortion due to other causes. There are a few other states in addition to Mexico City where abortion is more available but still only within certain limited and permissible legal stipulations. This more liberal group includes in order from the most state allowances to the fewest: Baja California Sur, Morelos, Veracruz, Chihuahua, San Luis Potosí and México.[97] Like both the US and Canada, although theoretically legal under certain legislated categories, in practice there continues to be severe limitations in accessing reproductive care. Please see Fig. 3.13 Abortion in Mexico for further details

## Barriers to Access

Due to Mexico's extremely restrictive abortion policies, women encounter a wide array of barriers when seeking abortion access. As was seen in the case of Paulina where although this young woman was legally allowed to receive an abortion, hospital staff, doctors, public servants and other anti-choice groups successfully obstructed and eventually prevented her from receiving the abortion she sought. Her case is just one example yet epitomizes the myriad obstacles women encounter daily seeking reproductive healthcare throughout Mexico.

In a randomized study about public opinions on abortion, 3,000 Mexicans were surveyed reflecting the general distribution of the Mexican population between urban and rural areas. Researchers noted that general attitudes and basic knowledge about abortion were low. They believe this probably reflects the inaccessibility of legal abortion. Less than half of those surveyed (45 percent) accurately knew under what circumstances abortion is legal in their state and of those 45 percent, 79 percent thought abortion was always illegal. An interesting result of their study revealed that correct information on abortion reflected certain demographic factors including the state where one lived, one's education level, one's sex, one's party affiliation and the frequency one attended religious services. If a person was less educated, lived in a rural area, attended religious services at least once a week and was between 41 and 65, statistically this person would be anti-choice. If a person did not know abortion was legal under certain circumstances, the chance this person was anti-choice was three times greater. On the other hand, if a man was of a higher socioeconomic level and knew someone who had had an abortion, there was a greater chance he would be pro-choice. Another interesting result of the survey demonstrates that 79 percent of the respondents identifying as Catholic believe abortion should be legal in some situations and 80 percent of self-identifying Catholics feel all public health institutions and hospitals should provide legal abortions.[98]

In another study focusing on prevalent attitudes and knowledge about medical abortions and emergency contraception, researchers conducted a series of focus groups with middle-class people of reproductive age in Mexico City. Although Mexico City has the most liberal abortion laws in Mexico, the study revealed gross misinformation and a lack of basic knowledge regarding abortion. Participants although familiar with different types of abortion, did not reveal specific knowledge and were misinformed about a fetus's development during the beginning stages of pregnancy. It was clear from the respondents that abortion was a common occurrence, obtaining an abortion is relatively easy but finding one that is safe is expensive. Almost every group discussed the case of Paulina and was aware of the difficult situation this young woman had endured. Additionally, young women were more informed than men about medical abortion. The study revealed prevalent dissatisfaction people felt with their healthcare providers. Most groups mentioned they thought their doctors were withholding information based on what the doctor felt was best for the patient, rather than encouraging the patient to participant in their own healthcare decisions.[99]

Another study conducted at three Mexico City public sector facilities further confirms how one's socioeconomic level can create obstacles for woman trying to access abortion. At the time of this survey, there were 17 public facilities offering abortion. Reflecting the demographic of public facilities in Mexico City and their patient profiles, the researchers conducted surveys at the highest volume sites including a general hospital, a maternity hospital and a primary health center. Unmarried women with a primary education or less were statistically more likely to encounter two or more obstacles in seeking an abortion. What I found most interesting in the study was the way in which the process to access abortion is implemented compared with that in the United States and Canada. An appointment is secured by arriving to a facility with proof of residency and government issued identification. Facility hours are only during the week and if lucky, a patient may receive an appointment the same day or if unlucky may have to wait up to 15 days with out-of-state patients receiving priority. Both medication and surgical abortions require two appointments.[100] Seeking an abortion is much more time intensive compared to that in the US and Canada where an appointment can be made over the phone. Requiring a woman to go to a provider's office in order to make an appointment takes more time, creates further obstacles and more difficulties in accessing reproductive health care.

Clearly with over 80 percent of the country identifying as Catholic, there is tremendous social and political pressure from Catholic doctrine not supporting any form of family planning. However, through feminist organizations such as GIRE and supporters such as Catholics for the Right to Decide (CDD) major progress has been made in countering Catholic doctrine. Yes, abortion is a choice but this choice is not made lightly or easily and in fact more harm and more suffering could result if an abortion is not accessed. These groups have also redirected the conversation towards one of abortion being a basic human right.[101] According to Human Rights Watch, "[a]uthoritative interpretations of international law recognize that abortion is vitally important to women's exercise of their human rights."[102] They further advocate that all governments have an "obligation to protect the full range of human rights for all women."[103]

Doctors are in large part the gatekeepers "to safe legal abortions in Mexico."[104] Unlike in both the US and Canada where independent clinics are easier points of access for women, it is through the public sector doctor that Mexican women are dependent upon reproductive healthcare. In a study of Mexican physicians, researchers were interested in determining what affects their willingness to provide abortions in cases of rape had on access. From their study, family and general practitioners were far more likely than ob/gyns to agree that abortion should be legal in case of rape and to provide abortion services. The older the doctor was the more likely s/he would be to provide abortions. Physicians identifying with a religion other than Catholic were less likely to agree to perform abortions. A doctor's religion influenced one's ideas on abortion legislation but did not influence the willingness to perform abortions. About one quarter of all 1,206 physicians surveyed did not know that women pregnant due to rape could legally seek abortions. About half of the physicians surveyed thought women were "irresponsible" if seeking an abortion. Also noted were physicians working in both public and private practices may be more inclined to provide abortions than those working only in the public sector due to monetary gain and those in the public sector may encounter insurmountable barriers to providing abortion services that private physicians do not experience.[105]

In a most recent survey of Mexican health providers, a few startling statistics regarding medical knowledge about abortion were discovered. Randomly surveying 418 health care providers of which 90 percent were ob/gyns at the Colegio Mexicano de Especialistas en Ginecologia y Obstetricia conference, the researchers found that only 54 percent of respondents correctly knew that abortion was legal if a woman was raped. Statistically doctors from Mexico City defend abortion in all cases. About 85 percent of all doctors surveyed noted abortion complications to be a concern in their practice. Most of the doctors knew that misoprostol was an abortifacient and that 90 percent stated it was easier for a woman to access a medical drug-induced abortion than a surgical abortion. However, 86 percent of doctors acknowledged that women do access the drug in pharmacies without a prescription. Another disturbing issue this survey revealed is that only 19 percent of doctors knew the appropriate range of dosage to administer for a medical abortion and there was clearly a significant lack of knowledge about the legalities of abortion and appropriate dosage for drug-induced abortions. Doctors providing medical abortion are more likely female, recently completed their residency requirement, are from Mexico City and have no strong religious affiliations. The researchers conclude that abortion training in Mexico must become more comprehensive and provide more accurate information in order to expand a woman's access.[106]

Another issue diminishing abortion access is through the use of conscientious objection by health care providers. Diego Portales University Law Professor Lidia Casas makes a clear case that although conscientious objectors should be accommodated for, there is both a professional and ethical responsibility for doctors to provide medical care and a doctor should not be able to exercise their right at the expense of health care for others. Through the imposition of one's religious beliefs onto another person with no alternative provided, a person is unable to access quality healthcare and her reproductive rights are being infringed upon and is "a violation of the bioethics principle of non-maleficence."[107] Further noted is how Mexican law tries to balance the interest of both sides. It stipulates that conscientious objection "cannot be claimed in emergency cases ... life and health must prevail over religious or personal belief."[108] It is observed in Canada, the US and Mexico conscientious objection is being used to further erode a woman's access to birth control, EC and abortion preventing her from receiving her full rights legally defined under law. She is not being treated as an equal citizen due to the fact she is unable to exercise her full rights to health care, as a citizen should. As Casas points out, this creates a society where some "are more equal than others."[109]

## Pharmacies, Contraception and Emergency Contraception

Contraception use has significantly increased in Mexico from 25 percent during the 1970s to 71 percent in 2006. Yet research reveals the need for preventing unintended pregnancy has still increased faster than contraceptive use. Adolescents do not receive sex education in Mexican schools and although the government began a national family planning program in 1973 and contraception is widely available, one in eight women have an unmet contraception need.[110] Emergency contraception was officially included in the family planning guidelines in 2004 requiring all public health and family planning clinics to provide it.[111]

A study of middle-class women and men in Mexico City revealed that similar to knowledge about abortion, participants' knowledge about family planning was moderate. Women knew more than men about contraception, adults more than youth and much misinformation was common especially in regards to modern contraception methods. Knowledge about EC was even less well known. One study showed that only 18 percent of people using family planning were aware of its existence.[112]

As I am arguing for in the United States, pharmacies provide an opportunity in helping prevent pregnancies if EC is easily acquired. In Latin America, pharmacies are a point of access for a much broader level of healthcare information, services and medication. Pharmacy workers are not pharmacists and can have only a minimum of the equivalent of high school education with no medical training. However, pharmacies are required to employ a *responsible sanitario*, a professional with pharmacy and health training, but in 2005 only 31 percent of all pharmacies in Mexico actually did so and most were not fully employed, working only part time. Another study using two mystery clients (MCs) to visit 169 pharmacies in one Mexican state, sought to discover what kind of information is being provided when using misoprostol, a known abortifacient. Although intended for the treatment of ulcers, misoprostol has proven incredibly effective as an abortifacient. A prescription is legally required to purchase the drug but in practice one can buy the drug over-the-counter at pharmacies either by bottle or by pill throughout Mexico. Misoprostol is a less expensive option to an illegal abortion costing on average $4.07 per pill or $83–$167 per bottle of 28 pills.

Researchers found no real differences in responses based on pharmacist's gender or location. Ninety percent of pharmacies discussed misoprostol and it was for sale in 61 percent out of the 153 pharmacies where mentioned. Interestingly 75 percent of all pharmacy workers did not request a prescription although legally required to do so. More disturbing is that 84 percent prescribed a much lower dosage than would work and did not recommend the most effective way to use the drug. When the MC prompted the discussion about misoprostol, 52 percent were either hesitant to interact or refused altogether. The study confirms the inaccurate knowledge pharmacy workers are providing when administering misoprostol over the counter. So although a woman may purchase the drug, she may not be provided accurate information about how to administer it rendering the drug ineffective.[113]

## Security

The United States Department of Justice Federal Bureau of Investigation (FBI) Terrorism report declares terrorism to be "the unlawful use of force and violence against persons or property to intimidate or coerce a government, the civilian population, or any segment thereof, in furtherance of political or social objectives."

It further defines domestic terrorism as "a group or individual based and operating entirely within the United States or Puerto Rico without foreign direction committed against persons or property to intimidate or coerce a government, the civilian population, or any segment thereof in furtherance of political or social objectives." "Eight out of the fourteen recorded terrorist preventions [from 2002 to 2005] stemmed from right-wing extremism and included disruptions to plotting by individuals involved with the militia, white supremacist, constitutionalist and tax protestor, and anti-abortion movements.[114]

Although the general public may consider anti-abortion protestors to be just exercising their first amendment rights, there is a segment of this protest population that the FBI considers to be domestic terrorists. This is an important distinction to be made and should be more publicly acknowledged. Although this group may be labeled as a radical subset within the larger anti-abortion movement, I would argue there is really a problematic and disturbing gray zone between domestic terrorism and what women and employees of reproductive health facilities encounter on an often daily basis in order to walk in the front door of a clinic. Protestors often use intimidation and coercion to further their political and social objectives. At what point is the line demarcating domestic terrorism crossed? How do we define this and know it when we see or experience it? When does the ongoing breaking of injunctions and subjection to a continual onslaught of demeaning and intimidating interrogation move from mere protesting to being subjected to domestic terrorism tactics?

When considering the larger topic of security for abortion clinics, women's shelters and hospitals, a number of overarching themes emerge. These include the distinction between exterior and interior security technologies, the scale of whom or what is being prevented access, distinguishing between the different layers of protection needed for separate programmatic spaces and the degrees to which materials offer protection. The issues, although vary in intensity and immediacy of concern for the three types of spaces being considered, are surprisingly not that dissimilar. Abortion clinics, women's shelters and various units of hospitals are deeply invested in providing a high level of protection for their patients, residents and employees. How visible or invisible systems of security should be is inherently a design concern greatly impacting the use and environment these spaces are hoping to cultivate and foster. As security continues to become a bigger public concern costing more and more money, these user groups are requiring more serious and secure systems to be installed throughout their properties. There must be a more holistic security approach between both the inside and outside of buildings to better protect all who enter and exit.

The Feminist Majority Foundation's Clinic Defense Project has created a list of considerations when reviewing a building's security against attack. The list of "areas of vulnerability" include such items as building location (complex versus free-standing building), buildings with flat roofs, clinics with weak points such as "unsubstantial" doors and uncovered windows, lack of an alarm system, heavy shrubs and vegetation and insufficient outdoor lighting. The list of "affirmative actions to reduce vulnerability" include such suggestions as installing outdoor floodlighting, alarm systems, entrance and exit doors with appropriate hardware preventing their removal, adequate window coverings like steel bars or solid shutters, heavy landscaping like vines and shrubs should be well manicured and low to the ground with large trees removed preventing their use as ladders, hire a security guard and educate all personnel about security protocols.[115]

Within security literature, considering protection as an integral part of design's initial phasing is referred to as Crime Prevention through Environmental Design (CPTED). Rather than retrofitting a space, it is far more preferable to integrate security considerations from the outset of a project's inception. It is argued that this process further enhances and builds upon a site's natural access of control, inherent surveillance possibilities and territorial reinforcement. A goal of CPTED is for a site's natural and normal uses to meet the equivalent security needs as technical protection devices and methods typically employed would.[116] Supporters of CPTED believe that these natural effects can be more successful than traditional artificial barriers such as locks, alarms, fences, and so on. In other words "[g]ood security design enhances the effective use of the space at the same time prevents crime and potential acts of terror."[117] CPTED extols a common-sense approach based on the idea that improving the quality of life can help deter crime. Jane Jacobs, a well-known urban planner and critic, developed a theory of the "eyes of the street" where residents and community members participate in making their neighborhoods safe places while helping to simultaneously reduce crime.[118] Although this appears to be a sensible idea, it is not without its critics who are concerned this is social engineering masked through form making. More importantly, many abortion clinics and women's shelters are located in repurposed buildings due to budgetary constraints and availability. Security is typically added into the spaces creating more visible layers of devices that must be camouflaged and hidden if possible.

An important difference to note regarding security literature focuses on the prevention of or deterrence of criminal acts. Always the assumption is that people do not want to be detected or seen in public; trespassers will go to great lengths not be seen or apprehended. Essentially people breaking the law do not want to be caught.[119] This is more than likely true when considering these security issues for women's shelters and hospitals. But abortion clinics do not follow this same logic. Protestors want to be seen in public, seeking media attention, trying to create more interference with access to these types of healthcare facilities. The standard logic for protection and crime prevention works only up to a certain point for abortion clinics since these people want to be seen, want to be caught and want the publicity that their actions attract.

## Exterior Design Concerns

Everyone I have spoken with associated with women's shelters, abortion clinics and hospitals has voiced a similar concern: they must have security, it is absolutely necessary yet do not want the visibility of security to negatively affect a patient or resident's experience. It is imperative that all of these facilities not appear bunker-like or fortified too heavily in their attempts to deter a person from entering. But on the other hand they must be secure enough so that the healing and supportive environments resonate beyond the security needed to protect all those inside. For an easier ability to control access, it is important to distinguish between both exterior and interior public zones as well as patient care spaces for security planning.[120]

In our post 9/11 world, heightened exterior and entrance security has proliferated. It is no longer unusual to be required to remove one's bags and coats, walk through a metal detector and even be physically frisked. The infrastructures required to enable this security to work have greatly denigrated our public spaces in government buildings and elsewhere. More concern for aesthetics must work to counter the oppressive spaces created through the onslaught of these security devices.[121]

Recommendations from federal agencies suggest buildings such as courthouses and government facilities create setbacks from streets in order to keep vehicles from entrances in case bombs are detonated nearby. Women's reproductive health centers should follow similar guidance. The FACE law does not specify a required protected distance from entering or exiting but as has been discussed in Chapter 3, some court rulings have designated precise distances when access was severely impeded by protestors.[122] FEMA recommends the layers of defense strategy to help prevent terrorist attacks against buildings. As described by the American Planning Association (APA), each layer is a "demarcation point for a different set of potential security strategies." The first layer of defense includes the buildings and other infrastructures outside the extents of the site; the second layer of defense is the area between the sidewalk and the building including any landscape features, parking, sidewalks, natural barriers, and so on; and the third layer of defense is the building itself.[123] FEMA also recommends accessing the immediate surroundings potential risks and vulnerabilities as they relate to your site and suggests determining if the zoning is subject to future change would directly alter the safety and security of the building. Another suggestion is to consider whether natural features already on site such as topography, landscaping or water could be used to provide more security. For example, do natural berms exist that already provide some further protection between the street and entrance? Do existing trees or shrubs provide more privacy from the traffic?[124]

Although this makes sense, I have had several abortion providers tell me that they received conflicting information on how much visible security to install. As mentioned, one provider remarked that she had intended to install a fence around the entire building site after being gravely attacked and the FBI explicitly told her not to do so. Their rational being the clinic would become even more of a target with a fence around it.[125] Another provider observed for years they were being urged by law enforcement to remove a mature privacy hedge and then later on to construct a fence around the clinic property. After finally doing both, these efforts have not helped reduce protestor activity whatsoever. If anything, the clinic feels more imprisoned by the fence and law enforcement are no better able to keep the peace than before.[126]

The most preferred site design would create unobstructed views to both parking and entrances. The more visibility around and through the site the more protection provided.[127] Ideally parking is located away yet not too far from the building. The lot should be designed as a one-way circuit in order to keep cars moving and afford more visibility, emergency communication intercoms and telephones should be provided and drop-off zones should be outside the stand-off zone, neither underneath nor within the building. All circulation should bring people through one secured entrance.[128] However, separate entrances for staff and public help create an additional line of security between the public and access points.

Another important feature is exterior lighting. It is imperative to have enough lighting, equivalent to full daylight, throughout the site in order for people to feel protected as they exit the building going towards their car or the sidewalk. Lighting should not create dark spots but overlap to ensure full illumination. Timers and automatic photoelectric cells should be used to ensure no one forgets to turn the lights on at night.

If fences are used, they should be at least six feet tall. There should be no trash, debris, adjacent trees or vines obscuring the view of the fence. Another concern is trash dumpsters and medical waste receptacles. These should all be located as far away from the building as possible and locked at all times.[129] It should also be mentioned that fences could have a variety of technologies. Besides the most common chain link fence, there can be an added electrical current or fiber optics running along, through or buried underneath the fence that when the light source is broken, an intruder is detected.[130]

There are several design objects, both minor and major, that can be added to a building's site to offer more control over movement and access. These include such devices as bollards, planters, fences, walls, benches, anti-ram devices, closed circuit television (CCTV) and lighting.[131] More extreme examples referred to as deployable barriers include rising bollards and rising wedges that activate to their full upright position in two seconds seriously stopping a vehicle, lifting it off the ground, and grab barriers or net systems using a high-strength aircraft cable that stop both vehicles and pedestrians. Irrigation systems deploying a field of sprinklers can be used to disrupt people's movement.[132] As mentioned earlier in this chapter, one of the providers I interviewed has had these installed in the front of the clinic along the sidewalk and uses them as needed.

Although not an area that is generally tampered with, a building's air ventilation system or what is more commonly referred to as to as the hvac, can often be broken into. If air intake and return vents are located close enough to the ground and are larger than 96 square inches, a person could easily access and even enter into them. FEMA advises that all exterior vents and louvers should be secured and under surveillance. Fencing could be used to prevent and restrict access.[133]

## Interior Design Concerns

As mentioned earlier, creative and strategic programmatic planning can significantly enhance protection and security. FEMA suggests some basic design recommendations including not mixing high-risk with lower-risk tenants, locating areas needing the highest degree of security farther back into the building, areas with the most public activity should be as far as possible from those requiring the most security, interior barriers or walls can be used creating varying degrees of security throughout the facility, constructing foyers out of reinforced concrete walls and staggering all doors to limit the effects of a blast.[134] In addition, the entrance, waiting and reception area of these facilities becomes an important line of defense and protection. The physical separation between these programmatic uses can prove instrumental in controlling the flow of people into and out of the building. Although not as common in hospitals, once entering into a hospital vestibule, people can be screened through metal detection devices and even asked to provide identification as one checks in and receives a temporary pass to allow visitor admittance into the hospital. After screening a person in an abortion clinic or women's shelter, she is then typically allowed into the waiting or reception area. Personal belongings may be required to be searched and stored. Additionally not bringing these items into the main space of the clinic creates yet another layer of security. Depending upon where located, hospitals and reproductive healthcare facilities will use bullet-resistant glass in reception areas and all exterior-facing windows. Bullet-resistant wall material should be used throughout the interior as needed. In two examples of Planned Parenthoods in Oakland, California, bullet-resistant wall material was used throughout various spaces separating public and semi-public zones.[135]

Interior spaces where more private programs occur such as resident or patient rooms, dining and kitchen areas, nurseries, operating rooms, or medical storage, should be less obvious for the public to locate and require more effort to reach. Additional layers of security can be created through surveillance by the nurses' stations, security guards or security cameras. Hospitals have had to take more extreme measures to protect newborns from infant abduction. The in-patient embedded rooms for mothers and their newborns create less secure zones in the hospital. It is more important in such areas to minimize traffic and create clear sight-lines from the nurses' station to better monitor all the comings and goings of people on this floor.[136] Now newborns are also outfitted with security anklets. In addition to considering the security of newborns, pediatric and adult patients should not be mixed. There may be sharing of support areas and even nurses' stations but children must be separated from adults.[137]

Hospital psychiatric areas require varying degrees of securitization as well. Not only must seclusion rooms be located within this area but also security single-bed rooms. All aspects of this unit must be tamper resistant. Dementia units also require a higher degree of security and surveillance to help protect the patients from wondering off and leaving the facilities. Egress must be controlled so that people cannot just freely leave without notice. Outpatient surgical facilities require unrestricted, semi-restricted and restricted zones each with their own degrees of security.[138]

There are several additional programmatic support spaces that need to remain shielded, guarded and or locked. These include X-ray rooms, hospital pharmacies with narcotics and controlled drugs and radiopharmacies. The latter requires a high degree of shielding to prohibit radioactive particles from escaping. Sterilizing areas need to be restricted and protected as well.[139]

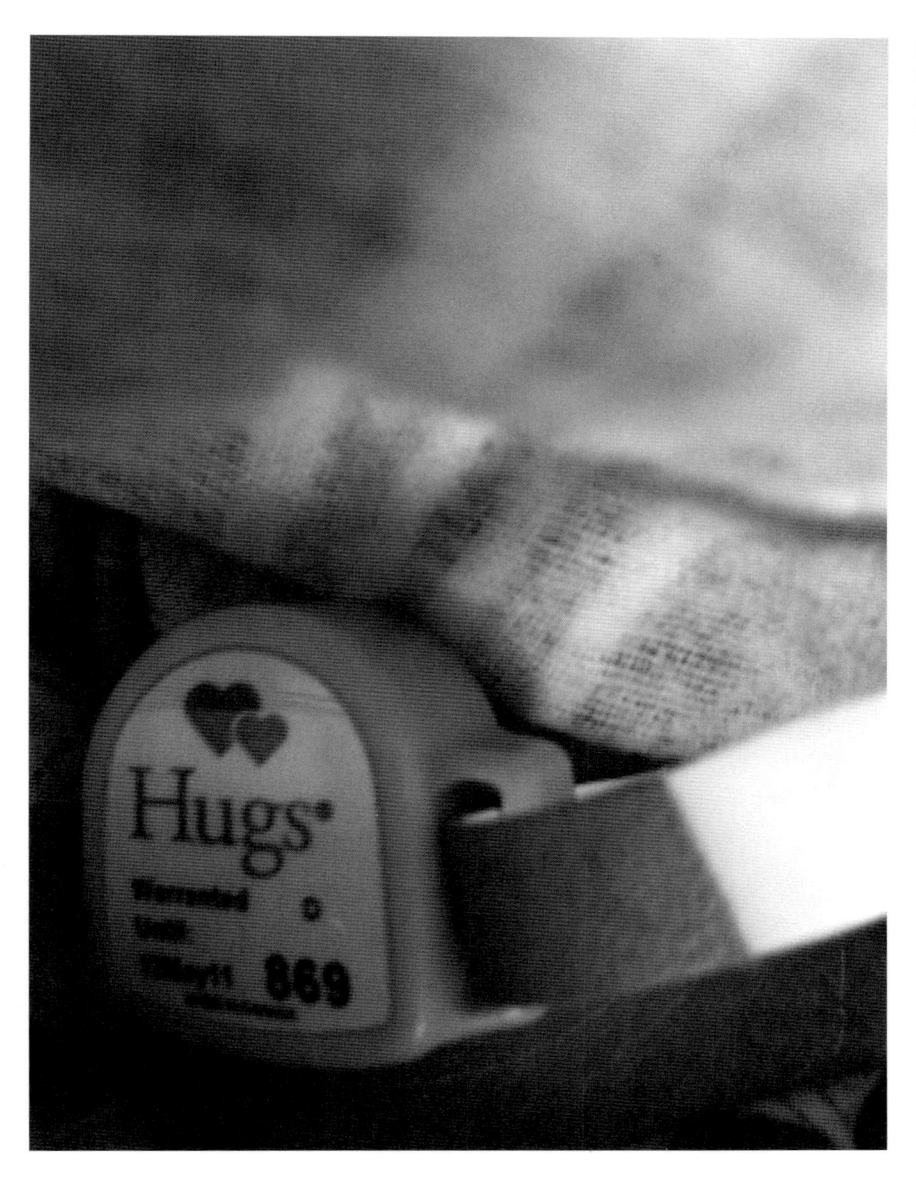

Fig. 5.25 Newborn security anklet
Source: Jennifer Hyndman 2011

Closed circuit televisions (CCTV) are used throughout all of these facilities. They provide a clear way to monitor and record activities both inside and outside the building. All cameras should have digital zoom capabilities and tape storage for at least one week.[140] I heard numerous examples when interviewing how clinics and women's shelters used their recorded footage to prove to the court someone had indeed trespassed although culprits were denying they had done so.

There are a diverse choice of locks that can be used throughout the facilities depending upon budgetary concerns and the speed of access needed. From regular keyed doors, to combination locks with codes, special keys that cannot be duplicated, to key card readers, a number of scenarios can be implemented. Another

Fig. 5.26 Detail, newborn security anklet
Source: Jennifer Hyndman 2011

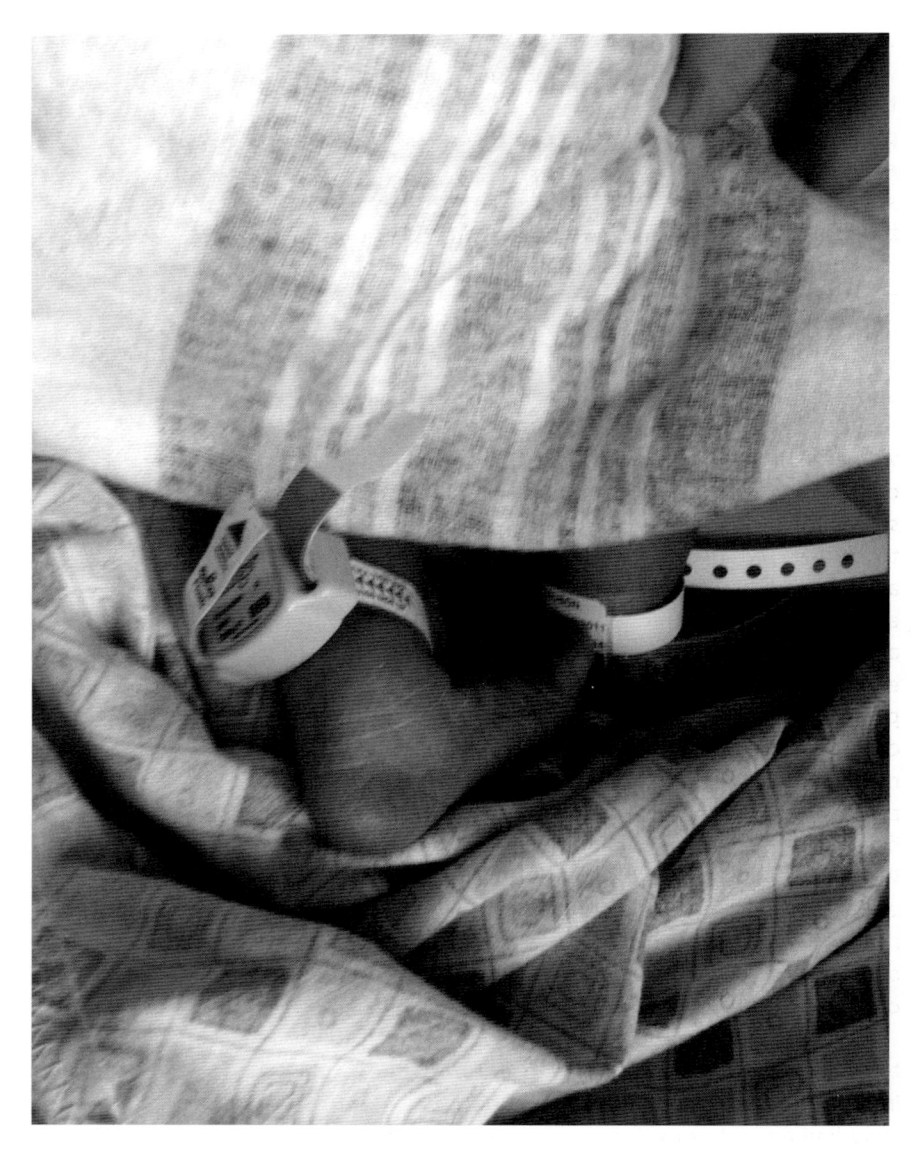

suggested component for doors going into private or semi-private spaces should include an automatic door closer to ensure doors do not remain open allowing anyone access. All of these facilities require some sort of alarm system preferably with motion sensors for both exterior and interior coverage. All reception areas should have a hidden emergency panic button that directly connects to a local law enforcement office.[141]

In addition to exterior and interior building considerations, another important component in creating a safe and protective environment includes evacuation planning and shelter preparation for staff. A clear plan should be in place that covers a range of protocols for identifying attempted and successful intrusions with response procedures outlined. These may include lines of safest egress with updated maps and floor plans to facilitate most direct exits visibly placed throughout the facility, a safe place to go once people have exited the building, protocol for staff and patients regarding protestors outside a clinic, protocol when experiencing harassment by patients and residents, an internal public address system used when an emergency occurs notifying all inside that security has been breached and what to do and where to go with delivered packages and mail that appear suspicious. Staff should not only be made aware of these protocols but also there should be regular practice drills to ensure people know their responsibilities during an emergency situation and these protocols are followed according to plan. Documenting and reporting all incidents to law enforcement and other appropriate organizations should also be a regular procedure followed by all.[142]

Maintaining a secure and safe environment is essential for abortion clinics, women's shelters and hospitals to function properly. As has been discussed, there are often difficult and complex issues that must be considered and put in place to do this successfully. A nuanced and multi-varied approach allows for security and protection to be handled through a variety of mechanisms ensuring as many concerns are addressed as possible. Spatial organization, security system infrastructures, educated and aware staff with well-rehearsed security plans and educated patients and residents are all critical for creating environments where residents, patients and employees feel protected. When reliable, law enforcement should be consulted as part of the security plans. From the clinics, shelters and hospitals I have visited and directors and doctors interviewed, visible security infrastructure does help mitigate many potential threats. There must be a balance maintained that provides both the perception and reality of protection while not creating a fortress-like facility. This is a fine line to maintain especially within the realm of abortion care and women's shelter. Where those clinics are under daily attack and suffer from a lack of substantial law enforcement support, more visible signs of protection are often the norm and are in place. At first it is not unusual for patients or residents to be surprised by the amount of security infrastructure. However, they also recognize and understand the necessity of why security is so visible.

Reproductive healthcare facilities have become twenty-first century equivalents to medieval cities where walls and moats were once used for security from intruders. Except now, protection depends upon advanced security systems including multiple surveillance cameras installed around and in entire properties and doctors' residences, multiple zones of bullet-proof glass at clinic entrances, the wearing of bullet-proof vests, and fulltime federal protection. After 5 bullets were fired into Dr. Warren Hern's Boulder Abortion Clinic in 1988, four sets of bullet-proof doors were installed at the entrance.[143]

How do clinics continue to ensure safety in the space of the everyday lives of those who come and go from such places? Dr. George Tiller's death illustrates that these domestic terrorists will go to any length to find their targets. Be it at work, at home or even at places of worship, the law's relationship to protection and public space must be rethought and the abortion bubble must evolve into a stronger and more protective space.

One clinic director was clear that she believes that abortion must seek broader support and become a part of the larger reproductive and social justice movement. One of their hopes in their sustainable renovation was to be able to connect with more environmental organizations. This has happened to varying degrees but not to the extent they had hoped. We know abortion cannot afford to remain isolated any longer. Many of the issues are the same when one looks beyond a woman's uterus: women do not have childcare, do not have decent education or equal job pay and do not have sufficient health care. In most cases, these are the larger contributing factors that must change.[144] Another doctor commented about the need for abortion to be integrated back into mainstream medical practices by locating clinics within larger medical and office park complexes. This ensures more anonymity and safety for all involved. By also providing a mix of obstetrician and gynecological services, it is far more difficult for others to ascertain what service a woman is seeking.[145] As advocated by a growing number of doctors and providers, abortion should be one of many reproductive healthcare services provided.

Another provider mentioned that in certain parts of the country it has become more and more difficult to find doctors willing to work in abortion care. It took her an entire year to find a back-up physician for her clinic. She relayed the current situation in her southern city where although young incoming pro-choice doctors would like to be able to refer patients to abortion clinics and provide services for local clinics, they ultimately cannot if they want to be employed there. New ob/gyn doctors are required to sign an agreement when entering into a practice in this city that they will "not refer to clinics and they won't provide any services whatsoever for clinics or clinic patients." No signing, no job. There is now a situation where no hospitals in this particular state will perform abortions. So if this clinic owner has a patient that needs a medically necessary abortion that her clinic cannot perform, the woman must go out of state to receive one.[146]

As Grimes et al. have argued, "[e]nding the silent pandemic of unsafe abortions is an urgent public-health and human-rights imperative." Although abortions occur frequently worldwide, unsafe abortions are still one of the most neglected public health challenges the world faces. When abortion is legal, safe and accessible, research has demonstrated that women's health improves.[147] Research has also demonstrated medical abortions are safe and reliable. Although misoprostol is a part of medical abortion regimes in North America, Western Europe, and several Asian and African countries, there needs to be more global availability especially in lower resource areas. This "would do more than any other realistically achievable, sustainable, large-scale intervention to save the lives of women at risk for death by maternal causes."[148] Although this research is focusing only on North America, the ability to more easily access emergency contraception would greatly help reduce abortions as demonstrated when this was made possible in British Columbia. Broadening access through pharmacies is clearly one of the easiest and least time consuming ways to do this. Something can be learned from Shippensburg University in Pennsylvania where EC, condoms, and pregnancy tests among other things are being sold out of a vending machine in the student health center for the past several years. Proposed by students and only accessible to students, the cost is about half of what it would be in a pharmacy and because all the students are older than 17, no prescription is needed.[149] *This* is unimpeded access.

## NOTES

1. Jones et al. 2008: 13.
2. Jones et al. 2008: 14.
3. Jones and Kooistra 2011: 45. In the Northeast 18 percent of women live in counties with no providers with 53 percent of counties having no providers with a minimum of 13 percent of counties in Connecticut and a maximum of 82 percent of counties in Pennsylvania with no providers; in the Midwest, 52 percent of women live in counties with no providers and 94 percent of counties are without providers with a minimum of 83 percent of counties in Michigan and a maximum of 98 percent of counties in South and North Dakota without providers; in the south 47 percent of women live in counties with no providers and 91 percent of counties are with no providers with a minimum of 0 percent in the District of Columbia and a maximum of 99 percent of counties in Mississippi without providers; and in the west 13 percent of women live in counties without providers and 74 percent of counties are without providers with a minimum of 20 percent of counties in Hawaii and a maximum of 97 percent of counties in Utah without providers.
4. Guttmacher Institute 2011.
5. National Abortion Federation (NAF) (b).
6. Steinauer et al. 2009: 74–80.
7. Crist 1996: 3–4.
8. Email correspondence with Medical Students for Choice, February 2012.
9. Interview with author, July 2011.
10. Interview with author, July 2011.
11. Interview with author, July 2011.
12. Interview with author, July 2011.
13. Interview with author, July 2011.
14. Email with author, October 2011.
15. Interview with author, July 2011.
16. Interview with author, July 2011.
17. Anderson and Zurek 2011.
18. Grossman et al. 2011.
19. Donaldson James 2011.
20. Interview with author, July 2011.
21. Interview with author, July 2011.
22. Interview with author, July 2011.
23. Interview with author, July 2011.

24  Hess 2012.
25  U.S. Census Bureau 1999.
26  NARAL Pro-Choice America (b).
27  ARAL Pro-Choice America (a).
28  U.S. Census Bureau 1999.
29  NARAL Pro-Choice America (b).
30  NARAL Pro-Choice America (a).
31  Interview with author, August 2011.
32  Interview with author, June 2011.
33  Please see http://coolscenics.com/index.php for an example of what is being described.
34  ICU (n.d.).
35  Interview with author, August 2011.
36  Interview with author, June 2011.
37  Interview with author, June 2011.
38  U.S. Census Bureau 1999.
39  Bazelon 2009.
40  NARAL Pro-Choice America (a) and http://www.guttmacher.org/pubs/sfaa/south_dakota.html.
41  Goodman 2006. Also please see Briggs 2006 and *The Economist* 2006.
42  National Park Service (n.d.).
43  Just this New Year's day January 2012, a clinic in Pensacola, Florida was arsoned without receiving any real national attention. This clinic has been the recipient of numerous acts of violence including the murder of Dr. John Britton and the wounding of his wife in 1984. Please see http://www.pnj.com/article/20120105/NEWS01/120105019/Florida-abortion-clinic-has-history-as-target-for-protests and http://www.rhrealitycheck.org/article/2012/01/03/abortion-clinic-burned-on-new-years-morning-%E2%80%93-into-streets-abortion-rights-on-r-0 for more information.
44  Interview with author, May 2008.
45  Interview with author, July 2011.
46  Interview with author, July 2011.
47  Interview with author, May 2008.
48  Hagerty 2010.
49  Please see ACLU letter 2010 and Kaplan 2010.
50  Bassett 2011b.
51  Interview with author, May 2008.
52  U.S. Census Bureau 1999.
53  NARAL Pro-Choice America (a).

54  Steinbrook 2012: 365–6.
55  Interview with author, May 2008.
56  Nather and Nocera 2011.
57  Planned Parenthood Federation of America 2009–2010 Annual Report (n.d.).
58  New *York Times* 2011.
59  Bassett 2011(a).
60  Clark 2011.
61  Interview with author, June 2011.
62  Interview with author, July 2011.
63  Interview with author, July 2011.
64  Sulzberger 2011.
65  Frontline 2005.
66  Interview with author, August 2011.
67  Feminist Majority Foundation (a).
68  Feminist Majority Foundation (b).
69  Videos can be found on Youtube: http://www.youtube.com/watch?v=L9Zj9yx2j0Y (New Jersey) and http://www.youtube.com/watch?v=0iMScbJJS2g (Virginia). Please see Schulman 2011 and Pareene 2011 for more detailed information. Both reported that Planned Parenthood alerted the attorney general and FBI immediately after these encounters.
70  Interview with author, July 2011 and follow-up email correspondence with author, October 2011.
71  Interview with author, July 2011.
72  Interview with author, July 2011.
73  Kishen and Stedman 2010: 573.
74  Sethna and Doull 2007: 643 and Eggerston 2001: 649.
75  Downie and Nassar 2007: 143–6.
76  Kishen and Stedman 2010: 571.
77  Downie and Nassar 2007: 162.
78  Downie and Nassar 2007: 170.
79  Downie and Nassar 2007: 170 and see also Blackmer 2007: 1310.
80  Downie and Nassar 2007: 147–9.
81  Sethna and Doull 2009: 170.
82  Downie and Nassar 2007: 150.
83  Sethna and Doull 2007: 645.
84  Sethna and Doull 2007: 643.
85  Sethna and Doull 2007: 640, 643–6.

86   Downie and Nassar 2007: 154–5.
87   Downie and Nassar 2007: 158.
88   Sibbald 2001: 849.
89   Soon et al. 2005: 870, 878.
90   CanWest News Service 2008.
91   Darabi 2009.
92   Sánchez-Fuentes et al. 2008: 348.
93   Sedgh et al. 2012.
94   Sánchez-Fuentes et al. 2008, 347.
95   Sánchez-Fuentes et al. 2008: 348.
96   Sánchez-Fuentes et al. 2008: 347–8, 352.
97   Grupo de Información en Reproducción Elegida GIRE 2007.
98   García et al. 2004: 65–71.
99   Gould et al. 2002: 417–24.
100  Becker et al. 2011: S16–18.
101  Sánchez-Fuentes et al. 2008: 352.
102  Human Rights Watch 2005.
103  Human Rights Watch 2005.
104  Silva et al. 2009: 56.
105  Silva et al. 2009: 61–2.
106  Dayananda et al. 2012: 304–8.
107  Casas 2009: 87.
108  Casas 2009: 81.
109  Casas 2009: 83.
110  Juarez et al. 2008: 163, 165–6.
111  Langer and Catino 2006: 483.
112  Gould et al. 2002: 417–18, 420.
113  Billings et al. 2009: 445–51.
114  U.S. Department of Justice Federal Bureau of Investigation (n.d.).
115  Feminist Majority Foundation 1994.
116  Atlas 2008a: 3.
117  Atlas 2008b: 24.
118  Sorensen et al. 2008: 53–4.
119  Sorensen et al. 2008: 55.
120  Jung 2004: 8.11–8.12.

121 Bershad and Phifer 2004: 16.1–16.2.

122 Nadel 2004: 21.3. For more information on the FACE law and the FBI's policies in enforcing it as well as other links, see http://www.fbi.gov/about-us/investigate/civilrights/face.

123 American Planning Association 2005.

124 Wible 2007: 142–3.

125 Interview with author, July 2011.

126 Email correspondence with author, October 2011.

127 Nadel 2004: 21.3.

128 Wible 2007: 146–7.

129 Anti-Defamation League 2004: 17.11–13.

130 Sewell 2004: 27.5.

131 Wible 2007: 144.

132 Norman 2007: 359–63, 368.

133 *Federal Emergency Management Agency* (FEMA) (b).

134 *Federal Emergency Management Agency* (FEMA) (a).

135 Nadel 2004: 21.4–6.

136 Nadel 2004: 8.19.

137 American Institute of Architects Academy of Architecture for Health et al. 2006: 57–61.

138 American Institute of Architects Academy of Architecture for Health et al. 2006: 113, 146, 221–3, 286.

139 American Institute of Architects Academy of Architecture for Health et al. 2006: 146–68, 221–30.

140 Nadel 2004: 17.4–17.7.

141 Nadel 2004: 17.6–17.9.

142 *Federal Emergency Management Agency* (FEMA) (c).

143 PBS NOW 2009.

144 Interview with author, August 2011.

145 Interview with author, May 2008.

146 Interview with author, July 2011.

147 Grimes et al. 2006: 1908.

148 Fernandez et al. 2009: 180.

149 Levy 2012.

# 6

## Conclusion

*Ultimately health is political because power is exercised over it as a part of a wider economic, social and political system.*[1]

Clearly we have to change the terms of the abortion debate. At what point does the ability to have free speech weigh differently or more importantly than someone being able to access an abortion clinic? Legally there has not been an outright ruling for access to an abortion clinic over free speech. Legal scholars are not addressing what this means for in-the-field application. From the many providers I have interviewed, it is clear that their rights are not being protected. At great expense to both patients and employees, the careful abstract dissection of free speech as it pertains to one's First Amendment rights is presented as being far more important than a woman's ability to legally and physically access her right to abortion. We should learn from situations such as when the Ontario NDP government filed an injunction limiting free speech around abortion clinics and hospitals in order to provide the highest level of safety and security for women seeking reproductive healthcare.[2] Courts and lawmakers need to consider whether anti-abortion speech constitutes a special class of speech. The US does make free speech exceptions around such spaces as polling places and military funerals.[3]

What has become clear to me over the time I have spent researching, visiting and interviewing abortion providers is that space, the actual space of clinics, the geography of location, is not being considered as a *real* concern. Court rulings try to make the argument for a "balanced" decision according to government interests as weighed against the right of someone to exercise their First Amendment or the right of someone to access abortion. But nothing is balanced or fair in abortion. As time passes and the perverse debate on abortion availability continues and as more states continue to pass more restrictive legislation, abortion becomes less and less balanced. Even as the United States' healthcare mandate is slowly moving forward, the issue of abortion has stymied passage. The most recent congressional contraception debacle combined with the Health and Human Services Secretary Kathleen Sebelius overruling the Food and Drug Administration's (FDA) recommendation to make emergency contraception a non-prescription drug regardless of age are two cases furthering this point.[4] Basic women's healthcare continues to be argued not as a universal right or human health necessity (as Canada and Mexico City believe) but one steeped in morality and religious politics. Both of these examples demonstrate to what extent politics is directly impacting medical access.

Anti-abortion groups have been successful in co-opting issues around choice, fetal pain and ideas of fetal personhood. But the far more important and larger issues surrounding access are not being discussed and debated. Access is a geographical and space-dependant issue. Access without availability is not access. Not acknowledging women's reproductive healthcare as a basic and fundamental human right is the most egregious of acts. "Abortion is becoming more of an economic good available for those who can afford it rather than a constitutional right assured to all who wish to exercise it."[5] This is the elephant in the room clearly at issue in all of the North American examples cited. What is not fore grounded is whom this is really impacting most: poor women of color. "[M]uch of the debate is conducted at too high a level of abstraction … debates … have to … examine *which women*, in *which contexts* suffer disadvantages … "[6] As Kimberly Mutcherson, Rutgers University School of Law Professor, has argued structural inequalities only continue to reproduce social inequalities and these directly influence a woman's ability for choice. She believes for women to have equal citizenship they must have real reproductive rights. These rights are integral to equal citizenry. Insurance is part of this causal relationship and access without means in meaningless.[7]

Abortion has been abandoned by the larger field of medicine. As cited earlier, 33 percent of all medical schools surveyed by Steinauer et al. do not include "any discussion of elective abortion procedures, pregnancy options counseling, post-elective abortion care or elective abortion law/policy/availability" and 44 percent of US schools offered "no formal preclinical elective abortion education."[8] In the US 70 percent of all abortions are performed in stand-alone abortion clinics not a part of comprehensive ob/gyn practices (378 clinics accounting for 21 percent of all abortion providers), with 24 percent of non-specialized clinics (473 clinics accounting for 26 percent of all abortion providers), 4 percent of hospitals (610 hospitals accounting for 34 percent of all abortion providers) and 1 percent of physician offices (332 offices accounting for 19 percent of all abortion providers) reported providing abortions.[9] As has been discussed in Chapter 5, if hospitals return to becoming another primary space of access, this greatly alters the physical landscape. However, it must be noted that now one in six hospitals are affiliated with the Catholic Church[10] comprising the "largest single group of not-for-profit hospitals in the country" and unlike other religiously affiliated hospitals generally operating in a non-sectarian manner, Catholic affiliated hospitals operate their facilities in line with Catholic doctrine allowing the denial of women's reproductive healthcare.[11] As University of Toronto Law Professor Bernard Dickens argues, a patient's rights should never be directly connected to a practitioner's rights and I would add by extension, a hospital's moral code. When women are being confronted with objections to provide healthcare, he argues hospitals are legal corporations and as such, they do not have spiritual obligations.[12]

Combine this with the fact that over 87 percent of all counties in the United States do not have an abortion provider. We are left with the very chilling reality that the ability to exercise one's right to abortion is dependent upon where in North America you live and how much money you have. Not only has the medical establishment segregated abortion care but also contraception and family planning are not typical phrases uttered out of most people's mouths. Our society, the US in particular, allows images of sex to be everywhere but does not want to discuss or allow age appropriate sex education in large parts of the country. As Sarah Brown from The National Campaign to Prevent Teen and Unplanned Pregnancy stated at a 2010 symposium, family planning is not integrated into women's health. The public is ignorant about contraception knowledge and this country has a non-system of family planning. Although family planning is part of public health in other countries, large constituencies within the US have popularized contraception as a moral and ethical issue.[13]

There is an argument put forth by Dr. Meera Kishen and others that abortion services should be provided by non-medical practitioners such as nurse practitioners (NP), nurse midwifes (NM), advanced practice clinicians (APC) and physician assistants (PA). Why should abortion not be included as one of the services under their purview especially since these groups continue to administer more of our health care these days?[14] It is one of the most common surgical procedures in the US today.[15] Because fewer doctors are being trained and are willing to perform abortions, this would substantially increase abortion access. Evidence demonstrates that there are no greater complications if abortions are provided by APCs, performing equally as well as doctors when providing abortions. In Vermont and Montana APCs have been providing abortions since 1973 when abortion became legal.[16] By 2004 APCs were providing medical and sometime surgical abortions in 14 states in the US but thus far California has been the only state to legally allow NPs and CNMs (certified nurse midwives) to provide medical abortions.[17]

Carol Joffe, long-time abortion supporter and sociologist, has written extensively on abortion. In her most recent book she discusses how the free-standing abortion clinic evolved into existence in New York state and Washington D.C. where in the early 1970s before *Roe v. Wade,* both had liberalized their abortion laws. Although clinics have excellent safety records, offer more flexible care and have helped to keep the cost of abortions as low as possible, the separation and dislocation of the service being situated outside ob/gyn practices and general medicine in stand-alone spaces has had a negative effect on the relationship between abortion to the rest of the medical profession. Not only through their professional separation but also through their individualized physical locations abortion clinics are much more visible and far more easily targeted by anti-abortion groups.[18] Joffe also argues for the normalization of abortion into healthcare. With the development of new technologies such as medical abortion, earlier abortion can be performed in a

# Mississippi_Composite Maps

VARIES FROM 55 MILES TO 217 MILES TO HOSPITALS

VARIES FROM 55 MILES TO 165 MILES TO CLINICS

5 FULL FUNDING FOR HOSPITAL AND CLINIC ABORTIONS

Mississippi_Composite Maps

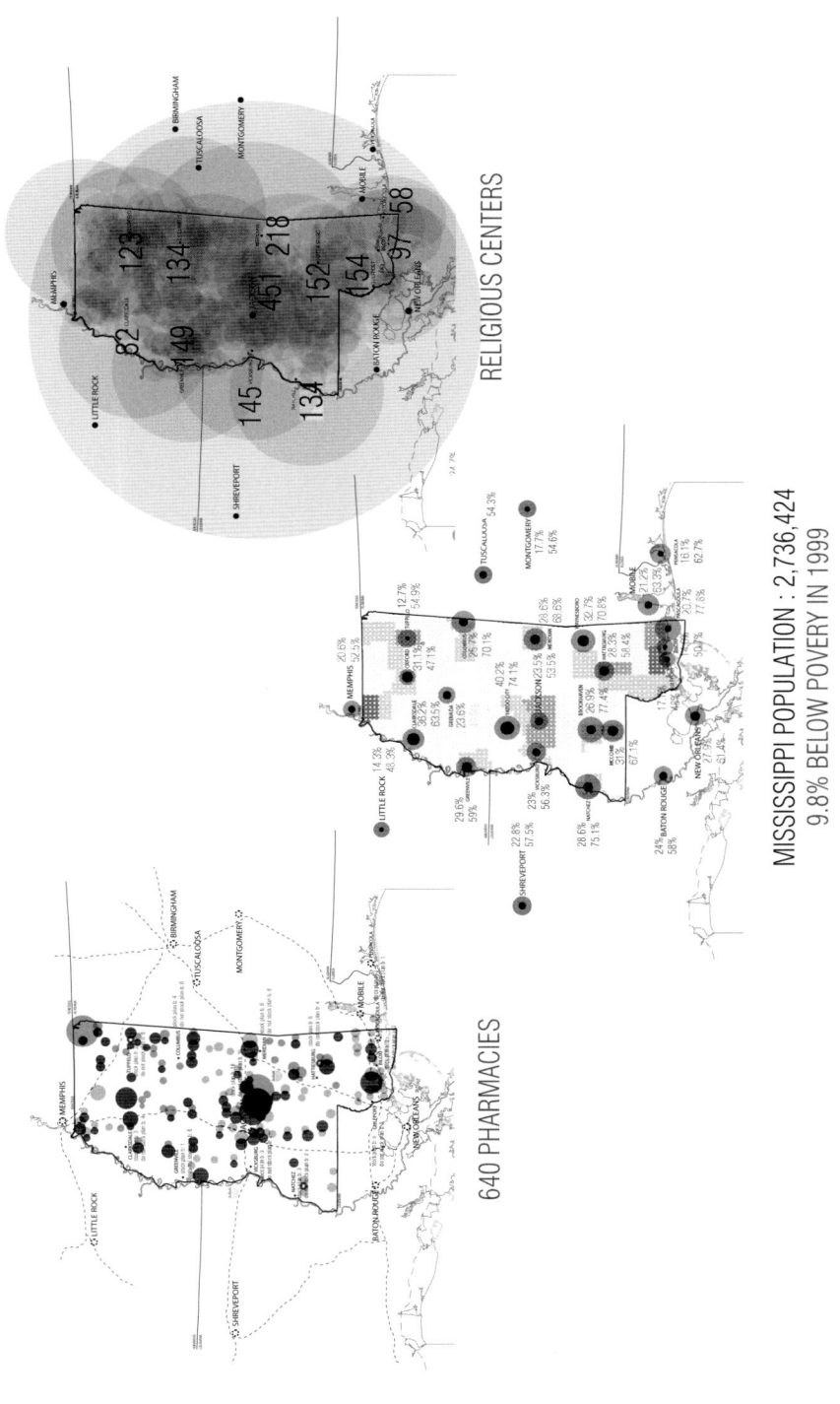

640 PHARMACIES

MISSISSIPPI POPULATION : 2,736,424
9.8% BELOW POVERTY IN 1999

RELIGIOUS CENTERS

Fig. 6.1   Composite maps for Mississippi

The drawings demonstrate the significant change expanding access would have if hospitals and pharmacies fully participate in providing coverage. In the second phase new clinics would be located in all cities and towns with populations over 10,000 people.

## Kentucky_Composite Map

VARIES FROM 41 MILES TO 272 MILES TO HOSPITALS

VARIES FROM 47 MILES TO 272 MILES TO CLINICS

17 FULL FUNDING FOR HOSPITAL AND CLINIC ABORTIONS

Kentucky_Composite Map

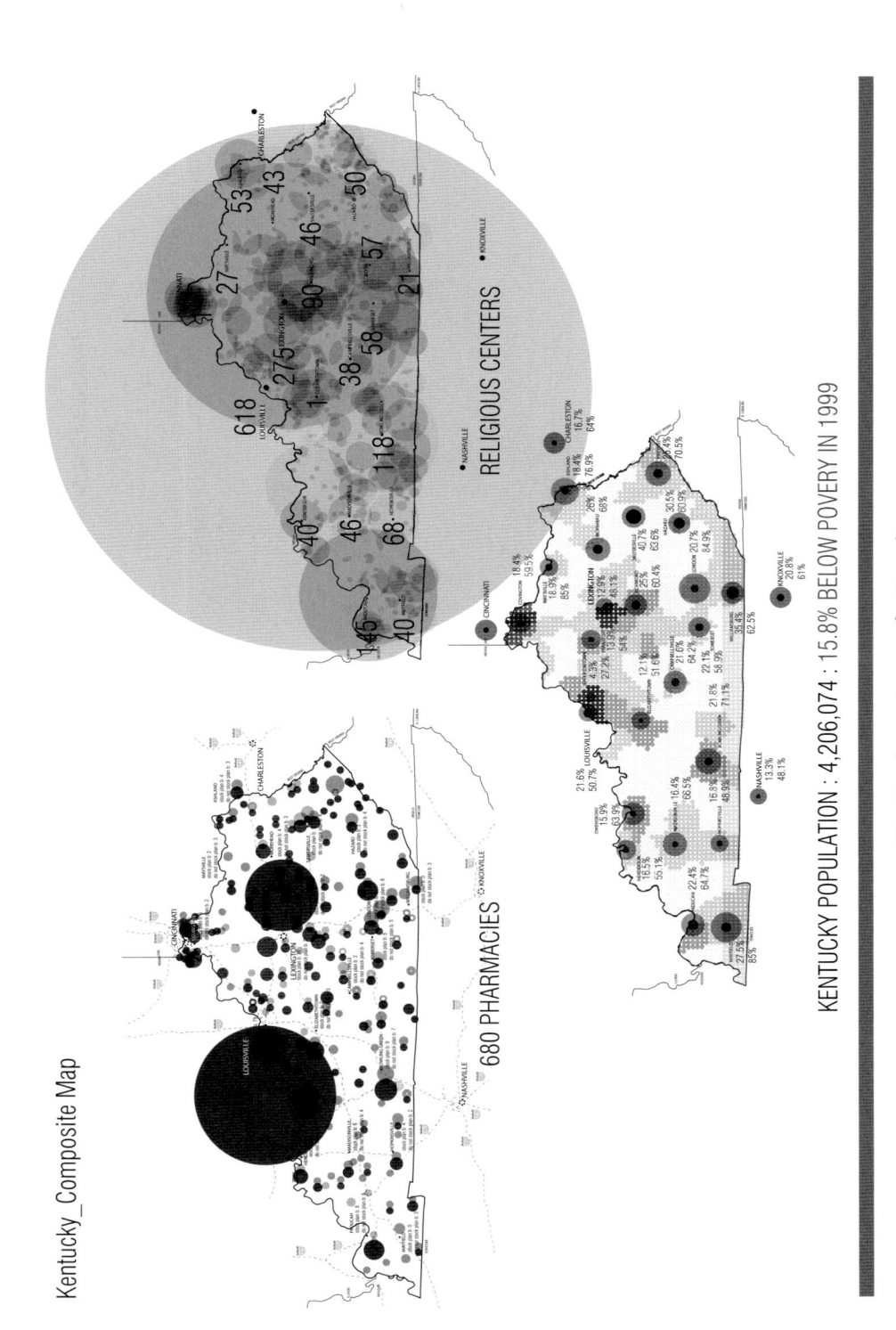

Fig. 6.2   Composite maps for Kentucky

KENTUCKY POPULATION : 4,206,074 : 15.8% BELOW POVERTY IN 1999

The drawings demonstrate the significant change expanding access would have if hospitals and pharmacies fully participate in providing coverage. In the second phase new clinics would be located in all cities and towns with populations over 10,000 people.

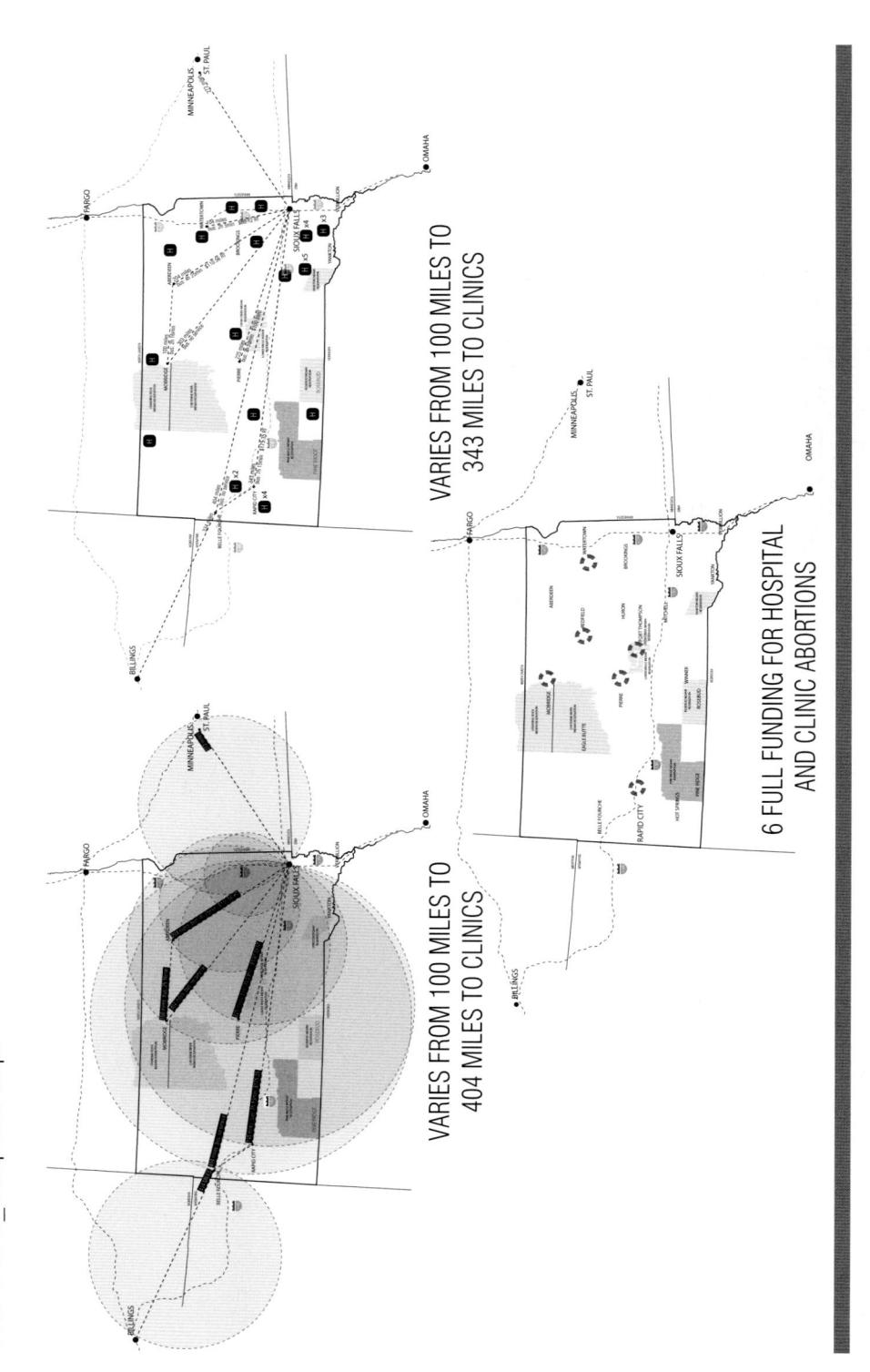

South Dakota_Composite Maps

VARIES FROM 100 MILES TO 343 MILES TO CLINICS

VARIES FROM 100 MILES TO 404 MILES TO CLINICS

6 FULL FUNDING FOR HOSPITAL AND CLINIC ABORTIONS

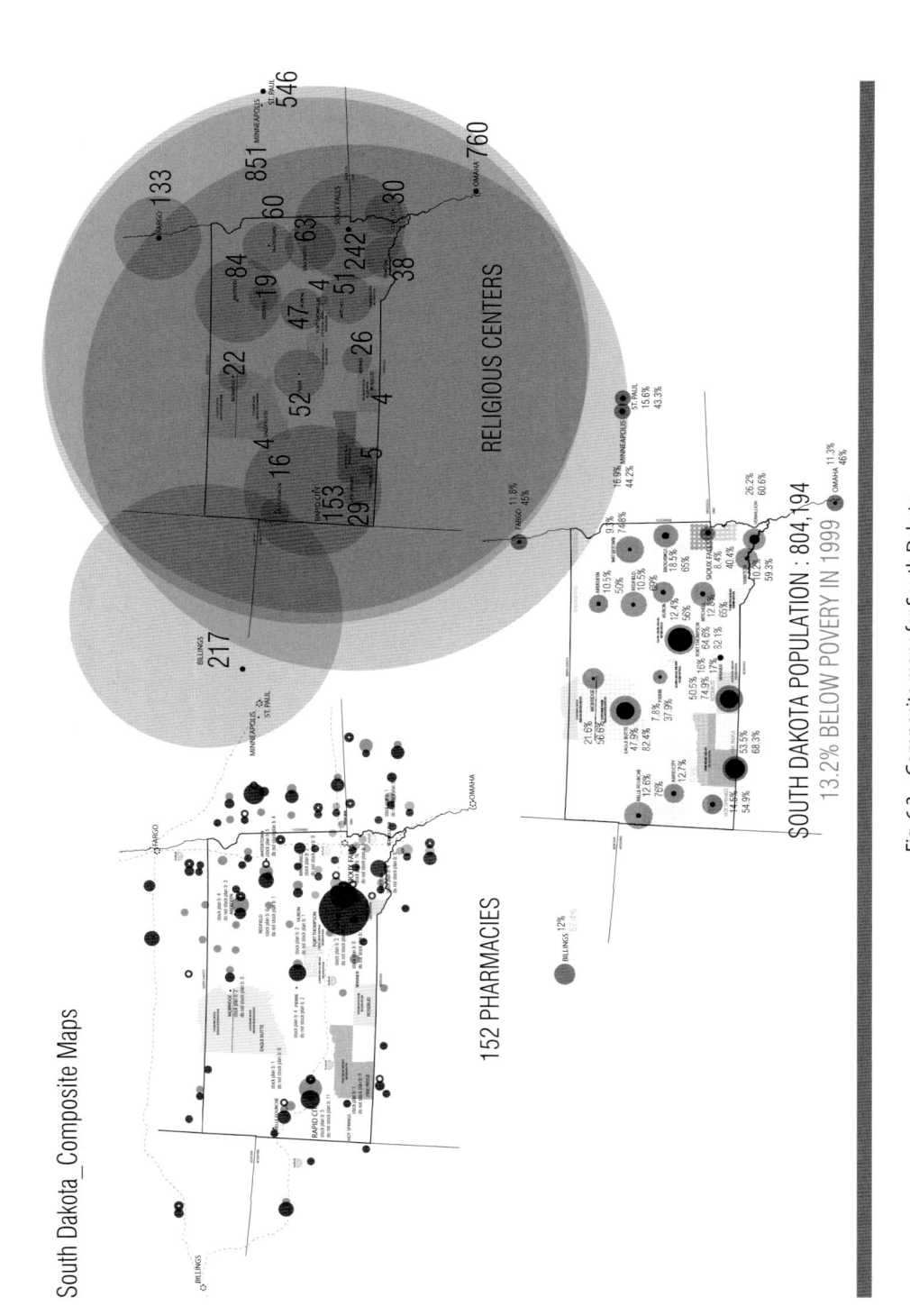

Fig. 6.3 Composite maps for South Dakota

The drawings demonstrate the significant change expanding access would have if hospitals and pharmacies fully participate in providing coverage. In the second phase new clinics would be located in all cities and towns with populations over 10,000 people.

Utah_Composite Maps

VARIES FROM 30 MILES TO 309 MILES TO HOSPITALS

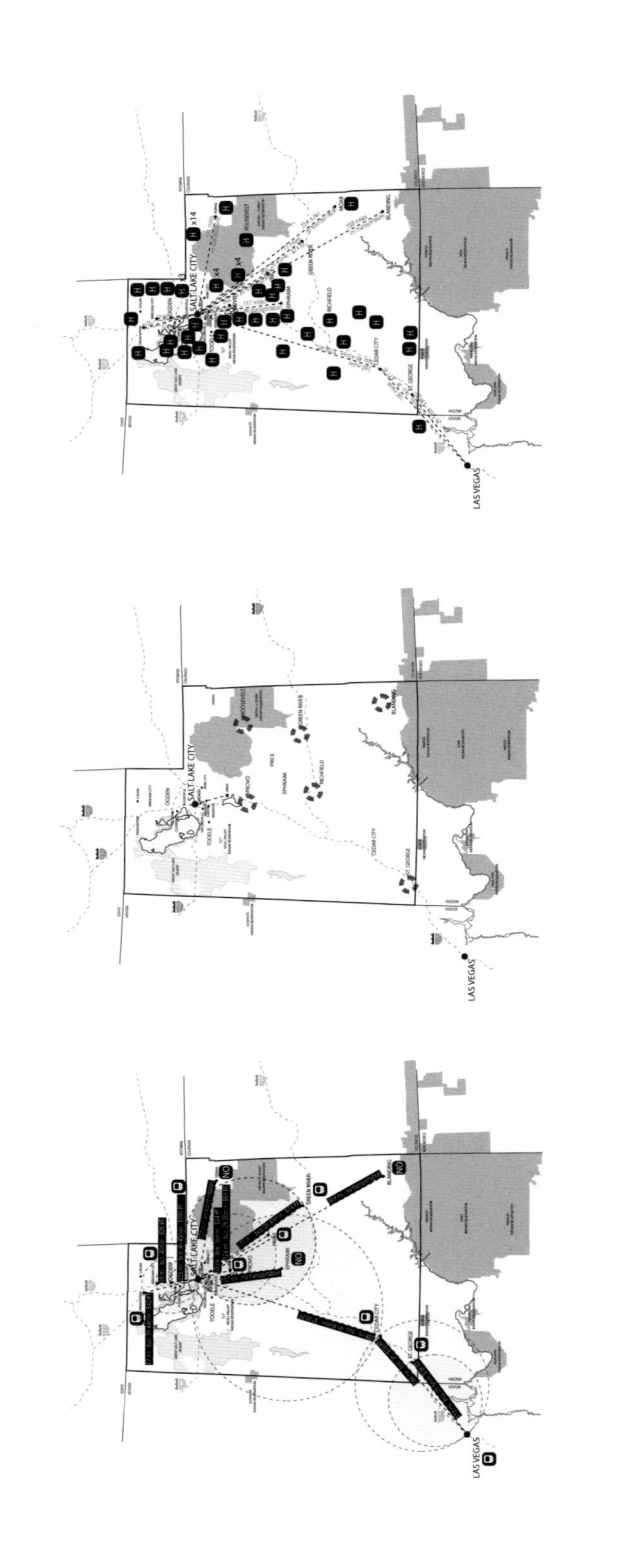

5 FULL FUNDING FOR HOSPITAL AND CLINIC ABORTIONS

VARIES FROM 30 MILES TO 309 MILES TO CLINICS

Utah_Composite Maps

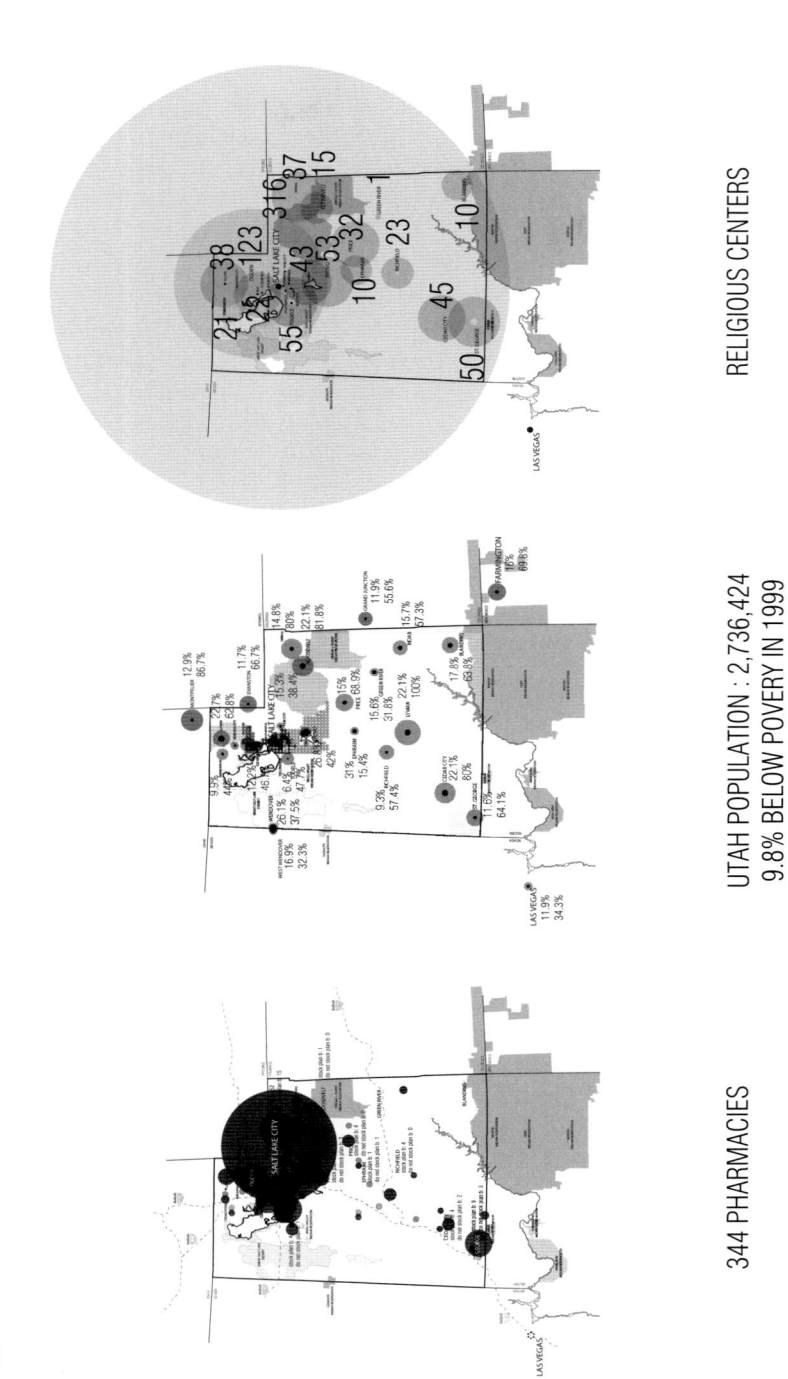

344 PHARMACIES

UTAH POPULATION : 2,736,424
9.8% BELOW POVERTY IN 1999

RELIGIOUS CENTERS

Fig. 6.4    Composite maps for Utah

The drawings demonstrate the significant change expanding access would have if hospitals and pharmacies fully participate in providing coverage. In the second phase new clinics would be located in all cities and towns with populations over 10,000 people.

primary care office by APCs.[19] Through integrating abortion into general medicine it decreases the stigma as well as allowing the process to be more anonymous.

The broader scope of this book is not one of policy but one concerned with space so I would like to conclude by speculating upon the issue of access from this vantage point. Because the courts present abortion more in terms of free speech, space is not commonly addressed or explicitly considered. Although dimensions of "protection" have been adjudicated, these remain abstract ideas applied to abstract space. Abortion is a federally protected right that requires a REAL space for this right to be exercised. Theory and practice are in direct conflict. What reads well on paper is not working out on-the-ground in real space. The use of First Amendment concerns around "speech" only mask and further camouflage the on-the-ground implications of the ever increasing list of state legislations. Sure bubble laws have been created as well as varying types of spatial zones but access only continues to be whittled away by individual state governments who are alarmingly more and more anti-woman and anti-healthcare as a basic human right. These new-founded (although not really new) types of spatial restrictions and demarcations have not made abortion access safer or easier. In fact, as I write, abortion access continues to be more difficult to procure and walking into a clinic is more and more a test of a woman's will and dexterity to not succumb to the hatred and outright domestic terrorism that many of these anti-abortion protestors exercise against both patients and employees going into clinics.

The argument must be redirected and changed. This project attempts to redirect the debate to the real space around real clinics that is not legislated equally. Why is it that the country and even continent has allowed the politics around abortion to completely control a woman's access to a medical procedure that is actually legal and safe? Space is central to these concerns as countless abortion clinics will attest. These clinics are not being protected, their spatial rights are not being guaranteed. Infringements take place daily.

In order to further foreground the issue, I am going to advocate a far more radical approach. Abortion clinics should not have to be hidden away somewhere in order to ensure privacy and protection. Such spatial isolation will not prevent protestors from gaining intimate details about a clinic and its staff. Some anti-choice websites have regularly posted photographs of people going into clinics. Other anti-choice websites have documented the areas in and around abortion clinics in order to better inform protestors how to physically access these spaces including precise locations of security cameras and the circulation paths patients use to enter and exit the building. The level of surveillance required to create these various websites is quite disturbing and the publicity created by the various groups' documentation calls into question how the FACE law is actually being enforced to protect those who are both providing and receiving reproductive health care services. FACE has the potential, if enforced, to actually protect these contested landscapes by targeting specific types of actions and creating "safe" zones around health and religious facilities.

Although in theory not a difficult process to undertake, the expansion of access through rethinking hospitals as possible places of access and the use of EC requires a shift in national and regional attitudes. The first phase would simply require all pharmacies in each state to actually stock AND sell EC and ALL hospitals would provide abortions as part of their basic outpatient surgery services. The second phase builds upon the first and essentially fills the geographic gaps produced by the first phase. This would include creating new clinics to be located in areas with high female head-of-household poverty rates typically intersecting major transportation networks.

I advocate for clinics to become more centrally located in our daily spatial lives. They need to be front and center in our society, not hidden away and difficult to access. Locate them in shopping malls where protests cannot happen due to malls not being public space. There is a spatial separation inscribed there. Already other types of medical practices have established themselves in malls including dermatologists, primary care practitioners, chiropractors, dentists and opticians to name a few.[20] Return abortion back into hospitals, back into general gynecology and obstetric care and back into part of regular primary care practices. Rather than continuing to be banished and excluded, abortion must be re-introduced into mainstream healthcare services.[21]

If one is to radicalize and open up reproductive health care services, then where else could these services be located? Why not fully democratize their locations and accessibility? What places attract large groups of people? By siting facilities in places that attract the demographics most needing these services, these "new" clinics would have a greater potential to help more women. In addition to malls,[22] let's consider military bases, jails, public high schools, and churches for starters. Some of these locations provide proximity to locations that could provide services and immediate educational outreach (public schools, military bases, shopping malls) while other locations provide potentially far more privacy because of their specific clientele (jails and churches).

Architecture has the ability to engage the larger political and social issues inherent within the abortion conflict. In order for architecture to reclaim its place in shaping our daily lives, it must again engage the many and conflicting factors influencing what *that* form can become. Through reconsidering the spatial implications of our First Amendment rights and the security now required to protect them, abortion clinics and women shelters provide an opportunity to both claim and defend space simultaneously. These decades-long conflicts create opportunities for architecture to re-insert itself into all aspects of design, from invisibly legislated protection zones to how and where someone enters a clinic, actually impacting everyday people's everyday lives. As architect Kim Dovey has written:

> *the relations of architecture to social behavior are complex and culturally embedded interactions ... Most people, most of the time, take the built environment for granted ... [the] relegation of built form to the unquestioned frame is the key to its relations to power. The more that the structures and representations of power can be embedded in the framework of everyday life, the less questionable they become and the more effectively they can work.*[23]

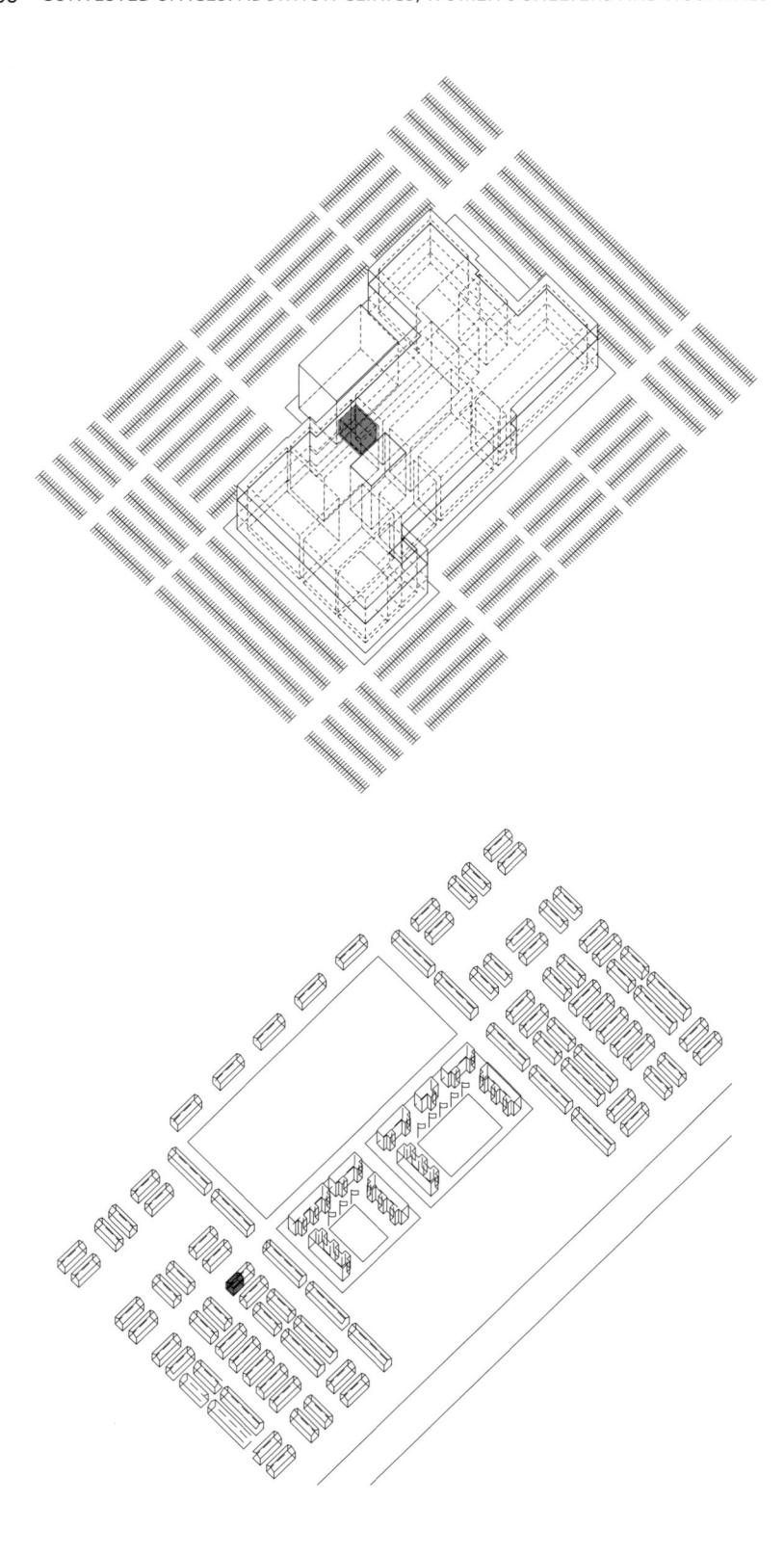

Figs. 6.5–6.8 New locations for clinics: Shopping malls, military bases, jails, public and high schools

CONCLUSION 207

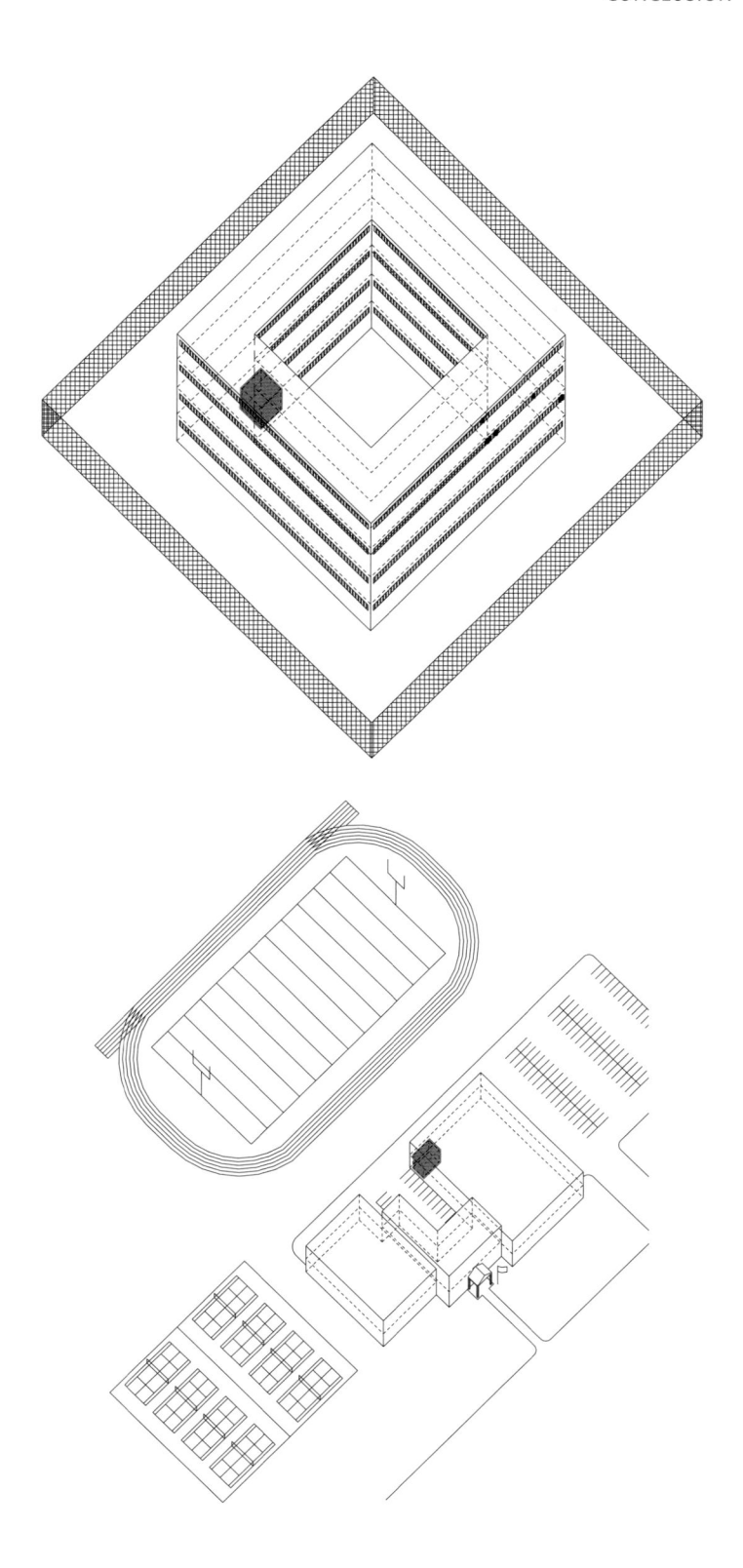

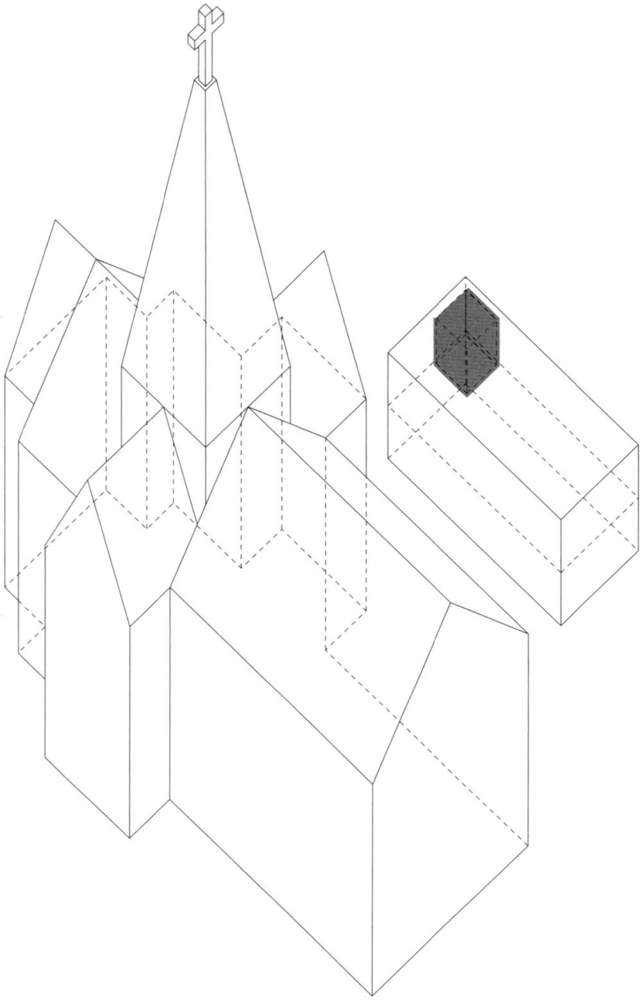

Fig. 6.9 New locations for clinics: churches

How to apply theory into practice? Where are the spaces of potential? As mentioned in Chapter 2, Homi Bhabha's ideas of third space as one that is fluid not fixed, something in between and is continually remaking boundaries and exposing limits seems to offer a possible way to consider these contested spaces. Although we speak of these spaces as fixed through legislation and the built environment, history continues to demonstrate there are those who have been able to operate in between, tactically and surreptitiously within and against the law. Through Elizabeth Grosz's questioning of architecture to think architecture differently without conforming to our standard practices, responses and modes of signification, architecture has the potential, I would argue the responsibility continuing her line of thought, to become something larger than mere form signified through building. What is at stake in this research is how do landscapes of access—spatial access, economic access, political access, gender access and racial access, become places of intervention? For contestation? If for Deleuze "thought as difference" freed from representation is a place of potential transformation, then we must continue to attack these issues by moving outside the bounded ways we have been engaging them. Architectural inquiry provides a way of thinking about these relationships outside the structures that hold them together, thus helping produce social change.

I believe by expanding the focus to include broader reproductive, social and environmental justice concerns builds more critical mass. As Rosalind Petchesky notes, "[f]eminist concepts of power and empowerment are closely related to their challenges to mainstream views of sustainable development."[24] We must connect to these larger movements both locally and globally. As one clinic has put into practice through their non-profit medical and sustainable clinic building, the group is focusing on this broader context in hopes of expanding the terms of the debate and those who are included in the debate. Through connecting at the local level in their community they are in fact changing the world, one step at a time.

## NOTES

1   Monk et al. 2009: 805.
2   AbortionInCanada.ca. (a).
3   I would like to thank Don Mitchell for his critical insights into this area of free speech.
4   Steinbrook 2012: 365.
5   Gober and Rosenberg 2001: 102.
6   Monk et al. 2009: 801.
7   Mutcherson 2010.
8   Steinauer et al. 2009: 75–6.
9   Jones and Kooistra 2011: 46.
10  Freedman 2010a.
11  Freedman 2010b: 119.
12  Dickens 2010. He also cites *Rodriguez v. Chicago* (1998) where a police officer requested an exemption from protecting an abortion clinic because of religious beliefs but the court denied him this exemption. See http://caselaw.lp.findlaw.com/scripts/getcase.pl?navby=search&case=/data2/circs/7th/973339.html.
13  Brown 2010. For a thought-provoking documentary demonstrating the effects of abstinence-only education and one young woman's fight to change this see *The Education of Shelby Knox*, directed by Marion Lipschutz and Rose Rosenblatt, 2005.
14  Kishen and Stedman 2010, 569–78.
15  Samora and Leslie 2007: 471.
16  Kishen and Stedman 2010: 569–78. See also Yarnall et al. 2009: 61–9.
17  Samora and Leslie 2007: 473.

18  Joffe 2009: 48–9.
19  Joffe 2009: 28, 43,157.
20  See for example Wonderland Medical Center 2012, Hayden 1989: 12–29, and Felix 1991: 30–57.
21  Even back in the late 1960–70s as an assistant professor in obstetrics and gynecology Dr. Takey Crist's "A Model for a Youth Family Planning Clinic in a Community without a University" recommended creating a family planning clinic within the Public Health Department of any county. Operating one night a week from six to eleven in the evening, the clinic would focus on serving young adults from 12 years old to 19 providing education and counseling combined with medical and contraceptive services. Please see Crist (n.d.).
22  The location of dermatologists' offices providing botox and other cosmetic medical procedures in shopping malls could be considered the beginning of a precedent locating medical offices in more retail-centered areas. See Natasha Singer 2006.
23  Dovey 2008: 2.
24  Petchesky 2003: 11.

# Bibliography

AbortionInCanada.ca. (a). "Abortion in Canada Timeline." http://www.abortionincanada.ca/history/Abortion_Canada_Timeline.html. Accessed January 30, 2012.

AbortionInCanada.ca. (b). "Legal Abortion in Canada." http://www.abortionincanada.ca/history/legal_abortion_canada.html. Accessed April 7, 2012.

ACLU letter 2010. Written by Laura Murphy, Vania Leveille, Brigitte Amiri, Alexa Kolbi-Molinas and Daniel Pochoda. July 1. http://www.aclu.org/reproductive-freedom/aclu-letter-centers-medicare-and-medicaid-regarding-denial-reproductive-health. Accessed January 14, 2012.

AGI. 1999. *Sharing Responsibility: Women, Society and Abortion Worldwide*. New York: AGI.

American Institute of Architects Academy of Architecture for Health, the Facility Guidelines Institute and U.S. Department of Health and Human Services. 2006. *Guidelines for Design and Construction of Health Care Facilities*. Washington, D.C.: American Institute of Architects.

American Planning Association. 2005. "Policy Guide on Security." http://www.planning.org/policy/guides/adopted/security.htm. Accessed February 18, 2012.

Anderson, Wyndi and Melanie Zurek. 2011. "Study Shows Telemedicine Abortion Is Safe and Effective; Politics Intervenes Nonetheless." RH Reality Check Reproductive & Sexual Health and Justice News Analysis & Commentary. http://www.rhrealitycheck.org/blog/2011/08/04/medical-abortion-telemedicine-keeping-technological-progress-open-fields-medicine. Accessed January 6, 2012.

Anti-Defamation League. 2004. "Religious Institutions and Community Centers." In *Building Security Handbook for Architectural Planning and Design*, edited by Barbara A. Nadel, 17.1–17.17. New York: McGraw-Hill.

"Atelier Van Lieshout." (n.d.) http://www.ateliervanlieshout.com/. Accessed November 25, 2011.

Atlas, Randall I. 2008a. "Background and Theory." In *21st Century Security and CPTED Designing for Critical Infrastructure Protection and Crime Prevention*, edited by Randall I. Atlas, 3–8. Boca Raton, FL: CRC Press Auerbach Publications.

Atlas, Randall I. 2008b. "The Challenge of Architecture in a Free Society." In *21st Century Security and CPTED Designing for Critical Infrastructure Protection and Crime Prevention*, 17–28. Boca Raton, FL: CRC Press Auerbach Publications.

Awan, Nishat, Tatjana Schneider and Jeremy Hill, eds. 2011. *Spatial Agency: Other Ways of Doing Architecture*. London: Routledge.

Baehr, Nina. 1990. *Abortion without Apology: A Radical History for the 1990s*. Boston: South End Press.

Ball, Donald W. 1967. "An Abortion Clinic Ethnography." *Social Problems* 14(3): 293–301.

Banham, Reyner. 1999. "A Black Box: The Secret Profession of Architecture." In *A Critic Writes*, edited by Mary Banham, Paul Barker, Sutherland Lyall and Cedric Price. Berkeley: University of California Press.

Bartlett, L.A. et al. 2004. "Risk Factors for Legal Induced Abortion-Related Mortality in the United States." *Obstetrics & Gynecology* 103(4): 729–37.

Bassett, Laura. 2011a. "Defunding Planned Parenthood Opposed by Most Americans: Polls." *HuffPost Pollster* July 29, 2011. http://www.huffingtonpost.com/2011/07/29/defunding-planned-parenthood-polls_n_913685.html. Accessed January 21, 2012.

Bassett, Laura. 2011b. "Protect Life Act, Controversial Anti-Abortion Bill, Passes House." *Huffington Post* October 13, 2011. http://www.huffingtonpost.com/2011/10/13/protect-life-act-passes-house-of-representatives_n_1009876.html. Accessed January 14, 2012.

Baumgardner, Jennifer. 2008. *Abortion & Life*. New York: Akashic Books.

Bazelon, Emily. 2007. "Is there a Post-Abortion Syndrome?" *New York Times Magazine*, January 21.

Bazelon, Emily. 2009. "The Place of Women on the Court." *New York Times Magazine*, July 12.

Bazelon, Emily. 2010. "The New Abortion Providers." *New York Times Magazine*, July 18.

Becker, Davida, Claudia Diaz-Olavarrieta, Clara Juarez, Sandra G. Garcia, Patricio Sanhueza Smith and Cynthia C. Harper. 2011. "Sociodemographic Factors Associated with Obstacles to Abortion Care: Findings from a Survey of Abortion Patients in Mexico City." *Women's Health Issues* 21–3S: S16–20.

Beckman, Linda J. and S. Marie Harvey, eds. 1998. *The New Civil War: The Psychology, Culture, and Politics of Abortion*. Washington, D.C.: American Psychological Association.

Bellafante, Gina. 2010. "Abortion in the Eyes of a Girl from Dillion." *New York Times*, July 9. http://www.nytimes.com/2010/07/10/arts/television/10lights.html?r=3. Accessed April 23, 2012.

Bershad, Deborah and Jean Parker Phifer. 2004. "Perimeter Security: The Aesthetics of Protection." In *Building Security Handbook for Architectural Planning and Design*, edited by Barbara A. Nadel, 16.1–16.9. New York: McGraw-Hill.

Billings, Deborah L., Claudia Moreno, Celia Ramos, Deyanira González de León, Rubén Ramírez, Leticia Villaseñor Martínez, and Mauricio Rivera Díaz. 2002. "Constructing Access to Legal Abortion Services in Mexico City." *Reproductive Health Matters* 10(19): 86–94.

Billings, Deborah L., Dilys Walker, Guadalupe Mainero del Paso, Kathryn Andersen Clark and Ila Dayananda. 2009. "Pharmacy Worker Practices Related to Use of Misoprostol for Abortion in One Mexican State." *Contraception* 79: 445–51.

Blackmer, Jeff. 2007. Letter to the Editor. *Canadian Medical Association Journal CMAJ* 176 (9) April 24.

Blomley, Nicholas. 2005. "Flowers in the Bathtub: Boundary Crossings at the Public-Private Divide." *Geoforum* 36: 281–96.

Blomley, Nicholas. 2011. *Rights of Passage: Sidewalks and the Regulation of Public Flow*. Abingdon, Oxon: Routledge.

Blunt, Alison and Robyn Dowling. 2006. *Home*. London: Routledge.

*Body Politic, The*. 1993. "The Overground Railroad Builds Up Head of Steam." 3(1): 13 http://www.publiceye.org/body_politic/mag/back/art/0301pg13.htm. Accessed April 27, 2012.

Boettcher, Mike. 1992. *NBC Nightly News*, April 25.

Boonstra, H. et al. 2006. *Abortion in Women's Lives*, New York: Guttmacher Institute.

*Boos v. Barry*, 485 U.S. 322

Boys, Jos. 1998. "Beyond Maps and Metaphors? Re-Thinking the Relationships between Architecture and Gender." In *New Frontiers of Space, Bodies and Gender*, edited by Rosa Ainley, 203–17. London: Routledge.

Briggs, Kara. 2006. "Pine Ridge Leader Faces Battle over Abortion Ban, *Womens enews.org*, June 27. http://womensenews.org/story/campaign-trail/060627/pine-ridge-leader-faces-battle-over-abortion-ban. Accessed April 18, 2012.

Brown, Lori A., ed. 2011. *Feminist Practices: Interdisciplinary Approaches to Women in Architecture*. Surrey, England: Ashgate Publishing Limited.

Brown, Lori A. and Özlem Erdoğdu Erkarslan. 2009. "A Study of Women's Shelters: Places of Transcendental Homelessness and Identity." In *Gender at the Crossroads: Multi-Disciplinary Perspectives*, edited by Nurten Kara, 295–303. Famagusta, North Cyprus: Eastern Mediterranean University Press.

Brown, Sarah. 2010. "Preventing Unintended Pregnancies." Participant at the Open Hearts, Open Minds and Fair Minded Words: A Conference on Life and Choice in the Abortion Debate, Princeton University Princeton, New Jersey, October 15–16.

Butler, J. Douglas and David F. Walbert, eds. 1992. *Abortion, Medicine, and the Law*. New York: Facts On File.

1892 Criminal Code of Canada Section 251.

Criminal Code Bill C-150 (1969).

CanWest News Service. 2008 "Morning-After Pill Approved for over-the-Counter Sales." May 16. http://www.canada.com/ottawacitizen/news/story.html?id=eb9a322c-0b86-414c-8a28-a21d22c8c6a3. Accessed February 1, 2012.

Carmen, Arlene and Howard Moody. 1973. *Abortion Counseling and Social Change from Illegal Act to Medical Practice: The Story of the Clergy Consultation Service on Abortion*. Valley Forge: Judson Press.

Casas, Lidia. 2009. "Invoking Conscientious Objection in Reproductive Health Care: Evolving Issues in Peru, Mexico and Chile." *Reproductive Health Matters* 17(34): 81–7.

CBC Digital Archives. 1969–1989. "Dr. Henry Morgantaler: Fighting Canada's Abortion Laws." http://archives.cbc.ca/health/reproductive_issues/topics/107/. Accessed January 30, 2012.

CBCnews Canada. 2009. "Abortion Rights: Significant Moments in Canadian History." CBC May 21. http://www.cbc.ca/news/canada/story/2009/01/13/f-abortion-timeline.html. Accessed January 30, 2012.

CBCnews Canada. 2011. "Abortion Crusader Deeply Divides Canadian Society." http://www.cbc.ca/news/canada/story/2008/07/02/f-morgentaler.html. Accessed November 26, 2011.

Centers for Disease Control. 2010. "The National Intimate Partner and Sexual Violence Survey." http://www.cdc.gov/violenceprevention/nisvs/. Accessed March 25, 2012.

Chalker, Rebecca and Carol Downer. 1992. *A Woman's Book of Choices Abortion, Menstrual Extraction, RU-486*. New York: Four Walls Eight Windows.

Chen, Alan. 2003. "Statutory Speech Bubbles, First Amendment Overbreadth, and Improper Legislative Purpose." *Harvard Civil Rights-Civil Liberties Law Review* 38, 31–90. Cambridge, MA: Harvard Law School.

Cherniak, Donna and Allan Feingold. 1972. "Birth Control Handbook 1971." In *Women Unite: An Anthology of the Canadian Women's Movement*. Toronto: Canadian Women's Educational Press.

Chicago Women's Liberation Union. (n.d.) "CWLU and the Women's Health Movement in Chicago 1969–1977." CWLU herstory project video, 20:30, http://www.cwluherstory.org/Women-s-Health/. Accessed April 20, 2012.

Choices West. 1995. January 19. Merle Hoffman Papers Box CH21 Correspondence, Duke University Sallie Bingham Center for Women's History and Culture.

Clark, Stephen. 2011. "Several States Take Up Fight over Defunding Planned Parenthood." *Fox News* State & Local Politics, April 26, 2011. http://www.foxnews.com/politics/2011/04/28/states-fight-defunding-planned-parenthood/. Accessed January 21, 2012.

Colomina, Beatriz. 1992. "Introduction." In *Sexuality & Space*, edited by Beatriz Colomina. New York: Princeton Architectural Press.

Cook, Rebecca. 2010. "Abortion in America: Should It Be a Constitutional Question?" Participant at the Open Hearts, Open Minds and Fair Minded Words: A Conference on Life and Choice in the Abortion Debate, Princeton University Princeton, New Jersey, October 15–16.

Crist, Takey. (n.d.) "A Model for a Youth Family Planning Clinic in a Community without a University." Takey Crist Papers 2004-098, Box 5. Duke University Sallie Bingham Center for Women's History and Culture.

Crist, Takey.1996. "Commentary." *North Carolina Medical Journal NCMJ* 57(1): 3–4. Takey Crist Papers 2006-098, Box 1. Duke University Sallie Bingham Center for Women's History and Culture.

CWLU herstory project (a). "Abortion: A Woman's Decision, a Woman's Right." Jane informational pamphlet. http://www.cwluherstory.org/abortiona-womans-decision-a-womans-right.html. Accessed December 7, 2011.

CWLU herstory project (b). "An Overview of the Abortion Counseling Service and How It Began." Hyde Park Kenwood Voices. http://www.cwluherstory.org/part-i.html. Accessed December 7, 2011.

CWLU herstory project (c). "CWLU and the Women's Health Movement in Chicago 1969–1977." Chicago Women's Liberation Union video, 20:30, http://www.cwluherstory.org/Women-s-Health/. Accessed April 20, 2012.

CWLU herstory project (d). "Doing More of the Abortions Themselves Leads to New Challenges for the Service." Hyde Park Kenwood Voices. http://www.cwluherstory.org/part-v.html. Accessed December 7, 2011.

CWLU herstory project (e). "Finding a Solution to the Problem of Long Term Pregnancies Leads the Service into Doing Actual Medical Procedures. Hyde Park Kenwood Voices. http://www.cwluherstory.org/part-iii.html. Accessed December 7, 2011.

CWLU herstory project (f). "The Service Has a Close Brush with Tragedy and Performs Its First Unassisted D&C." Hyde Park Kenwood Voices. http://www.cwluherstory.org/part-iv.html. Accessed December 7, 2011.

CWLU herstory project (g). "The Service Learns How to Obtain Medical Instruments and Drugs While Trying to Avoid Police Attention." Hyde Park Kenwood Voices. http://www.cwluherstory.org/part-vi.html. Accessed December 7, 2011.

Darabi, Leila. 2009. "Despite Being Largely Illegal, Abortion in Mexico Is far More Prevalent Than in the United States." Guttmacher Institute February 9. http://www.guttmacher.org/media/nr/2009/02/02/index.html. Accessed February 12, 2012.

Dayananda, Ila, Dilys Walker, Erica E. Atienzo and Sadia Haider. 2012. "Abortion Practice in Mexico: A Survey of Health Care Providers." *Contraception* 85: 304–310.

de Certeau, Michel. 1984. *The Practice of Everyday Life*. Translated by Steven Rendall. Berkeley: University of California Press.

Dickens, Bernard. 2010. "How Far Does the Right of Conscientious Refusal Extend?" Participant in Open Hearts, Open Minds and Fair Minded Words: A Conference on Life and Choice in the Abortion Debate. Princeton University Princeton, New Jersey, October 15–16.

Donaldson James, Susan. 2011. "Abortion without Doctor On-Site Gets High Grades in Iowa." ABC News July 27. http://abcnews.go.com/Health/iowa-study-shows-telemedicine-abortion-safe-women-access/story?id=14166312#.Twd40UpGicp. Accessed January 6, 2012.

Douglas, Jack D. 1970. *Observations of Deviance*, New York: Random House.

Dovey, Kim. 2008. *Framing Spaces Mediating Power in Built Form*. 2nd ed. London: Routledge.

Downie, Jocelyn and Carla Nassar. 2007. "Barriers to Access to Abortion through a Legal Lens." *Health Law Journal* 15. 143–73. Ottawa: University of Ottawa.

Duncan, Nancy. 1996. "Renegotiating Gender and Sexuality in Public and Private Spaces." In *BodySpace Destabilizing Geographies of Gender and Sexuality*, edited by Nancy Duncan, 127–45. London: Routledge.

Dwyer Julia and Anne Thorne. 2007. "Evaluating Matrix: Notes from inside the Collective." In *Altering Practices Feminist Politics and Poetics of Space*, edited by Doina Petrescu, 41–56. London: Routledge.

Eckholm, Erick. 2012. "Ultrasound: A Pawn in the Abortion Wars." *New York Times*, February 25. http://www.nytimes.com/2012/02/26/sunday-review/ultrasound-a-pawn-in-the-abortion-wars.html?_r=2&ref=opinion. Accessed March 14, 2012.

*Economist, The*. 2006. "Fire Thunder's Lightening Turning to Tribal Sovereignty as a Way, Perhaps, to Get around the Law." June 29. http://www.economist.com/node/7119415. Accessed April 19, 2012.

Eggerston, Laura. 2001. "Abortion Services in Canada: A Patchwork Quilt with Many Holes." *Canadian Medical Association Journal* 164 (6), March 20, 847–9. Ottawa: Canadian Medical Association.

*Erznoznik v. Jacksonville,* 422 U.S. 205 (1975).

*Everysaturdaymorning Blog*. 2012. http://everysaturdaymorning.net/. Accessed April 6.

Fatima Juarez, Susheela Singh, Sandra G. Garcia and Claudio Diaz Olavarrieta. 2008. "Estimates of Induced Abortion in Mexico: What's Changed between 1990 and 2006?" *International Family Planning Perspectives* 34(4): 158–68.

*Federal Emergency Management Agency* (FEMA) (a). "Building Design Guidance." In *Reference Manual to Mitigate Potential Terrorist Attacks Against Buildings* 426. http://www.fema.gov/library/viewRecord.do?id=1559. Accessed February 22, 2012.

*Federal Emergency Management Agency* (FEMA) (b). "Principles of Design for Risk Reduction Related to Operational Security Measures." In *Incremental Protection for Existing Commercial Buildings from Terrorist Attack* 459. http://www.fema.gov/library/viewRecord.do?id=3270. Accessed February 22, 2012.

*Federal Emergency Management Agency* (FEMA) (c). *Incremental Protection for Existing Commercial Buildings from Terrorist Attack: Providing Protection to People and Buildings* 459. http://www.fema.gov/library/viewRecord.do?id=3270. Accessed February 22, 2012.

*Federal Emergency Management Agency* (FEMA) (d). *Reference Manual to Mitigate Potential Terrorist Attacks against Buildings* 426. http://www.fema.gov/library/viewRecord.do?id=1559. Accessed February 22, 2012.

Feldberg, Georgina, Molly Ladd-Taylor, Alison Li, and Kathryn McPherson. 2003. "Comparative Perspectives on Canadian and American Women's Health Care since 1945." In *Women, Health, and Nation Canada and the United States since 1945*, edited by Georgina Feldberg, Molly Ladd-Taylor, Alison Li, and Kathryn McPherson, 15–37. Montreal: McGill-Queen's University Press.

Felix, R.A. 1991. "Beyond the Physician's Office – The Medical Mall." *College Review* Fall 8(2): 30–57.

Feminist Majority Foundation. 1994. Clinic Defense Project Security Considerations. Merle Hoffman Papers, Box CH21. Duke University Sallie Bingham Center for Women's History and Culture.

Feminist Majority Foundation. (a.)."2010 National Clinic Violence Survey." http://feminist.org/rrights/clinicsurvey.html. Accessed January 18, 2012.

Feminist Majority Foundation. (b). "National Clinic Access Project." http://feminist.org/rrights/ncapabout.asp. Accessed January 22, 2012.

Feminist Majority Foundation and NOW Legal Defense and Education Fund. 1996. "Drawing the Line against Anti-Abortion Violence and Harassment." Arlington, VA: The Feminist Majority Foundation.

Fernandez, Maria M., Francine Coeytaux, Rodolfo Gomez Ponce de León and Denise L. Harrison. 2009. "Assessing the Global Availability of Misoprostol." *International Journal of Gynecology and Obstetrics* 105 (2009): 180–86. doi: 10.1016/j.ijgo.2008.12.016. Accessed January 25, 2012.

Fessler, Ann. 2006. *The Girls Who Went Away: The Hidden History of Women Who Surrendered Children for Adoption in the Decades before Roe v. Wade*. New York: The Penguin Press.

FindLAw for Legal Professionals. (a). "Hill et al. v. COLORADO et al." http://caselaw.lp.findlaw.com/cgi bin/getcase.pl?court=US&navby=case&vol=000&invol=98-1856. Accessed July 29, 2009.

FindLAw for Legal Professionals. (b). *Schenck v. Pro Choice Network of Western New York*, footnote 9, http://caselaw.lp.findlaw.com/cgi-bin/getcase.pl?navby=case&court=US&vol=519&invol=357. Accessed July 29, 2009.

Findley, Lisa. 2005. *Building Change Architecture, Politics and Cultural Agency*. London: Routledge.

Finer, Lawrence B. and Stanley K. Henshaw. 2003. "Abortion Incidence and Services in the United States in 2000." *Perspectives on Sexual and Reproductive Health* 35(1): 6–15.

Finer, Lawrence B., Lori F. Frohwirth, Lindsay A. Dauphinee, Susheela Singh and Ann M. Moore. 2005. "Reasons U.S. Women Have Abortions: Quantitative and Qualitative Perspectives." *Perspectives on Sexual and Reproductive Health* 37(3): 110–18.

Finer, Lawrence B. and Stanley K. Henshaw. 2005. "Estimates of U.S. Abortion Incidence in 2001 and 2002." The Alan Guttmacher Institute (AGI), http://www.guttmacher.org/pubs/2005/05/18/ab_incidence.pdf. Accessed May 17, 2005.

Finer, Lawrence B. and Stanley K. Henshaw. 2006. "Disparities in Unintended Pregnancy in the United States, 1994 and 2001." *Perspectives on Sexual and Reproductive Health* 38(2): 90–96.

Fisher, Thomas. 2008. "Public-Interest Architecture: A Needed and Inevitable Change." In *Expanding Architecture: Design as Activism*, edited by Bryan Bell and Katie Wakeford, 8-13. New York: Metropolis Books.

Fiske, Edward B. 1967. "Clergymen Offer Abortion Advice." *New York Times*, May 22. http://select.nytimes.com/gst/abstract.html?res=F50917F7385C117B93C0AB178ED85F438685F9. Accessed April 28, 2012.

Fraser, Nancy. 1990. "Rethinking the Public Sphere: A Contribution to the Critique of Actually Existing Democracy." *Social Text* Number 25/26, 56–80.

Freedman, Lori. 2010a. "How Far Does the Right of Conscientious Refusal Extend? Discussion Session." Open Hearts, Open Minds and Fair Minded Words: A Conference on Life and Choice in the Abortion Debate, Princeton University Princeton, New Jersey, October 15–16.

Freedman, Lori. 2010b. *Willing and Unable: Doctor's Constraints in Abortion Care*. Nashville: Vanderbilt University Press.

Frontline. 2005. *The Last Abortion Clinic* (Boston: WGBH Educational Foundation, November 8), DVD.

Gajdušek, Petr. 2004. "Quickening Doctrine." *Common Law Review*, Issue 5 Medical Law. http://review.society.cz/index.php?option=com_content&task=view&id=78&Itemid=2. Accessed July 22, 2009.

García, Sandra G., Carrie Tatum, Davida Becker, Karen A. Swanson, Karin Lockwood and Charlotte Ellertson. 2004. "Policy Implications of a National Public Opinion Survey on Abortion in Mexico." *Reproductive Health Matters* 12(24 Supplement): 65–74.

Garrow, David J. 1998. *Liberty and Sexuality: The Right to Privacy and the Making of Roe v. Wade*. Berkeley: University of California Press.

Githens, Marianne and Dorothy McBride Stetson, eds. 1996. *Abortion Politics: Public Policy in Cross-Cultural Perspective*. New York: Routledge.

Gober, Patricia and Mark W. Rosenberg. 2001. "Looking Back, Looking Around, Looking Forward: A woman's Right to Choose." In *Geographies of Women's Health*, edited by Isabel Dyck, Nancy Davis Lewis and Sara McLafferty, 88–102. London: Routledge.

Goodman, Amy. 2006. "South Dakota Abortion Ban Draws Fiery Opposition from Native Americans." Interview with Charon Asetoyer and Sarah Stoesz. *Democracy Now*. March 28. http://www.democracynow.org/2006/3/28/south_dakota_abortion_ban_draws_fiery.

Goodstein, Laurie. 2012. "Obama Shift on Providing Contraception Splits Critics." *New York Times*, February 14. http://www.nytimes.com/2012/02/15/us/obama-shift-on-contraception-splits-catholics.html?scp=36&sq=contraception%20coverage&st=cse. Accessed March 14, 2012.

Gorney, Cynthia. 2004. "Gambling with Abortion Why Both Sides Think They Have Everything to Lose." *Harper's*, November.

Gottfried, Heidi. 1996. "Introduction Engaging Women's Communities: Dilemmas and Contradictions in Feminist Research." In *Feminism and Social Change Bridging Theory and Practice*, edited by Heidi Gottfried, 1–20. Urbana: University of Illinois Press.

Gould, Heather, Charlotte Ellerston and Georgina Corona. 2002. "Knowledge and Attitudes about the Differences between Emergency Contraception and Medical Abortion among Middle Class Women and Men of Reproductive Age in Mexico City." *Contraception* 66: 417–26.

Grady, Denise. 2012. "Ruling on Contraception Draws Battle Lines at Catholic Colleges. *New York Times*, January 29. http://www.nytimes.com/2012/01/30/health/policy/law-fuels-contraception-controversy-on-catholic-campuses.html?_r=1&scp=1&sq=contraception&st=cse. Accessed March 14, 2012.

Grady, Rachel and Heidi Ewing. 2010. *12th & Delaware*. DVD. HBO Documentary Films with Loki Films.

Grimes, David A., Janie Benson, Susheela Singh, Marianna Romero, Bela Ganatra, Friday E. Okonofua and Iqbal H. Shah. 2006. "Unsafe Abortion: The Preventable Pandemic." *Lancet* 368: 1908–19. doi:10.1016/S0140- 6736(06)69481-6. Accessed January 25, 2012.

Grossman, D., J. Kingston, S. Schweikert, E. Troncoso, S. Falquier and D.L. Billings. 2005. "Crossing to Safety: The Experience of Mexican Women who Access Safe, Legal Abortion Services in San Diego." *Contraception* Abstracts 72 (2005): 236.

Grossman, Daniel, Kate Grindlay MSPH, Todd Buchacker RN, Kathleen Lane and Kelly Blanchard MSc. 2011. "Effectiveness and Acceptability of Medical Abortion Provided through Telemedicine." *Obstetrics & Gynecology* 118(2:1): 296-303. http://journals.lww.com/greenjournal/Abstract/2011/08000/Effectiveness_and_Acceptability_of_Medical.14.aspx. Accessed January 6, 2012.

Grosz, Elizabeth. 1992. "Bodies-Cities." In *Sexuality & Space*, edited by Beatriz Colomina, 241–53. New York: Princeton Architectural Press.

Grosz, Elizabeth. 2001. *Architecture from the Outside Essays on Virtual and Real Space*. Massachusetts: MIT Press.

Grupo de Información en Reproducción Elegida GIRE. 2007. "Abortion in State Penal Codes." June. http://www.gire.org.mx/contenido.php?informacion=196. Accessed February 12, 2012.

Guttmacher Institute. 2006a. "An Overview of Abortion Laws, State Policies in Brief." June. http://www.guttmacher.org/statecenter/spibs/spib_PIMA.pdf. Accessed June 23, 2006.

Guttmacher Institute (n.d.)"Are You IN THE KNOW? Characteristics of Women Having Abortions." http://www.guttmacher.org/presentations/ab_slides.html. Accessed April 9, 2012.

Guttmacher Institute. 2006b. "State Funding of Abortion under Medicaid: State Policies in Brief." April. http://www.guttmacher.org/statecenter/spibs/spib_SFAM.pdf. Accessed April 28, 2006.

Guttmacher Institute. 2009. "State Policies in Brief: Protecting Access to Clinics." *Guttmacher Institute*, August 1. http://www.guttmacher.org/. Accessed August 15, 2009.

Guttmacher Institute. 2012. "States Enact Record Number of Abortion Restrictions in 2011." January 5. http://www.guttmacher.org/media/inthenews/2012/01/05/endofyear.html. Accessed March 14, 2012.

Habermas, Jürgen. 1989. "Preliminary Demarcation of a Type of Bourgeois Public Sphere." *The Structural Transformation of the Public Sphere: An Inquiry into a Category of Bourgeois Society*. Translated by Thomas Burger and Frederick Lawrence. Cambridge, MA: MIT Press.

Hagerty, Barbara Bradley. 2010. "Nun Excommunicated for Allowing Abortion." *All Things Considered National Public Radio*, May 19. http://www.npr.org/templates/story/story.php?storyId=126985072. Accessed January 14, 2012.

Hall, Catherine. 1992. *White, Male and Middle-Class Explorations in Feminism and History*. New York: Routledge.

Hames, Margie Pitts. 1993. "A Brief History of Abortion Laws in the United States: Will We Return to Pre-*Roe* Legislation?", edited by Jane B. Wishner, *Abortion and the States: Political Change and Future Regulation Section of Urban, State, and Local Government Law*, 54. Chicago, American Bar Association, Section of Urban, State and Local Government Law.

Harding, Sandra. 1987a. "Conclusion Epistemolgoical Questions." In *Feminism & Methodology Social Science Issue*, edited by Sandra Harding, 181–90. Bloomington: Indiana University Press.

Harding, Sandra. 1987b. "Introduction: Is There a Feminist Method?" In *Feminism & Methodology Social Science Issue*, edited by Sandra Harding, 1–14. Bloomington: Indiana University Press.

Harris, Lynn. 2010. "MTV's Shockingly Good Abortion Special." *Salon.com*, Wednesday December 29. http://www.salon.com/2010/12/29/mtv_abortion_show_no_easy_choice/. Accessed April 23, 2012.

Hayden, Dolores. 2000. "What Would a Non-Sexist City Be Like? Speculations on Housing, Urban Design, and Human Work." In *The City Reader*, 2nd ed, edited by Richard T. Legates and Frederic Stout, 503–18. London: Routledge, Originally published in Catharine R. Stimpson, ed., *Women and the American City* (Chicago: University of Chicago Press, 1981).

Hayden, K.R. 1989. "The Delivery of Medical Services in a Retail Shopping Mall: A Strategy for Growth." *College Review* Fall 6(2): 12–29.

Hendershott, Anne. 2006. *The Politics of Abortion*, New York: Encounter Books.

Henshaw, Stanely K. and Lawrence B. Finer. 2003. "The Accessibility of Abortion Services in the United States, 2001." *Perspectives on Sexual and Reproductive Health* 35(1): 16–24.

Henshaw, Stanley K., Susheela Singh and Taylor Haas. 1999. "Recent Trends in Abortion Rates Worldwide." *International Family Planning Perspectives* 25(1): 44–8.

Henshaw, Stanley K., Susheela Singh and Taylor Haas. 1999. "The Incidence of Abortion Worldwide." *International Family Planning Perspectives* 25 (suppl): S30–S38.

Hern, Dr. Warren M. 2000. "Abortion 'Bubble Bill' Going before U.S. Supreme Court." June 11. http://www.drhern.com/bubblelaw.htm. Accessed July 29, 2009.

Hess, Jeffrey. 2012. "Mississippi Legislature Passes Abortion Clinic Bill." *Kaiser Health News* April 4. http://www.kaiserhealthnews.org/Stories/2012/April/05/Mississippi-Abortion-Clinic-Bill.aspx. Accessed April 9, 2012.

*Hill v. Colorado*, 530 U.S. 703 (2000).

Hill, Jeremy. 2005. "The Negotiation of Hope." In *Architecture and Participation*, edited by Peter Blundell Jones, Doina Petrescu and Jeremy Hill, 23–41. London: Spon Press.

Hobart, Margaret. 2011. Washington State Coalition against Domestic Violence. Interview with author.

Hoffman, Merle. 1995. Choices West January 19. Merle Hoffman Papers, Box CH21, Correspondence. Duke University Sallie Bingham Center for Women's History and Culture.

Hoffman, Nathaniel. 2005. "Middle-class Mexican Women Come to U.S. for Safer Abortions." *Chicago Tribune*, July 27. http://articles.chicagotribune.com/2005-07-27/features/0507260329_1_abortions-mexican-women-population-council. Accessed February 17, 2012.

Human Rights Watch. 2005. "International Human Rights Law and Abortion in Latin America." http://www.hrw.org/legacy/backgrounder/wrd/wrd0106/. Accessed February 13, 2012.

ICU. (n.d.) "Why We Go … the ICU Mobile Mission." http://icumobile.org/site/. Accessed January 11, 2012.

*Implementation of the Freedom of Access to Clinic Entrances Act of 1993*. 1994. Hearing before the Subcommittee on Crime and Criminal Justice of the committee on the Judiciary House of Representatives 103rd Congress 2nd session September 22, 1994 Serial No. 83, Washington: U.S. Government Printing Office, 1994 Y4.J 89/1: 103/83

*Implementation of the Freedom of Access to Clinic Entrances Act of 1993*. 1993. Hearing before the committee on Labor and Human Resources United States Senate 103rd Congress 2nd session May 12, 1993 Serial No. 636, Washington: U.S. Government Printing Office, 1994 Y4.J 89/1: 103/83

Jelen, Ted G. and Marthe A. Chandler, eds. 1994. *Abortion Politics in the United States and Canada Studies in Public Opinion*. Westport, Connecticut: Praeger.

Joffe, Carole. 2009. *Dispatches from the Abortion War: The Costs of Fanaticism to Doctors, Patients, and the Rest of Us*. Boston: Beacon Press.

Jones, Peter Blundell, Doina Petrescu and Jeremy Hill, eds. 2005. *Architecture and Participation*. London: Spon Press.

Jones, Rachel K., Jacqueline E. Darroch and Stanley K. Henshaw. 2002. "Patterns in the Socioeconomic Characteristics of Women Obtaining Abortions in 2000–2001." *Perspectives on Sexual and Reproductive Health* 34(5): 226–35.

Jones, Rachel K. and Kathryn Kooistra. 2011. "Abortion Incidence and Access to Services in the United States, 2008." *Perspectives on Sexual and Reproductive Health* 43(1): 41–50. Doi: 10.1363/4304111.

Jones, Rachel K., Mia R.S. Zolna, Stanley K. Henshaw and Lawrence B. Finer. 2008. "Abortion in the United States: Incidence and Access to Services, 2005." *Perspectives on Sexual and Reproductive Health* 40(1): 6–16. Doi: 10.1363/4000608.

Juarez, Fatima, Susheela Singh, Sandra G. Garcia and Claudia Diaz-Olavarrieta. 2008. "Estimates of Induced Abortion in Mexico: What's Changed between 1990 and 2006?" *International Family Planning Perspectives* 34(4): 158–68.

Jung, Thomas M. 2004. "Health Care Security." In *Building Security Handbook for Architectural Planning and Design*, edited by Barbara A. Nadel, 8.1–8.31. New York: McGraw-Hill.

Kaplan, Karen. 2010. "Religion Shouldn't Influence Medical Care in Hospitals That Get Medicare Funds, the ACLU Says." Health, *Los Angeles Times*, July 3. http://latimesblogs.latimes.com/booster_shots/2010/07/aclu-letter-to-cms-regarding-abortion-rights.html. Accessed January 14, 2012.

Kaplan, Laura. 1995. *The Story of Jane: The Legendary Underground Feminist Abortion Service*. New York: Pantheon Books.

Kaufman, K. 1997. *The Abortion Resource Handbook*. New York: Simon & Schuster.

Kishen, Meera and Yvonne Stedman. 2010. "The role of Advanced Nurse Practitioners in the availability of abortion services." *Best Practice & Research Clinical Obstetrics and Gynaecology* 24: 569–78.

Kossak, Florian Doina Petrescu, Tatjana Schneider, Renata Tyszczuk and Stephen Walker. 2010. *Agency: Working with Uncertain Architectures*. London: Routledge.

Lamas, Marta. 1997. "The Feminist Movement and the Development of Political Discourse on Voluntary Motherhood in Mexico." *Reproductive Health Matters* 10 November: 58–67.

Lamas, Marta and Sharon Bissell. 2000. "Abortion and Politics in Mexico: 'Context is All.'" *Reproductive Health Matters* 8(16): 10–23.

Lambert-Beatty, Carrie. 2008. "Twelve Miles: Boundaries of the New Art/Activism." *Signs: Journal of Women in Culture and Society* 33(2): 309–27.

Langer, Ana and Jennifer Catino. 2006. "The Health of Women in Mexico Opportunities and Challenges." In *Changing Structure of Mexico Political, Social, and Economic Prospects*, edited by Laura Randall, 475–88. Armonk, New York: M.E. Sharpe.

Lefebvre, Henri. 1991. *The Production of Space*. Translator by Donald Nicholson-Smith Oxford: Blackwell.

Lepik, Andres and Barry Bergdoll, eds. 2010. *Small Scale, Big Change: New Architectures of Social Engagement*. New York: MOMA.

Lepore, Jill. 2011. "Birthright: What's next for Planned Parenthood?" *New Yorker*, November 14, 44-55.

Levy, Rachel. 2012. "University Selling "Morning-After" Pill from Vending Machine." *The Slatest*, Tuesday February 7. http://slatest.slate.com/posts/2012/02/07/shippensburg_university_sells_emergency_contraceptive_from_vending_machine.html?from=rss/&wpisrc=newsletter_slatest. Accessed April 25, 2012.

Lewis, Karen J. and Jon O. Shimabukuro. 2002. "Abortion Law Development: A Brief Overview." Almanac of Policy Issues Congressional Research Service. www.policyalmanac.org/culture/archive/crs_abortion_overview.shtml. Accessed July 22, 2009.

Ley Robles or Robles Law (2000).

Lipschutz, Marion and Rose Rosenblatt, dir. 2005. *The Education of Shelby Knox*.

LiveActionFilms. 2011a. "Planned Parenthood Manager Offers to Help Sex Ring, Gets Fired." YouTube video, 10:58. February 1. http://www.youtube.com/watch?v=L9Zj9yx2j0Y.

LiveActionFilms. 2011b. "Second Planned Parenthood Aids Pimp's Underage Sex Ring." YouTube video, 7:00. February 3. http://www.youtube.com/watch?v=0iMScbJJS2g.

Longhurst, Robyn. 1998. "(Re)Presenting Shopping Centres and Bodies: Questions of pregnancy." In *New Frontiers: Space of Bodies and Gender*, edited by Rosa Ainley, 20–34. London: Routledge.

Longhurst, Robyn. 1999. "Pregnant Bodies: Public Scrutiny 'Giving' Advice to Pregnant Women." In *Embodied Geographies: Spaces, Bodies and Rites of Passage*, edited by Elizabeth Kenworthy Teather, 78–90. London: Routledge.

Longhurst, Robyn. 2001. *Bodies: Exploring Fluid Boundaries*. London: Routledge.

Longhurst, Robyn. 2008. *Maternities: Gender, Bodies and Space*. New York: Routledge.

*Los Angeles Times*. 1992. "Abortion 'Railroad' Readied to Cope with Possible Restrictions." June 7. http://articles.latimes.com/1992-06-07/news/mn-186_1_underground-railroad. Accessed April 27, 2012.

Low, Setha M. 1988. "Cultural Aspects of Design: An Introduction to the Field." *Architectural Behavior* 4(3): 187–90.

Luker, Kristin. 1984. *Abortion & the Politics of Motherhood*. Berkeley: University of California Press.

Madrazo, Alejandro. 2009. "The Evolution of Mexico City's Abortion Laws: From Public Morality to Women's Autonomy." *International Journal of Gynecology and Obstetrics* 106: 266–9. doi: 10.1016/j.ijgo.2009.05.004. Accessed February 1, 2012.

*Madsen v. Women's Health Center*, 512 U.S. 753 (1994).

Matrix Feminist Design Co-operative. (n.d.) http://www.spatialagency.net/database/matrix.feminist.design.co-operative. Accessed March 28, 2012.

McDowell, Linda. 1996. "Spatializing Feminism Geographic perspectives." In *BodySpace Destabilizing Geographies of Gender and Sexuality*, edited by Nancy Duncan, 28–44. London: Routledge.

McDowell, Linda. 1999. *Gender, Identity & Place Understanding Feminist Geographies*. Minneapolis: University of Minnesota Press.

McLaren, Angus and Arlene Tigar McLaren. 1997. *The Bedroom and the State: The Changing Practices and Politics of Contraception and Abortion in Canada, 1880–1997*. 2nd ed. Toronto: Oxford University Press.

Messer, Ellen and Kathryn E. May. 1994. *Back Rooms: Voices from the Illegal Abortion Era*. Buffalo: Prometheus Books.

Mexican Constitution of 1917. Mexican Constitution was amended in 1973.

Mexico City's Health Law (2004), (2007).

Mexico General Health Act in 1984.

Mexican Reform Laws of 1859.

Mitchell, Don. 2005. "The S.U.V. Model of citizenship: Floating Bubbles, Buffer Zones, and the Rise of the "Purely Atomic" Individual." *Political Geography* 24: 77–100.

Monk, Janice, Patricia Manning, Catalina Denman and Elsa Cornejo. 2009. "Place, positionality, and priorities: Expert's Views on Women's Health at the Mexico-US border." *Health & Place* 15: 799–806.

Moss, Pamela. 2002. "Taking on, Thinking about, and Doing Feminist Research in Geography." In *Feminist Geography in Practice Research and Methods*, edited by Pamela Moss, 1–17. Oxford: Blackwell Publishers.

Mutcherson, Kimberly. 2010. "Preventing Unintended Pregnancies." Participant at the Open Hearts, Open Minds and Fair Minded Words: A Conference on Life and Choice in the Abortion Debate, Princeton University Princeton, New Jersey, October 15–16.

Nadel, Barbara A. 2004. "Women's Health Centers: Workplace Safety and Security." In *Building Security Handbook for Architectural Planning and Design*, edited by Barbara A. Nadel, 21.1–21.15. New York: McGraw-Hill.

NARAL Pro-Choice America (a). "Who Decides? The Status of Women's Reproductive Rights in the United States." http://www.prochoiceamerica.org/choice-action-center/in_your_state/who-decides/state-profiles/. Accessed January 8, 2012.

NARAL Pro-Choice America (b). "Who Decides? The Status of Women's Reproductive Rights in the United States Kentucky." http://www.prochoiceamerica.org/choice-action-center/in_your_state/who-decides/state-profiles/kentucky.html. Accessed January 8, 2012.

NARAL Pro-Choice America. 2004. Who Decides? A State-by-State Report on the Status of Women's Reproductive Rights. http://www.prochoiceamerica.org/media/publications/. Accessed June 6, 2004.

NARAL Pro-Choice America. 2012. Who Decides? A State-by-State Report on the Status of Women's Reproductive Rights. http://www.prochoiceamerica.org/media/publications/. Accessed February 1, 2012.

Nathan, Debbie. 2000. "Abortion Stories on the Border." In *Gender through the Prism of Difference*, 2nd ed, edited by Maxine Baca Zinn, Pierrette Hondagneu-Sotelo and Michaael A. Messner, 123–5. Boston: Allyn and Bacon.

Nather, David and Kate Nocera. 2011. "House Votes to Defund Planned Parenthood." *Politico*, February 18. http://www.politico.com/news/stories/0211/49830.html. Accessed January 21, 2012.

National Abortion Federation (NAF) (a). "In the Courts Court Cases/*Hill v. Colorado*." http://www.prochoice.org/policy/courts/hill_v_colorado.html. Accessed July 29, 2009.

National Abortion Federation (NAF) (b). "NAF Violence and Disruption Statistics." http://www.prochoice.org/about_abortion/violence/violence_statistics.html. Accessed April 9, 2012.

National Abortion Federation (NAF) (c). "Public Funding for Abortion: Medicaid and the Hyde Amendment." http://www.prochoice.org/about_abortion/facts/public_funding.html. Accessed July 23, 2009.

National Abortion Federation (NAF) and the American College of Obstetrics and Gynecology (ACOG). 1991. Who Will Provide Abortions? Ensuring the Availability of Qualified Practitioners, Washington, D.C.

National Network to End Domestic Violence. (n.d.) http://www.nnedv.org/. Accessed December 13, 2011.

National Park Service. (n.d.) "Indian Reservation in the Continental United States." http://www.nps.gov/history/nagpra/documents/ResMapIndex.htm. Accessed July 25, 2009.

National Right to Life. (n.d.) "Abortion History Timeline." http://www.nrlc.org/abortion/facts/abortiontimeline.html. Accessed July 23, 2009.

*New York Times*. 2011. Editorial "The War on Women." February 25. http://www.nytimes.com/2011/02/26/opinion/26sat1.html?scp=9&sq=defunding%20planned%20parenthood&st=cse. Accessed January 21, 2012.

Norman, Thomas. 2007. *Integrated Security Systems Design Concepts, Specifications, and Implementation*. Amsterdam: Butterworth-Heinemann.

NOVA. (n.d.) "The Hippocratic Oath: Classical Version." http://www.pbs.org/wgbh/nova/doctors/oath_classical.html. Accessed July 22, 2009.

NOW Legal Defense and Education Fund and the Feminist Majority Foundation. (n.d.) *Drawing the Line against Anti-Abortion Violence and Harassment*. http://feminist.org/searchresults.htm?q=drawing%20the%20line. Accessed July 2, 2009.

O'Connor, Karen. 1996. *No Neutral Ground? Abortion Politics in an Age of Absolutes*. Boulder, Colorado: Westview Press.

Ojeda, Norma. 2006. "Abortion in a Transborder Context." In *Women and Change at the U.S.-Mexico Border Mobility, Labor, and Activism*, edited by Doreen J. Mattingly and Ellen R. Hansen, 53–69. Tucson: The University of Arizona Press.

On the Move. 2012. "Places and Non-Places – A Conversation with Marc Augé, January 26, 2009. http://onthemove.autogrill.com/gen/lieux-non-lieux/news/2009-01-26/places-and-non-places-a-conversation-with-marc-auge. Accessed March 14 2012.

Ortiz-Ortega, Adriana. 2007. "Law and the Politics of Abortion." In *Decoding Gender Law and Practice in Contemporary Mexico*, ed. Helga Baitenmann, Victoria Chenaut and Ann Varley, 197–212. New Brunswick, New Jersey: Rutgers University Press.

Ortiz-Ortega, Adriana and Mercedes Barquet. 2010. "Gendering Transition to Democracy in Mexico." *Latin American Research Review* Special Issue: 108–37.

Ortiz-Ortega, Adriana, Ana Amuchástegui and Marta Rivas. 1998. "'Because They Were Born From Me': Negotiating Women's Rights in Mexico." In *Negotiating Reproductive Rights Women's Perspectives across Countries and Cultures* International Reproductive Rights Research Action Group, edited by Rosalind P. Petchesky and Karen Judd, 145–79. London: Zed Books.

Overground Railroad. (n.d.) Merle Hoffman Papers, Box CH2. Duke University Sallie Bingham Center for Women's History and Culture.

Pain, Rachel. 1999. "Women's Experiences of Violence over the Life-Course." In *Embodied Geographies Spaces, Bodies and Rites of Passage*, edited by Elizabeth Kenworthy Teather, 126–41. London: Routledge.

Pareene, Alex. 2011. "The Weird, Failed Planned Parenthood 'Sting.'" *Salon*, February 1. http://www.salon.com/2011/02/01/planned_parenthood_sting/. Accessed January 22, 2012.

PBS NOW. 2009. "Abortion Providers under Siege." *Life Now Women and Men in the Twenty-First Century* video 25:38. June 12. http://www.pbs.org/now/shows/524/.

Pear, Robert. 2012a. "Obama Reaffirms Insurers Must Cover Contraception." *New York Times*, January 20. http://www.nytimes.com/2012/01/21/health/policy/administration-rules-insurers-must-cover contraceptives.html?scp=5&sq=health%20care%20mandate%20and%20contraception%20coverage&st=cse. Accessed March 14, 2012.

Pear, Robert. 2012b. "Passions Flare as House Debates Birth Control Rule." *New York Times*, February 16. http://www.nytimes.com/2012/02/17/us/politics/birth-control-coverage-rule-debated-at-house-hearing.html?scp=3&sq=congressional%20hearing%20on%20contraception&st=cse. Accessed March 14, 2012.

Pearson, Cindy. (n.d.) "Self Help Clinic Celebrates 25 Years." Accessed November 24, 2011. http://www.fwhc.org/selfhelp.htm.

Petchesky, Rosalind P. 1990. *Abortion and Woman's Choice: The State, Sexuality, and Reproductive Freedom*. Boston: Northeastern University Press.

Petchesky, Rosalind Pollack. 2003. *Global Prescriptions Gendering Health and Human Rights*. London: Zed Books in association with United Nations Research Institute for Social Development.

Petrescu, Doina, ed. 2007. *Altering Practices: Feminist Politics and Poetics of Space*, London: Routledge.

Piazza, Jo. 2011. "Abortion No Longer Taboo Topic on Prime Time Television." *FoxNews.com*, November 2. http://www.foxnews.com/entertainment/2011/11/01/abortion-no-longer-taboo-topic-on-prime-time-television/. Accessed April 23, 2012.

Pinsky, Drew. 2010. *No Easy Decision*. MTV video, 29:32. December 28. http://www.mtv.com/videos/no-easy-decision-special/1654990/playlist.jhtml.

Planned Parenthood Federation of America 2009–2010 Annual Report. (n.d.) http://www.plannedparenthood.org/about-us/annual-report-4661.htm. Accessed January 21, 2012.

Pollock, Griselda. 1996. "Preface." *Generations and Geographies in the Visual Arts Feminist Readings*, edited by Griselda Pollock, xii–xx. London: Routledge.

Power, Doris. 1972. "Statement to the Abortion Caravan 1970." In *Women Unite: An Anthology of the Canadian Women's Movement*. Toronto: Canadian Women's Educational Press.

Press, Eyal. 2006. *Absolute Convictions: My Father, a City, and the Conflict That Divided America*, New York: Henry Holt and Company.

*R v. Morgantaler* (1988).

Reagan, Leslie J. 2003. "Crossing the Border for Abortions: California Activists, Mexican Clinics, and the Creation of a Feminist Health Agency in the 1960s." In *Women, Health, and Nation Canada and the United States since 1945*, edited by Georgina Feldberg, Molly Ladd-Taylor, Alison Li, and Kathryn McPherson, 355–78. Montreal: McGill-Queen's University Press.

Religious Coalition for Reproductive Choice. (n.d.) "A Proud History as a Voice of Conscience." http://rcrc.org/about/history.cfm. Accessed April 28, 2012.

Rendell, Jane. 2000. "Introduction: 'Gender, Space, Architecture.'" In *Gender Space Architecture: An Interdisciplinary Introduction*, edited by Jane Rendell, Barbara Penner and Iain Borden, 225–39. London: Routledge.

Rendell, Jane. 2006. *Art and Architecture: A Place Between*. London: I.B. Tauris. Originally published in Joan Ockman, ed., *Architecture, Criticism, Ideology* (Princeton: Princeton Architectural Press, 1995).

Rendell, Jane. 2011. "Critical Spatial Practices: Setting Out a Feminist Approach to Some Modes and What Matters in Architecture." In *Feminist Practices: Interdisciplinary Approaches to Women in Architecture*, edited by Lori A. Brown, 17–55. Surrey, England: Ashgate Publishing Limited.

*Rodriguez v. Chicago* (1998). http://caselaw.lp.findlaw.com/scripts/getcase.pl?navby=search&case=/data2/circs/7th/973339.html. Accessed April 28, 2012.

Rose India Technologies Pvt, Ltd. 2011. "GPS Services in Mobile Phones." http://www.roseindia.net/technology/gps/gps-services-mobile-phones.shtml. Accessed December 5.

Rose, Melody. 2007. *Safe, Legal and Unavailable? Abortion Politics in the United States*. Washington, D.C.: CQ Press.

Rubin, Eva R. 1994. *The Abortion Controversy: A Documentary History*. Westport, Connecticut: Greenwood Press.

Salter, Rosa. 1992. "Overground Railroad Volunteer Network to Help Women Elude State's Restrictions." *The Morning Call*, July 27. http://articles.mcall.com/1992-07-27/features/2874878_1_pennsylvania-s-abortion-control-act-abortion-clinics-denise-neary. Accessed April 27, 2012.

Samora, Julie Balch and Nan Leslie. 2007. "The Role of Advanced Practice Clinicians in the Availability of Abortion Services in the United States." *Journal of Obstetric, Gynecologic, & Neonatal Nursing* 36(5): 471–6. doi: 10.111/J.1552-6909.2007.00169.x. Accessed April 9, 2012.

Sánchez-Fuentes, Maria Luísa, Jennifer Paine and Brook Elliott-Buettner. 2008. "The Decriminalization of Abortion in Mexico City: How Did Abortion Rights Become a Political Priority?" *Gender & Development*, 16: 2: 345–60.

Scheidler, Joseph M. 1985. *Closed: 99 Ways to Stop Abortion*, San Francisco: Ignatius Press.

Schiavon, Raffaela, Maria Elena Collado, Erika Troncoso, José Ezequiel Soto Sánchez, Gabriela Otero Zorrilla and Tia Palermo. 2010. "Characteristics of Private Abortion Services in Mexico City after Legalization." *Reproductive Health Matters* 18(36): 127–35.

*Schenck v. Pro Choice Network of Western New York*, 519 U.S. 357 (1997).

Schulman, Jeremy. 2011. "HOAX VIDEO EXPOSE: Planned Parenthood *Already* Reported "Sex Trafficking" to FBI." *Media Matters for America*, February 1. http://mediamatters.org/blog/201102010014. Accessed January 22, 2012.

Sedgh, Gilda, Susheela Singh, Iqbal H. Shah, Elisabeth Åhman, Stanley K. Henshaw and Akinrinola Bankole. 2012. "Induced Abortion: Incidence and Trends Worldwide from 1995 to 2008." *The Lancet* January 19: 1–8. Accessed February 1, 2012. doi: 10.1016/S0140-6736(11)61786-8.

Sethna, Christabelle. 2011. "All Aboard? Canadian Women's Abortion Tourism, 1960–1980." In *Gender, Health, and Popular Culture Historical Perspectives*, edited by Cheryl Krasnick Warsh, 89–108. Waterloo, Ontario: Wilfrid Laurier University Press.

Sethna, Christabelle and Marion Doull. 2007. "Far from Home? A Pilot Study Tracking Women's Journeys to a Canadian Abortion Clinic." *Journal of Obstetrics and Gynaecology Canada*. Vancouver: Society of Obstetricians and Gynaecologists of Canada 27(8): 640–47.

Sethna, Christabelle and Marion Doull. 2009. "Journeys of Choice? Abortion, Travel, and Women's Autonomy." In *Critical Interventions in the Ethics of Healthcare Challenging the Principle of Autonomy in Bioethics*, edited by Stuart J. Murray and Dave Holmes, 163–79. United Kingdom: Ashgate Publishing Group.

Sethna, Christabelle and Steve Hewitt. 2009. "Clandestine Operations: The Vancouver Women's Caucus, the Abortion Caravan, and the RCMP." *The Canadian Historical Review* 90(3) September, 463–95.

Sewell, William G. 2004. "Security Technology." In *Building Security Handbook for Architectural Planning and Design*, edited by Barbara A. Nadel, 27.3–27.19. New York: McGraw-Hill.

Shorto, Russell. 2006. "Contra-Contraception." *New York Times Magazine*, May 7.

Shrage, Laurie. 2003. *Abortion and Social Responsibility Depolarizing the Debate*, Oxford: Oxford University Press.

Sibbald, Barbara. 2001. "Over-the-Counter Emergency Contraception Available soon across Country." *Canadian Medical Association Journal CMAJ* 164: 6 (March 6): 849.

Silva, Martha, Deborah L. Billings, Sandra G. García and Liana Lara. 2009. "Physicians' Agreement with and Willingness to Provide Abortion Services in the Case of Pregnancy from Rape in Mexico." *Contraception* 79: 56–64.

Silverstein, Helena. 2007. *Girls on the Stand: How Courts Fail Pregnant Minors*. New York: New York University Press.

Simonds, Wendy. 1996. *Abortion at Work Ideology and Practice in a Feminist Clinic*. New Brunswick, New Jersey: Rutgers University Press.

Singer, Natasha. 2006. "Skin Deep; Love the New Lips! From the Mall?" *The New York Times* October 26. http://www.nytimes.com/2006/10/26/fashion/26skin.html?scp=1&sq=Skin%20Deep;%20Love%20the%20New%20Lips!%20From%20the%20Mall?&st=cse. Accessed July 30, 2009.

Singer, Peter. 2010. "Abortion in America: Should it be a Constitutional Question?" Participant at the Open Hearts, Open Minds and Fair Minded Words: A Conference on Life and Choice in the Abortion Debate, Princeton University Princeton, New Jersey, October 15–16.

Solinger, Rickie. 1994. *The Abortionist: A Woman against the Law*. New York: Free Press.

Solinger, Rickie, ed. 1998. *Abortion Wars: A Half Century of Struggle 1950 – 2000*. Berkeley: University of California Press.

Solinger, Rickie. 2005. *Pregnancy and Power: A Short History of Reproductive Politics in America*. New York: New York University Press.

Soon, Judith A., Marc Levine, Brenda L. Osmond, Mary H.H. Ensom and David W. Fielding. 2005. "Effects of Making Emergency Contraception Available without a Physician's Prescription: A Population-Based Study." *Canadian Medical Association Journal CMAJ* 172: 7 (29 March): 878–83.

Soraghan, Mike. 2000. "DeGette Celebrates Decision: Ruling Upholds Law." *Denver Post*, June 29, A-09.

Sorensen, Severin, John G. Hayes and Randy Atlas. 2008. "Understanding CPTED and Situational Crime Prevention." In *21st Century Security and CPTED Designing for Critical Infrastructure Protection and Crime Prevention*, edited by Randall I. Atlas, 53–78. Boca Raton, FL: CRC Press Auerbach Publications.

Sparke, Matthew. 1996. "Displacing the Field in Fieldwork Masculinity, Metaphor and Space." In *BodySpace Destabilizing Geographies of Gender and Sexuality*, edited by Nancy Duncan, 212–33. London: Routledge.

*Spokeswoman, The*. 1971. "Feminists Discover and Patent the Do-It-Yourself Abortion!" December 1. Takey Crist Papers 2007-043 Duke University Sallie Bingham Center for Women's History and Culture.

Steinauer, Jody, Flynn LaRochelle, Marta Rowh, Lois Backus, Yarrow Sandahl and Angel Foster. 2009. "First Impressions: What Are Preclinical Medical Students in the U.S. and Canada Learning about Sexual and Reproductive Health?" *Contraception* 80: 74–80.

Steinbrook, Robert. 2012. "Science, Politics, and Over-the-Counter Emergency Contraception." *Journal of American Medical Association* JAMA 307: 4, 365–6.

Stratigakos, Despina. 2012. "Why Architects Need Feminism." *The Design Observer Places*, September 12. Accessed September 12, 2012.

Strauss, L.T. et al. 2004. "Abortion Surveillance–United States, 1999", *Morbidity and Mortality Weekly Report*, 2004(53): SS-9.

Stumpe, Joe and Monica Davey. 2009. "Abortion Doctor Shot to Death in Kansas Church." *New York Times*, May 31. http://www.nytimes.com/2009/06/01/us/01tiller.html?scp=10&sq=dr.+george+tiller%27s+death&st=nyt. Accessed November 27, 2011.

Sulzberger, A.G. 2011. "Kansas Gives License to One Abortion Clinic." *The New York Times*, June 30. http://www.nytimes.com/2011/07/01/us/01kansas.html?_r=1&ref=todayspaper. Accessed January 21, 2012.

Taracena, Rosario. 2002. "Social Actors and Discourse on Abortion in the Mexican Press: The Paulina Case." *Reproductive Health Matters* 10(19): 103–10.

Taylor, Affrica. 1998. "Lesbian Space: More Than One Imagined Territory." In *New Frontiers of Space, Bodies and Gender*, edited by Rosa Ainley, 129–41. London: Routledge.

Teather, Elizabeth Kenworthy. 1999. "Introduction: Geographies of Personal Discovery." In *Embodied Geographies Spaces, Bodies and Rites of Passage*, edited by Elizabeth Kenworthy Teather, 1–26. London: Routledge.

Ter Hor, Cheryl. 1999. "Abortion and the Underground." WomanNews section of the *Chicago Tribune* Online September. http://www.cwluherstory.org/abortion-and-the-underground.html. Accessed December 7, 2011.

Tillman, Laura. 2010. "Crossing the Line." *The Nation*, September 13. http://www.thenation.com/article/154166/crossing-line?page=full. Accessed February 17, 2012.

Torres, A. and Forrest, J.D. 1988. "Why Do Women Have Abortions?" *Family Planning Perspectives* 20(4):169–76.

Tremeear, W.J. 1908. *The Criminal Code and the Law of Criminal Evidence in Canada: Being an Annotation of the Criminal Code of Canada, and of the Canada Evidence Act with ... Justices and on Certiorari and Habeas Corpus*. 2nd ed. Philadelphia: Cromarty Law Book Company.

U.S. Census Bureau. 1999. "State & County QuickFacts." http://www.census.gov/. Accessed July 2009 and February 2012.

U.S. Department of Justice Federal Bureau of Investigation. (n.d.) "Terrorism 2002–2005." http://www.fbi.gov/stats-services/publications/terrorism-2002-2005. Accessed February 19, 2012.

"United States Constitution, The." 1789. http://www.usconstitution.net/const.html#Am1. Accessed March 14, 2012.

United States Court cases referenced.

United States Department of Justice Civil Rights Division. (n.d.) "Freedom of Access to Clinics Act." Title 18, USC., Section 248, http://www.usdoj.gov/crt/crim/248fin.php. Accessed July 29, 2009.

van Dijk, Marieke G., Luis Jorge Arellano Mendoza, Ana Gabriela Arangure Peraza, Aldo Alberto Toriz Prado, Abigail Krumholz and Eileen A. Yam. 2011. "Women's Experiences with Legal Abortion in Mexico City: A Qualitative Study." *Studies in Family Planning* 42(3): 167–74.

Verhagen, Sophie. 2001. "Rights of Women Bulletin: Rebecca Gomperts, Women on Waves." http://www.sophieverhagen.com/writing.htm. Accessed November 25, 2011.

Weinbar, Rebecca. 2007. "Bodies and Power: Access to Abortion in South Dakota." Masters Thesis, Syracuse University.

Weisman, Leslie Kanes. 1992. *Discrimination by Design: A Feminist Critique of the Man-Made Environment*. Urbana: University of Illinois Press.

Weisman, Leslie Kanes. 2000. "Prologue: Leslie Kanes Weisman Women's Environmental Rights: A Manifesto." In *Gender Space Architecture: An Interdisciplinary Introduction*, edited by Jane Rendell, Barbara Penner and Iain Borden, 1–5. London: Routledge. Originally published in *Heresies: A Feminist Publication on Art and Politics* (1981), 3(3), issue 11.

Wible, Robert C. 2007. *Architectural Security Codes and Guidelines Best Practices for Today's Construction Challenges*. New York: McGraw-Hill.

Wicklund, Susan with Alan Kesselheim. 2007. *This Common Secret: My Journey as an Abortion Doctor*. New York: PublicAffairs.

Wishner, Jane B., ed. 1993. *Abortion and the States: Political Change and Future Regulation Section of Urban, State, and Local Government Law*. American Bar Association.

Woman's Building, The. n.d. "Brief History." http://womansbuilding.org/history.htm. Accessed March 28, 2012.

Women on Waves. 2012. "About us." http://www.womenonwaves.nl/. Accessed November 11, 2012.

Women on Waves. 2012. "Campaigns." http://www.womenonwaves.nl/. Accessed November 11, 2012.

*Women Unite: An Anthology of the Canadian Women's Movement*. 1972. Toronto: Canadian Women's Educational Press.

WomensLaw.org. (n.d.) "Domestic Violence." http://www.womenslaw.org/simple.php?sitemap_id=39. Accessed March 24, 2012.

Wonderland Medical Center. 2012. http://wonderlandamericas.com/leasing-medical-center.html. Accessed April 4, 2012.

World's Columbian Exposition of 1893. "The Woman's Building." http://columbus.gl.iit.edu/dreamcity/00024006.html. Accessed March 28, 2012.

Yarnall, Jillian, Yael Swica and Beverly Winikoff. 2009. "Non-Physician Clinicians Can Safely Provide First Trimester Medical Abortion." *Reproductive Health Matters* 17(33): 61–9.

Young, Iris Marion. 1990. *Throwing Like a Girl and Other Essays in Feminist Philosophy and Social Theory*, Bloomington: Indiana University Press.

Young, Iris Marion. 2000. *Inclusion and Democracy*, Oxford: Oxford University Press.

Zinn, Janet H. 2001. "Pro-Choice Work under Siege: Politicization, Mobilization and Commitment in Three Urban Communities." PhD diss., Syracuse University.

Zukin, Sharon. 1991. *Landscapes of Power: From Detroit to Disney World*. Berkeley: University of California Press.

# Index

Page numbers in **bold** refer to illustrations, maps and charts. Page numbers with a suffix of 'n' followed by a number refer to endnotes.

abortion
  case studies 71, 72–85
  classes 72–3
  doctors and 44, 153, 170, 175–6, 186
  entertainment media portrayal of 71–2
  history of 43–4
  hospitals as providers 152, 159–64, 194–5
  integration into mainstream practice 186
  medical education 97, 170–71, 194
  Mexico 173
  non-medical practitioners 195
  and poverty 111, **114**, 121, **124**, 135–40, **138**, 154, **157**
  pregnancy, social and spatial effects of 24–6
  public-private nature of 24, 25, 26
  United States (US) 95, **98–9**, 104–6, 110
abortion, access to
  availability 194–204
  Canada **60**, **61**, 169–72
  and free speech 193
  integration into mainstream practice 186
  Mexico **64**, **65**, 174–6
  and space 204–9
  United States (US) 95, **96**, **98–9**, **105**, **112–13**, **122–3**, **131–2**, 135, **136–7**, 154, **155–6**, 187n3, **196–203**
Abortion Caravan 84

abortion clinics
  exterior design considerations 179–81
  interior design considerations 181–5
  location of 149–52, 204–5, **206–8**
  planning regulations 165
  as politicized spaces 1–2, 11–13, 23
  protests at **3**, **4**, 108–10, 134–5
  and public space 7–8
  security 166–9, 178–9, 188n43
  spatial experiences 107–8, 133, 149–52
  stand-alone clinics 194–5
  telemedicine 108
  violence against 95–7, 188n43
  *see also* security
Abortion Counseling Service of Women's Liberation (Jane) 74–8, **75**, **77**, 82–3
abortion law
  bubble laws 47–57, **50**, **51**, **52**, **54**, 59
  Canadian abortion law 57–61, 67, 169–70
  Mexican abortion law 62–8
  restrictions, US **102–3**, 111–20, 121–9, **132**, 140, 154
  state-level regulation of abortion 1, 6, **102–3**, 104–6, 111–20, 121–9
  US abortion law 43–57, 67, 111–20, 193–4
abortion tourism 85
Alaíde Foppa 86–7
Alcoff, Linda 23
American Civil Liberties Union (ACLU) 153
American Law Institute (ALI) 44
American Medical Association (AMA) 25, 44
American Planning Association (APA) 180
architecture
  contemporary culture 3–5

contested landscapes 11–13
donor expectations in the voluntary sector 32
and feminism 32–5
and gender 21–2
intersections of representational space 13–15
meaning of 12
politicized spaces 1–2, 11–13, 23
role of 3, 35–8, 205–9
spatial possibilities 35–8, 205–9
*Architecture and Participation* (Blundell Jones, Petrescu & Till) 5
Arizona **96**, **98–9**, 152–3
Army of Three 72–3
Association to Repeal Abortion Laws (ARAL) 73
Atelier Van Lieshout 82
Augé, Marc 3

Badgley Report (*Report of the Committee on the Operation of the Abortion Law*) 58
Banham, Reyner 5, 12
Benhabib, Seyla 28, 31
Bhabha, Homi 27–8, 208
Blackmer, Jeff 170
Blackmun J 45
Bloomer, Jennifer 34
Blundell Jones, Peter 5
body, the 21–6
*BodySpace Destabilizing Geographies of Gender and Sexuality* (Duncan) 22–3
*Boos v Barry* (1988) 48
Boys, Jos 37
Britain 9, 172–3
Britton, John 188n43
Brown, Sarah 195
bubble laws 47–57, **50**, **51**, **52**, **54**, 59
buffer zones 54, **54**
*Building Change Architecture, Politics and Cultural Agency* (Findley) 35–6
Butler, Judith 23

California 45, 72–4, **96**, **98–9**, 195
Canada
  abortion, access to **60**, **61**, 169–72
  abortion law 57–61, 67, 169–70
  case studies 84
  conscientious objectors 176
  emergency contraception (EC) 59, 172–3, 186

fetal rights 59
free speech 193
in this research 6
Canfield, Elizabeth 85
Casas, Lidia 176
Catholic Church 62, 152–3, 175, 194–5
Catholics for the Right to Decide (CDD) 175
Certeau, Michel de 13
Chicago 74–8, 82–3
Chicago, Judy 33
Chicago Women's Liberation Union (CWLU) 74–8, **75**, **77**
Chile 82
Christianity 43
cities, and bodies 21–2
Clergy Consultation Service (CCS) 78–80
clinics, *see* abortion clinics
closed-circuit television (CCTV) 183
Colomina, Beatriz 21
Colorado 44–5, 47, 48–9, **50**, 55–6, **96**, **98–9**
colour, use of 87–8
Common Law 43
Connecticut 95, **96**, **98–9**, 187n3
conscientious objectors 176
contraception
  access to 186–7
  Canada 59, 172–3, 186
  Mexico 62, 176–7
  pharmacies, availability from **119**, **129**, **144**, **146**, **148**, 159, **163**, 204–5
  United States (US) 1, 16, **119**, **129**, **144–6**, **148**, 159, **163**
Convention on the Elimination of all Forms of Discrimination Against Women (CEDAW) 173
Cook, Rebecca 67
Crime Prevention through Environmental Design (CPTED) 179
Crist, Takey 97, 210n21
cultural representation 11–13
cultural space 27–8, 35–6

de Bretteville, Sheila Levrant 33
DeGette, Diana 48–9
Deleuze, Gilles 37, 209
dementia units, security in 182
democracy, and public space 7–11
demonstrations 108–10, 134–5
design
  details improve environment 87–8

exterior design considerations 179–81
interior design considerations 181–5
meaning of 12
quiet reflective spaces 83–4
security 178–9
Women on Waves **81**, 82
Dickens, Bernard 194
Dickson CJ 58–9
*Dispatches from the Abortion Wars: The Costs of Fanaticism to Doctors, Patients, and the Rest of Us* (Joffe) 83
Diversa 86–7
doctors 44, 153, 170, 175–6, 186
*Doe v. Bolton* (1973) 45
domestic space 28–32, 73, 77
domestic violence 24, 29–32
Doull, Marion 171
Dovey, Kim 35, 205
Downer, Carol 73–4
Downie, Jocelyn 170, 172
Duncan, Nancy 8, 22–3, 27, 28, 29, 31

Ecuador 82
Ehrich, John 153
emergency contraception (EC)
  access to 186–7
  Canada 59, 172–3, 186
  Mexico 176–7
  pharmacies, availability from **119**, **129**, **144–8**, 159, **163**, 204–5
  United States (US) **119**, **129**, **144–6**, **148**, 159, **163**
entertainment media portrayal of abortion 71–2
environmentally friendly design 130–33
evacuation planning 184–5
*Everysaturdaymorning* blog 56–7

Face Law (Freedom of Access to Clinic Entrance Act, 1994) 55, 180, 204
Federal Bureau of Investigation (FBI) 177–8, 180
Federal Emergency Management Agency (FEMA) 180, 181–2
Feeley, Mike 48–9
feminism 14–15, 32–5
Feminist Majority Foundation 178–9
Feminist Women's Health Center 73–4
fetal rights 59
Fifth Street Women 33
Findley, Lisa 35–6
Fire Thunder, Cecilia 140

Fisher, Thomas 5
floating zones 54, **54**
Florida 49–53, **51**, **96**, **98–9**, 188n43
Foucault, Michel 24, 29
*4 months, 3 weeks and 2 days* (film) 72
*Framing Places: Mediating Power in Built Form* (Dovey) 35
France 9
Fraser, Nancy 9–10, 27, 30–31, 56
free speech 47–8, 193
Freedom of Access to Clinic Entrance Act ('Face Law', 1994) 55, 180, 204
*Friday Night Lights* (TV series) 72

gender, and space 21–4
*Gender, Identity and Place: Understanding Feminist Geographies* (McDowell) 19n59
Germany 9
GIRE (Grupo de Información en Reproducción Elegida) 85–6, 175
Gomperts, Rebecca 80, 82
Gottfried, Heidi 15
*Gray's Anatomy* (TV series) 72
Greene, Gayle 15
Grimes, David A. 186
Grosz, Elizabeth 21–2, 36–7, 208
Grupo de Información en Reproducción Elegida (GIRE) 85–6, 175
Gurner, Rowena 72–3

Habermas, Jürgen 8–11
Harding, Sandra 14–15
Harvey, David 36
Hawaii **96**, **98–9**, 187n3
Hayden, Dolores 34
Hern, Warren 55–6, 185
*Hill v. Colorado* (2000) 49, **50**
Hippocratic Oath 43
Hobart, Margaret 88–9
home 28–32, 73, 77
hospitals
  as abortion providers 152, 159–64, 194–5
  exterior design considerations 179–81
  interior design considerations 181–5, **183**, **184**
  location of 7, **116**, 120, **126**, **141**, **160**
  religious affiliations 152–3, 194–5
  security 178–9
human rights 173, 175
Human Rights Watch (HRW) 175

Hyde Amendment 45–6
Hyndman, Jennifer 16

Illinois 74–8, 82–3, **96**, **98–9**
Image Clear Ultrasound (ICU) 134
India 173
Indiana **96**, **98–9**, 164
insurance 171–2
Inter-Provincial Health Insurance Agreement Coordinating Committee (IHIACC) 172
intersections 13–15
Iowa **96**, **98–9**, 108
Ireland 82

Jacobs, Jane 179
Jane (Abortion Counseling Service of Women's Liberation) 74–8, **75**, **77**, 82–3
Joffe, Carole 83, 195
Johnston, Lynda 29
Jones, Bonnie Scott 165
Judson Memorial Church, New York 78–80
*Juno* (film) 71

Kansas 83–4, **96**, **98–9**, 134, 164, 165
Kentucky
  abortion, access to **122–3**, **198–9**
  abortion provision **96**, **98–9**, 120–29
  abortion restrictions 121–9
  contraception, provision of 16
  hospitals **126**
  pharmacies **127–9**, **199**
  poverty 121, **124**
  religious centers **125**, **199**
  women attending clinic, treatment of 56–7
Kishen, Meera 195
*Knocked Up* (film) 71

Lambert-Beatty, Carrie 82
landscapes, contested 11–13
law
  bubble laws 47–57, **50**, **51**, **52**, **54**, 59
  Canadian abortion law 57–61, 67
  Mexican abortion law 62–8
  spatial terms in 54, **54**
  US abortion law 43–57, 67, 111–20
Lefebvre, Henri 13, 36
lighting 87, 133, 181
location

  of abortion clinics 149–52, 204–5, 206–8
  of hospitals 7, **116**, 120, **126**, **141**, **160**
  of pharmacies **117–18**, 120, **127–8**, **142–3**, **145**, **147**, **161–2**, **197**, **199**, **201**, **203**
  of women's shelters 7, 88–90
Locke, John 27
London Matrix Feminist Design Co-operative 33
Longhurst, Robyn 23–4, 26, 29
Love, John A. 44–5
Low, Setha 12

McDowell, Linda 19n59, 23, 24, 27, 28, 32
*Madsen* v. *Women's Health Center* (1994) 49–53, **51**
Maginnis, Patricia 72–3
March for Women's Lives **2**
Markus, Thomas 35
Massachusetts 47, **96**, **98–9**
maternity units, security in 182, **183**, **184**
Matilda Joslyn Gage Foundation 1–2
Matrix Feminist Design Co-operative, London 33
McBride, Margaret 153
media, *see* entertainment media portrayal of abortion
Medicaid 45–6
medical education 97, 170–71, 194
Medical Students for Choice (MSFC) 97
medical therapy 25–6
menstrual extraction 74
Mexico
  abortion, access to **64**, **65**, 174–6
  abortion law 62–8
  abortion provision 173
  abortion tourism 85
  case studies 85–7
  conscientious objectors 176
  emergency contraception (EC) 62, 176–7
  pharmacies 177
  religion 62, 175
  in this research 6
Mexico City 63–8, 86, 174–5, 177
Michigan **96**, **98–9**, 187n3
midwestern United States (US) 130–33, **131–2**, 134–48, 187n3
misoprostol 176, 177, 186
Mississippi
  abortion, access to 95, **112–13**, 187n3, **196–7**

abortion provision **96, 98–9**, 110–20
abortion restrictions 111–20
contraception, provision of 16
hospitals **116**, 120
pharmacies **117–19**, 120, **197**
poverty 111, **114**
religious centers **115**, **197**
state-level regulation of abortion 6
Mitchell, Don 47
Monsiváis, Carlos 87
Montana 47, **96, 98–9**, 195
Moody, Howard 78
morbidity and abortion 173
Morgantaler, Henry 58–9, 84, 172
morning-after pill, *see* emergency contraception (EC)
mortality and abortion 173
Moss, Pamela 14
Mutcherson, Kimberley 194

Nassar, Carla 170, 172
National Abortion Rights Action League 73
National Association for the Repeal of Abortion Laws (NARAL) 73
National Network to End Domestic Violence (NNEDV) 88
National Organization of Women (NOW) 73
Native American reservations 140
Nebraska 16, **96, 98–9, 145**
Netherlands 80–83, 173
New Hampshire **96, 98–9**, 164
New York **52**, 53–4, 56, 78–80, **96, 98–9**
*No Easy Decision* (TV programme) 72
no-approach zones 54, **54**
noise and image zones 54, **54**
non-medical practitioners 195
North Carolina 45, **96, 98–9**, 164
North Dakota 16, **96, 98–9, 147–8**, 187n3
northeastern United States (US) 187n3
Norway 173

Oregon 45, **96, 98–9**
Overground Railroad 80

Pain, Rachel 30
Pakistan 82
Pennsylvania **96, 98–9**, 186–7, 187n3
Peru 82
Petchesky, Rosalind 209
Petrescu, Doina 5
pharmacies

emergency contraception (EC), availability of **119, 129, 144–8, 163**, 204–5
Kentucky **127–9, 199**
location of **117–18**, 120, **127–8, 142–3**, 145, **147, 161–2, 197, 199, 201, 203**
Mexico 177
Mississippi **117–19**, 120, **197**
Nebraska **145**
North Dakota **147–8**
South Dakota **142–4, 146, 201**
Utah **161–3, 203**
Phelan, Lana Clarke 72–3
place, meaning of 12
Plan B (emergency contraception)
access to 186–7
Canada 59, 172–3, 186
Mexico 176–7
pharmacies, availability from **119, 129, 144–8, 163**, 204–5
United States (US) **119, 129, 144–6, 148**, 159, **163**
Planned Parenthood 6, 164–6, 182
Poland 82
police action 108–10
politicized spaces 1–2, 11–13, 23
Pollock, Griselda 14
Portugal 82
poverty 111, **114**, 121, **124**, 135–40, **138**, 154, **157**
power, and architecture 35–6
Pozner, Jennifer L. 71
pregnancy 24–6
private space 29
protests **3, 4**, 108–10, 134–5
psychiatric units, security in 182
public space 7–11, 24–6
public-private dichotomies 26–8, 31
Pythagoreans 43

Quakers 80
quickening (fetal movement) 43–4

*R v. Morgantaler* (1988) 58–9, 84
Ramírez Jacinto, Paulina del Carmen 86–7, 174
Raven, Arlene 33
religion
Clergy Consultation Service (CCS) 78–80
hospitals with religious affiliations 152–3, 194–5

Kentucky **125**, **199**
Mexico 62, 175
Mississippi **115**, **197**
Overground Railroad 80
South Dakota **139**, **201**
Utah **158**, **203**
Rendell, Jane 34, 38
research project
　contested landscapes 11–13
　emergence of 6–7
　feminism, influence of 14–15
　intersections of representational space 13–15
　interviews 104
　methodology 15–17, 100–101
　public space, role of 7–11
Robles Law (Ley Robles) 66
Rockefeller, Nelson A. 45
*Roe v. Wade* (1973) 6, 8, 45, 72, 140
Roeder, Scott 83
Roman law 43
Rothman, Lorraine 74
Rounds, Mike 140
Ruskin, John 28–9
Ryan, Mary 9–10

safety 88–90
St. Joseph's Hospital and Medical Center, Phoenix, Arizona 152–3
*Schenk v. Pro-Choice Network of Western New York* (1997) **52**, 53–4, 56
Scott Jones, Bonnie 165
Sebelius, Kathleen 59, 193
security
　abortion clinics 166–9, 178–9, 188n43
　considerations 178–9
　exterior design considerations 179–81
　interior design considerations 181–5
　terrorism acts 177–8
　United States (US) 134–5, 149–52
　visibility of attacks 179
　women's shelters 88–90, 178–9
*Sesame and Lilies* (Ruskin) 28–9
Sethna, Christabelle 171
sexuality, and home 29
*Sexuality and Space* (Colomina) 21
shelters, *see* women's shelters
Shippensburg University 186–7
Singer, Peter 67
situated knowledge 22–3
*16 and pregnant* (TV series) 71
social relations

architecture, role of 35–8
and the body 24
domestic violence in the home 29–32
home, concept of 28–9
and pregnancy 24–6
and public-private dichotomies 26–8
and space 22–4
socio-economic group, and abortion 174
South Dakota
　abortion, access to 135, **136–7**, 187n3, **200–201**
　abortion provision **96**, **98–9**
　abortion restrictions 140
　contraception, provision of 16, **144**, **146**
　hospitals **141**
　pharmacies **142–4**, **146**, **201**
　poverty 135–40, **138**
　religious centers **139**, **201**
　state-level regulation of abortion 6
southern United States (US)
　abortion, access to **105**
　abortion provision 104–6, 110
　Kentucky 16, 56–7, 96, **98–9**, 120–29, **198–9**
　Mississippi 16, 95, **96**, **98–9**, 110–20, 187n3, **196–7**
　protests at clinics 108–10
　spatial experiences 107–8
　telemedicine 108
space
　abortion, access to 204–9
　abortion case studies 71, 72–85
　abortion clinic experience 107–8, 133, 149–52
　architecture, role of 35–8, 205–9
　and the body 21–4
　bubble laws 47–57, **50**, **51**, **52**, **54**, 59
　contested landscapes 11–13
　design and environment 87–8
　domestic violence in the home 24, 29–32
　and gender 21–4
　home, concept of 28–9
　intersections 13–15
　in the law 54, **54**
　political nature of 1–2, 11–13, 23
　pregnancy, effects of 24–6
　public space 7–11, 24–6
　and public-private dichotomies 26–8, 31
　quiet reflective spaces 83–4

representational space 13
and social relations 22–4
Spain 82
stand-alone clinics 194–5
state-level regulation of abortion, US
   bubble laws 47–57
   history of 44–5
   restrictions 1, 6, **102–3**, 104–6, 111–20, 121–9
Steinauer, Jody 194
Stoics 43
Sweden 173
Syracuse Housing Authority 2

tactics 13
Taft, Charlotte 107
Taracena, Rosario 86
Taylor, Affrica 23
Teather, Elizabeth Kenworthy 23
technology, use of 108
*Teen Mom* (TV series) 71
telemedicine 108
terrorism acts 177–8
Texas **96**, **98–9**, 164
third space 27–8
Thomas, Aquinas, Saint 43
Three Crusaders 72–3
Till, Jeremy 5
Tiller, George 83–4, 134, 185
Trudeau, Pierre 57, 84

United Nations Convention on the Elimination of all Forms of Discrimination Against Women (CEDAW) 173
United States (US)
   abortion, access to 95, **96**, **98–9**, **105**, **112–13**, **122–3**, **131–2**, 135, **136–7**, 154, **155–6**, 187n3, **196–203**
   abortion law 43–57, 67, 111–20, 193–4
   abortion provision **96**, **98–9**, 104–6, 110–29
   abortion restrictions **102–3**, 111–20, 121–9, 140
   abortion tourism 85
   bubble laws 47–57
   case studies 72–80, 83–4
   conscientious objectors 176
   Constitutional rights 46, 47–8, 51, 53–4, 193
   contraception, provision of 1, 16, **119**, **129**, **144–6**, **148**, 159, **163**

fetal rights 59
hospitals **116**, 120, **126**, **141**, **159–64**
medical education 97, 194
pharmacies **117–19**, 120, **127–9**, **142–8**, **161–3**, 177, **197**, **199**, **201**, **203**
poverty 111, **114**, 121, **124**, 135–40, **138**, 154, **157**
protests at clinics 108–10, 134–5
public space 7–8
religious centers **115**, **125**, **139**, **158**, **197**, **199**, **201**, **203**
security of clinics 134–5, 149–52
spatial experiences 107–8, 133, 149–52
state-level regulation of abortion 1, 6, 44–5, **102–3**, 104–6, 111–20, 121–9
telemedicine 108
violence against clinics 95–7
Utah
   abortion, access to 154, **155–6**, 187n3, **202–3**
   abortion provision **96**, **98–9**
   abortion restrictions 154
   contraception, provision of 16, **163**
   hospitals **160**
   pharmacies **161–3**, **203**
   poverty 154, **157**
   religious centers **158**, **203**

Vancouver Women's Caucus (VWC) 84
Venezuela 82
*Vera Drake* (film) 72
Vermont **96**, **98–9**, 195
voluntary sector 31–2

Washington DC (District of Columbia) **96**, **98–9**, 187n3
*Webster* v. *Reproductive Health Services* (1989) 80
Weisman, Leslie Kanes 33–4
western United States (US) 149–52, 154–8
Woman's Building, Los Angeles 33
Women on Waves 80–83, **81**
women's shelters
   exterior design considerations 179–81
   interior design considerations 181–5
   location of 7, 88–90
   public-private dichotomies 31
   security 88–90, 178–9
   voluntary sector 31–2

Young, Iris Marion  10–11, 25, 27, 56

Zukin, Sharon  12